P9-CFC-417

GRACE LIBRARY CARLOW COLLEGE
PITTSBURGH PA 15213

PREVENTION
The Etiology
of
Communicative Disorders
in
Children

Sanford E. Gerber

University of California at Santa Barbara

RJ
496
C67
G47
1990

PRENTICE HALL, Englewood Cliffs, New Jersey 07632

CATALOGUED

Library of Congress Cataloging-in-Publication Data

Gerber, Sanford E.
    Prevention : the etiology of communicative disorders in children /
  Sanford E. Gerber.
       p.   cm.
    Includes bibliographical references.
    ISBN 0-13-711110-X
    1. Communicative disorders in children--Prevention.
    2. Communicative disorders in children--Etiology.   I. Title.
  RJ496.C67G47   1990
  618.92'855071--dc20   89-16152
                                                                CIP

Editorial/production supervision
and interior design: Serena Hoffman
Cover design: Lorraine Mullaney
Manufacturing buyer: Peter Havens

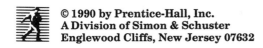 © 1990 by Prentice-Hall, Inc.
A Division of Simon & Schuster
Englewood Cliffs, New Jersey 07632

*All rights reserved. No part of this book may be
reproduced, in any form or by any means,
without permission in writing from the publisher.*

Printed in the United States of America
10 9 8 7 6 5 4 3 2 1

ISBN 0-13-711110-X

Prentice-Hall International (UK) Limited, *London*
Prentice-Hall of Australia Pty. Limited, *Sydney*
Prentice-Hall Canada Inc., *Toronto*
Prentice-Hall Hispanoamericana, S.A., *Mexico*
Prentice-Hall of India Private Limited, *New Delhi*
Prentice-Hall of Japan, Inc., *Tokyo*
Simon & Schuster Asia Pte. Ltd., *Singapore*
Editora Prentice-Hall do Brasil, Ltda., *Rio de Janeiro*

Maxima debetur puero reverentia

"The greatest respect is owed to a child"
Juvenal

Contents

3

Disorders of Genetic Origin 54

4

Teratogens, Mutagens, Infections, and Iatrogens 108

5

Trauma 162

6

Complex Craniofacial Disorders 183

7

Respiratory Disorders 255

8

Metabolic Disorders 275

9

Prevention Programs 293

Foreword

I have wished for a long time that someone would prepare a treatise on the etiology and prevention of communicative disorders. There is a great need for it, and the volume that Professor Gerber has prepared goes a long way toward meeting this need. The problems of communicative disorders and their etiologies are multitudinous, and Sanford Gerber has taken on the enormous task of preparing this volume in an ordered fashion that will be very helpful to those of us who are interested in the problem. I believe that the organization of this volume is excellent, and I am confident that the reader who seeks information about etiology and prevention will get as much out of it as I have.

The subject of communicative disorders is difficult to cover satisfactorily. I know of no other treatise that gives such organized information on this subject; and, therefore, I welcome this work with a great deal of enthusiasm. I compliment Professor Gerber on presenting this material in a fashion that is understandable and has a sense of order with respect to the various etiologies of communicative disorders. Much of what we know about the etiology and prevention of communicative disorders has come to us through many sources, with no attempt to assemble the information into one volume, as has been done here. I know of no one more able to do this than Sanford Gerber, as he has been dealing with these matters for many years and has a broad knowledge of communicative disorders. I know this book will be met with sincere enthusiasm.

Aram Glorig, M.D.

Preface

I have spent more than twenty years doing what I have now learned to call "secondary prevention." It occurs to me that far too little understanding about prevention exists among those of us who claim to be specialists in the study, diagnosis, and treatment of communicative disorders. Indeed, the American Speech–Language–Hearing Association (ASHA) does have a Committee on Prevention. That committee has done very good work, and that very good work has been published. But virtually no one has done anything about it. As late as 1980, Rolland Van Hattum, a former president of ASHA, commented that there "is still little emphasis on prevention." I agree with Van Hattum's prediction that "prevention will ultimately prove to be more productive" than curing.

I have been inspired by advertising sponsored by the Association for Retarded Citizens–United States. This advertising tells us, correctly, that 50 percent of mental retardation *could be prevented*. In my opinion, this is a conservative estimate. Mental retardation is itself a major communicative disorder. For most persons who are retarded, what sets them apart from the rest of the community is the absence or oddity of their communication skills.

The U.S. Environmental Protection Agency has issued rulings to diminish and eventually prohibit the use of tetraethyl lead in gasoline. Some optimists have predicted that this act alone would raise the U.S. national IQ by five points. Although this is obviously a misunderstanding of intelligence and the tests that purport to measure it, it also fails to account for many other things. No matter. The fact remains that some proportion of retardation and other neurological disorders can be prevented by removing lead from gasoline. This is a form of primary prevention.

Most of my own clinical activities for many years have been in the area of secondary prevention; that is, I have been concerned with early identification. Repeatedly, my colleagues and I have pointed out that early identification and intervention constitute a major means of reducing handicaps. For example, if a child is born deaf due to a dominantly inherited gene, I cannot keep him from being deaf. However, I can do my utmost to minimize the handicap that results from the deafness. In that sense, then, early identification is secondary prevention.

Historically, those of us who work in the speech and hearing sciences have been concerned with tertiary prevention; that is, we are fixers. Tertiary prevention is habilitation or rehabilitation. It would certainly be desirable if the ratio of our patients receiving tertiary prevention to those receiving secondary prevention could be substantially reduced. It would be even better if we could increase the rate of primary prevention.

This volume may not cause those improvements to occur, but perhaps it will inspire some of us to think more carefully, more actively, and in more detail about these issues. Although many communicative disorders are not yet available for primary or secondary prevention—that is, they are not predictable at the present state of the art—many such disorders are amenable to primary prevention. Genetic counseling, for example, may cause some prospective parents to decide against producing children who have a high risk of handicap. The use of seat belts and other restraints in automobiles is well established as a major means to prevent head injury. Immunization programs can prevent the deafness that results from prenatal rubella or the voice disorders that sometimes follow bulbar poliomyelitis. Ruben (1980) commented that we have "a certain amount . . . of knowledge . . . in the area of prevention. . . . " He included only vaccines, understanding of toxic substances, and genetic counseling. Such is the state of our knowledge and our ability to act on our knowledge.

Of course, primary prevention activities require an understanding of underlying etiologies, and this understanding is lacking for many communicative disorders. Nevertheless, we can make educated guesses, behave accordingly, and monitor the results. For example, probably the most frequent problems we encounter in a speech clinic are those involving the phonologic or articulatory system in the absence of speech organ pathology and/or observable neuromotor disability. We don't know what causes them, but the state of our knowledge should lead us to examine genetic factors, nongenetic prenatal conditions, and the consequences of early disease.

The dichotomy that some of our colleagues try to make between so-called *psychogenic* (or functional) disorders and so-called *biogenic* disorders is a false one. There is no behavior without an organism to do the behaving; there is no organism free of behavior. Hence, the notions of "functional" and "organic" disorders are empty notions. Grobstein (1988) commented that function means activity "to maintain the integrity of the organism," and behavior is the function "that relates the organism to its environment." I trust that this view is evident throughout this book.

Many programs of secondary prevention are already in place. For example, certain states (Florida, New Jersey, and Tennessee, among them) have programs mandating the screening of hearing of newborns who are at risk for deafness. In California, the Child Health and Disability Prevention program mandates (among other things) speech, language, hearing, and dental screening prior to entrance to the public schools. The overwhelming majority of states (all but two) mandate PKU screening.

Meanwhile, tertiary prevention (habilitation or rehabilitation) has been emphasized. I certainly don't wish to de-emphasize tertiary prevention. However, this is not a book on habilitation; it is a book on primary and secondary prevention and, consequently, on etiology.

We have learned that infant morbidity has diminished with infant mortality. Although that is true, it is also true that there has been no diminution of the incidence of severe or moderate congenital anomalies. The reduction in morbidity seems to be limited to mild handicaps or to mild developmental delay. This suggests that, although the prevalence of communicative disorders may diminish correspondingly, the severity of disorders that present for tertiary prevention may increase relatively. It is my opinion that we must turn our attention to understanding this process. Consequently, I have been bold enough to write this book. To the extent that any reader may be influenced positively by it to act, then I have succeeded. It is my wish and my hope that we who specialize in the understanding of communicative disorders direct our efforts also to preventing them.

I have debts to several people who have cooperated in many ways in this endeavor. I am indebted to Bob Shprintzen for writing Chapter 6, in which he demonstrates again that he knows much more than I do about the topic. My colleague, Dr. Hsiu-Zu Ho, spent valuable time reading Chapters 2 and 3 to minimize my errors. The mistakes that remain are mine. And I am especially indebted to Dr. Aram Glorig, who gave me my first job, for writing the foreword.

Sanford E. Gerber

References

Grobstein, Clifford, 1988. *Science and the Unborn.* New York: Basic Books, Inc.

Ruben, Robert J., 1980. "Research Priorities in Auditory Science: The Otologist's View," *Ann. Otol., Rhinol., Laryngol.,* 89, Suppl. 74, 132-33.

Van Hattum, Rolland J., (1980). "Research Priorities in Speech," *Ann. Otol., Rhinol., Laryngol.,* 89, Suppl. 74, 161-64.

1

Introduction

Until the 1950s, our understanding of prevention was largely limited to infectious diseases. This was certainly a good thing for attention to infectious diseases has improved the health of people in most parts of the world and has had an ameliorative effect on the caseloads of communicative disorders specialists. For example, in the first half of this century, we saw relatively large numbers of cases of profound congenital deafness due to prenatal rubella, chronic voice disorders that were the result of bulbar poliomyelitis, children who had both dysarthria and hearing impairment due to Rh incompatibility, and children who were profoundly deaf as a result of meningitis.

A number of years ago, McCabe (1963) investigated the causes of deafness among children who were not born deaf but were in public residential schools for the deaf. At that time, the most frequently occurring cause of profound acquired childhood deafness was good old-fashioned measles (rubeola). Certainly that is not true today, and it is a tribute to the worldwide efforts to prevent infectious diseases. The last major rubella epidemic in the United States was in the 1960s. There has not been another. And, undoubtedly, the most outstanding example of the prevention of infectious disease is the fact that smallpox does not exist anywhere in the world today.

Communicative disorders—including those caused by infectious diseases—have long been the most frequently occurring handicaps in the United States. Furthermore, profoundly handicapping communicative disorders are widespread in other parts of the world (Wilson 1984). Yet an emphasis on primary and secondary prevention of communicative

1

disorders is a fairly new concept in our profession. The Committee on Prevention of the American Speech–Language–Hearing Association (ASHA) published reports in 1982, 1984, and 1987. What is interesting, and somewhat distressing, is that not until the last quarter of this century had extensive attention been addressed to prevention. When I was a student, there was a heavy emphasis on etiology; that emphasis is (in essence) a kind of prevention. Simply stated, in many cases, if we know what causes the disorder, we may be able to prevent it. Sometimes we cannot prevent the occurrence, but we can prevent or minimize the handicap that results from it.

The first problem is to find out what counts as a communicative disorder. That is, how can we tell if someone has one? A general answer to that question is, if I cannot understand what you say, one or both of us has a communicative disorder. It may be that I don't hear well, it may be that you don't speak well, it may be that you don't hear well, or it may be all of these. This is certainly not a new idea; the founders of the profession now known as speech-language pathology had essentially the same notion. Even Alexander Graham Bell (1916) considered abnormal variation "a defect sufficient to attract the attention of anyone. . . . " If it attracted your attention or mine, one might think of it as defective. The consensus among the founders was that "speech is defective when it deviates so far from the speech of other people that it calls attention to itself, interferes with communication, or causes its possessor to be maladjusted" (Van Riper 1963).

This matter of attention being drawn to the speech rather than to the message was observed by others: "An individual's speech is defective if more attention is paid to how he speaks than to what he says" (Berry and Eisenson 1956). Johnson, in 1967, stated that "a child's speech presents a problem for himself and for others when his listeners pay critical or anxious or disapproving attention to how he speaks, or are distracted from what he is saying by the way he is saying it." In other words, "the audience, the speaker, or both may be reacting to the process of speech in such a way as to interfere with the communication of the content" (Milisen 1957).

Defective communication, however, extends beyond problems of articulation. West, Ansberry, and Carr (1957) called attention to a voice that is not loud enough to be heard, unintelligible speech because of "inaccurate articulation," speech that is unintelligible "by reason of serious lapses of grammar, syntax, or word use," or speech that is unpleasant to listen to or deviates in what we now would call the suprasegmental features. They also pointed out that hearing is defective "when it is inadequate to the individual's educational, vocational, and social needs." This last is an important observation; one need not be deaf to be communicatively impaired by a failure of audition. Hearing disorders are more easily quantifiable than are speech or language disorders except, perhaps, in the extreme. By "the extreme" is meant reference to the patient whose physical or intellectual impairment is so enormous that the production of spoken language is impossible. This also includes those with the most profound hearing impairments as well.

In 1979 the U.S. National Institute of Child Health and Human Development reported that communicative disorders of all degrees affect approximately 10 percent of the population. That is, some 20 million people in the United States alone had disorders of human communication of sufficient severity to interfere with their normal social or vocational activities. In 1982 Anastasiow reported that there were 1,187,000 handicapped children in the United States, of whom just 35 percent were receiving services. Moreover, there were nearly 600,000 births each year to teenage mothers, a group that gives birth to *four times* as many handicapped infants as the general population—and that number continues to rise.

In 1984 the U.S. Department of Education issued its sixth annual report on Public Law 94-142, the Education for All Handicapped Children Act. For the school year 1982–83, 4,298,327 children were identified as handicapped in public schools in the United States. The three most common handicapping conditions found among these schoolchildren were learning disabilities (4.4 percent of total school enrollment), speech impairment (2.86 percent), and mental retardation (1.92 percent).

EPIDEMIOLOGY

Epidemiologists view prevention as occurring at three levels. *Primary prevention* refers to prevention in the usual sense: The disease or event doesn't appear in the first place. Inoculations against rubella or polio would be examples of primary prevention. *Secondary prevention* is the early detection of a disorder including the prompt treatment of disease. For example, the many years of effort of the national Joint Committee on Infant Hearing should result in successful secondary prevention of deafness that appears early in life. However, tertiary prevention has been our history. *Tertiary prevention* is simply habilitation or rehabilitation. Habilitation is a good thing, but it would be wonderful if the need for habilitation were to be quantitatively diminished. That is to say, it would be a good thing for humankind were we to have more primary and secondary prevention resulting in a diminished need for tertiary prevention.

Primary prevention of communicative disorders, as well as any other kinds of disorders, falls into two general categories: the promotion of better health in general and the prevention of specific diseases. It is indeed likely that we can prevent certain communicative disorders by improving the health of the species. Obviously, if we would all stop smoking, the incidence of cancer of the larynx would diminish markedly and so would the need for laryngectomy and the need for the services that speech pathologists render to such patients. Improvement in the diet should eventually lead to a diminution in the prevalence of coronary heart disease and cardiovascular disease, which, in turn, should lead to a significant reduction in the incidence of cerebral vascular accidents with their accompanying aphasias. The wearing of seat belts in automobiles ought to prevent head injuries and that should also reduce the incidence of dysphasias and dysarthrias. Women who smoke during pregnancy have small babies and, although they seem to catch up by about the age of eight months, it would be better to have somewhat larger babies at birth. Women who drink often have small babies who don't catch up and have many problems.

Furthermore, primary prevention can be something more specific than the improvement of general health. Today we have immunization against many infectious diseases that existed when I was a child. I had pertussis (whooping cough); that disease has virtually disappeared. Prenatal rubella was once a major cause of deafness (cf. Bordley et al. 1967), but not any more. The incidence of congenital deafness has diminished as the incidence of prenatal rubella has diminished; yet prenatal rubella still accounts for about 18 percent of cases of congenital deafness (Barr 1982). Syphilis in a pregnant woman may be treated without consequence for her child if it is cured before the fifth month of pregnancy. If it is not, the risk of congenital syphilis is very high and the concomitant risk of severe sensory-neural hearing loss and eventual death is correspondingly high. Genital herpes is known to cause hearing impairment in the child of a woman who has the disease. The incidence of birth defects of all kinds in children born to mothers with diabetes is approximately double what it is in the general population. Consequently, the control and (when it becomes possible) cure of diabetes is again a form of primary prevention. Even genetic counseling is a kind of primary prevention because high-risk families may decide that it is disadvantageous to produce more children.

Secondary prevention consists of early detection and intervention. Our colleagues in special education have become outspoken advocates of early detection, especially of conditions that may lead to learning disabilities. There is evidence that the early detection of many disorders with consequences for communication can diminish the severity of those consequences. For example, the early provision of amplification for the severely hearing impaired infant has long been known to enhance that child's educational achievement. The analogy to eyeglasses for the visually impaired child is obvious. Certainly, prompt and efficacious treatment of disease should be expected to reduce the prevalence of resulting disorders. Interestingly, however, this has sometimes had beneficial, yet negative, consequences. Years ago, children would die of meningitis; today, they survive as very severely hearing impaired. Hence, the prevalence of meningitic deafness in early childhood has increased as the incidence of meningitis itself has decreased.

Although tertiary prevention is not a primary focus in this book, we should observe that it has also undergone a change among those who are concerned with communicative disorders. Not very many years ago, the majority of speech and language clinics would not see children under the age of three years on the supposition that there wasn't anything that could be done for them. In fact, this is the opposite of what we now know to be true. We enroll children in clinics at any age, and we are confident that the payoff over the long term will be beneficial.

The trend from tertiary to secondary to primary prevention is widespread. Geismar (1969) stressed the trend from remedial (i.e., tertiary) intervention to what he called "preventive intervention." He pointed out that remedial services are problem oriented, whereas preventive intervention addresses "problems that have not yet occurred or which have not become a serious threat to family welfare and unity." However, he also reminded us that it is important to establish that the service we render is, in fact, an effective preventive agent. That is, we must know that the community will suffer without this prevention and that, having introduced the prevention, it does not suffer. A stunning instance of that state is smoking; lung cancer occurs 1,000 times as often in males who smoke as it does in males who don't smoke. We know that the community suffers.

Wilson and Crouch (1987) have observed that society seems to be willing to spend more on prevention than on treatment, given that the community views the prevention as worthwhile. They calculated that, in the United States, we spend over $1 million per life to prevent cancer but about $50,000 per life to cure it.

We must eventually come to the state that Venkatesan (1978) described as "preventive behavior." He was talking about the behavior of the patient who either is or is not well, but it behooves us eventually to talk about the behavior of the health care delivery system and the professionals in it. Hence, we must do what was suggested by Marge (1984), which is to reduce the incidence of communicative disorders— that is, to reduce the number of new cases. Van Hattum (1980) also required "predictive formulations" for study and delivery leading to early detection and prevention.

SOME TERMINOLOGY

We must understand the difference between incidence and prevalence. Earlier, we said that it is important to reduce the incidence of communicative disorders. The assumption is that, by reducing the incidence, we will reduce the prevalence. What does that mean?

The *prevalence* of a disorder is the number of cases that exists at any given time. *Incidence* refers to the number of new cases. If incidence were to increase, one might assume that prevalence would also increase. Consider smoking: If we don't smoke, we reduce the incidence of lung and larynx cancer, and we reduce the prevalence of lung cancer. But it isn't true that incidence and prevalence must vary together. For example, there could be (heaven forbid!) a significantly increased incidence of a disorder that is always fatal. In such a case, while the incidence would go up, the prevalence would remain at zero because all patients died. A less bizarre example might be one in which the incidence increased in a given community and simultaneously decreased in another; then the prevalence, over all, would remain constant.

This could be a significant issue for communicative disorders specialists and special educators. Consider the following: The incidence of neonatal *mortality* (the ratio of children who die in the first 28 days of life to all births) has diminished considerably in the United States in the past decade (see Figure 1–1 and Table 1–1). One would suppose, therefore, that the incidence of *morbidity*—that is, the proportion of children being born who have some kind of disorder—would diminish accordingly. It has and it hasn't. Shapiro et al. (1983) observed that, indeed, the incidence of neonatal mortality has diminished, but the incidence of postneonatal mortality has not. Furthermore, they observed that the incidence of mild to moderate handicapping conditions or developmental disorders (i.e., morbidity) has declined, whereas the incidence of severe disorders has not. Therefore, it may be the case that the prevalence of communicative disorders in very young children has shrunk and the relative prevalence of severe disorders has grown. In fact, Gerber and Mencher (1983) had raised the question of the possibility of an increase in the incidence of congenital deafness. Perhaps it is the case, or was for a while, that the incidence of deafness in infants increased at the same time that hearing impairments in infants decreased. Was there a brief epidemic?

We must now understand the distinction between the terms "epidemic" and "endemic." Remember that the prefix *epi* means "on top of ",

FIGURE 1–1. Infant mortality rates by race and sex, United States, 1950–85

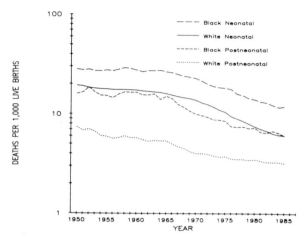

SOURCE: Myron E. Wegman, "Annual Summary of Vital Statistics," *Pediatrics*, 80, no. 6 (1987), 825. Reproduced by permission of *Pediatrics*. Copyright 1988.

as in epiglottis or epidermis. Hence, an *epidemic* is a situation in which there is a significantly increased incidence of a disorder. That is, the incidence happens "on top of" the prevalence of a given condition in a society, culture, or community; we suffered an epidemic of rubella in the United States in 1964–65. *Endemic,* on the other hand, refers to an unusually high prevalence in a given community or group as compared to other communities or groups. For example, the prevalence of otitis media in native American populations is much greater than in the urban population of the United States. Therefore, it is said that recurrent otitis media is endemic among native Americans.

Similarly, if we are to understand etiology (and therefore prevention), we must master some other distinctions. First, we must distinguish among a syndrome, a sequence, and an association. Then we must distinguish between a malformation and a deformation. These discriminations are essential, not only for diagnosis but also for prognosis and thus prevention.

Although a *syndrome* is a distinct collection of symptoms, it is more than that. A syndrome consists of multiple symptoms, multiple anomalies, or multiple signs, all of which have a common cause, a single etiology. The common cold is a familiar syndrome—runny nose, cough, perhaps fever, and the like—arising from a particular (unidentifiable) virus at a given time. Some communicative disorders are syndromes of genetic origin, Waardenburg syndrome, for example. In this case, the patient may exhibit sensory-neural hearing impairment, different col-

TABLE 1-1. Live births and Infant and Neonatal Mortality: Each State and Region*

State and Region	Live Births (No.)		Deaths of infants < 1 yr of Age		Mortality Rate†			
					Age < 1 yr			Age <28 d
	1987‡	1986‡	1987‡	1986§	1987‡	1986‡	1986§	(1986)§
New England	187,816	174,505	1,426	1,601	7.6	8.4	8.8	6.2
Maine	16,155	16,022	103	147	6.4	7.7	8.8	5.6
New Hampshire	16,435	16,361	119	144	7.2	7.2	9.1	5.9
Vermont	7,226	7,529	66	81	9.1	8.2	10.0	7.5
Massachusetts	86,934	80,063	678	697	7.8	7.9	8.5	5.8
Rhode Island	14,519	13,935	121	126	8.3	9.9	9.4	6.5
Connecticut	46,547	40,595	339	406	7.3	9.4	9.1	6.8
Middle Atlantic	548,021	529,720	5,597	5,526	10.2	10.4	10.4	7.0
New York	270,390	264,844	2,898	2,824	10.7	10.7	10.7	7.3
New Jersey	111,344	104,506	893	1,062	8.0	8.4	9.8	6.6
Pennsylvania	166,287	160,440	1,806	1,640	10.9	11.0	10.2	6.8
East North Central	618,999	618,696	6,322	6,951	10.2	10.7	11.1	7.4
Ohio	156,900	158,277	1,455	1,680	9.3	9.8	10.6	6.9
Indiana	77,694	79,630	768	895	9.9	10.8	11.3	7.5
Illinois	177,564	172,321	2,003	2,144	11.3	11.8	12.1	8.1
Michigan	136,374	136,198	1,477	1,564	10.8	11.4	11.4	7.8
Wisconsin	70,467	72,270	619	668	8.8	8.9	9.2	5.7
West North Central	262,637	265,986	2,564	2,583	9.8	9.8	9.7	5.9
Minnesota	64,068	64,819	555	606	8.7	9.3	9.2	5.5
Iowa	38,736	39,794	307	329	7.9	7.9	8.5	5.6
Missouri	75,950	76,224	934	805	12.3	11.4	10.7	6.8
North Dakota	11,545	11,900	102	91	8.8	9.5	8.4	4.1
South Dakota	11,514	11,714	116	155	10.1	11.6	13.3	7.1
Nebraska	23,657	24,433	234	247	9.9	10.2	10.1	6.6
Kansas	37,167	38,102	316	350	8.5	8.3	8.9	5.1
South Atlantic	629,371	606,735	7,061	7,130	11.2	11.7	11.7	7.9
Delaware	10,032	9,768	91	112	9.1	11.2	11.5	8.8
Maryland	64,692	61,953	631	816	9.8	10.3	11.7	8.3
District of Columbia	20,406	20,368	415	212	20.3	19.6	21.1	16.1

Virginia	87,002	84,209	850	881	965	9.8	10.5	11.1	7.5
West Virginia	23,572	24,195	215	253	238	9.1	10.5	10.2	6.6
North Carolina	93,405	90,597	1,064	1,058	1,042	11.4	11.7	11.5	7.7
South Carolina	50,693	49,604	653	649	684	12.9	13.1	13.2	8.8
Georgia	104,881	98,786	1,275	1,220	1,224	12.2	12.3	12.5	8.5
Florida	174,688	167,255	1,867	1,892	1,837	10.7	11.3	11.0	7.3
East South Central	222,131	221,525	2,557	2,561	2,544	11.5	11.6	11.6	7.5
Kentucky	51,075	51,682	410	477	509	8.0	9.2	9.8	6.4
Tennessee	71,343	71,890	887	820	727	12.4	11.4	11.0	6.9
Alabama	59,207	56,417	749	786	790	12.7	13.9	13.3	9.1
Mississippi	40,506	41,536	511	478	518	12.6	11.5	12.4	7.7
West South Central	209,856	210,959	4,443	4,948	4,728	9.6	10.4	10.1	6.3
Arkansas	23,464	23,896	286	326	355	8.6	9.6	10.3	5.7
Louisiana	75,313	77,953	883	943	927	11.7	12.1	11.9	7.8
Oklahoma	45,535	48,061	447	508	525	9.8	10.6	10.4	6.2
Texas	308,229	314,760	2,827	3,171	2,921	9.2	10.1	9.5	6.0
Mountain	235,177	229,868	2,076	2,210	2,167	8.8	9.6	9.3	5.4
Montana	11,976	12,372	90	86	122	7.5	7.0	9.6	5.6
Idaho	15,956	16,329	125	177	186	7.8	10.8	11.3	6.7
Wyoming	7,107	8,011	39	55	94	5.5	6.9	10.9	5.8
Colorado	54,314	55,724	557	529	476	10.3	9.5	8.6	5.3
New Mexico	30,169	23,952	207	256	261	6.9	10.7	9.5	5.4
Arizona	63,449	60,890	558	595	571	8.8	9.8	9.4	5.5
Utah	35,927	37,368	352	365	312	9.8	9.8	8.6	5.1
Nevada	16,279	15,222	148	147	145	9.1	9.7	9.1	4.9
Pacific	637,640	618,563	5,876	5,555	5,661	9.2	9.2	9.1	5.6
Washington	73,836	68,754	669	694	678	9.1	10.1	9.8	5.4
Oregon	39,708	40,356	387	360	366	9.7	8.9	9.4	4.7
California	494,053	478,822	4,528	4,205	4,315	9.2	9.1	8.9	5.6
Alaska	11,441	12,368	110	124	131	9.6	10.0	10.8	6.2
Hawaii	18,602	18,263	182	172	171	9.8	9.4	9.3	6.3

SOURCE: Myron E. Wegman, "Annual Summary of Vital Statistics—1987," Pediatrics, 82 (1988), 820. Reproduced by permission of Pediatrics. Copyright 1988.

* Data from National Center for Health Statistics. [2,6]
† Per 1,000 live births.
‡ Provisional, by state of occurrence.
§ Final, by state of residence.

ored eyes, a depigmented streak in the hair, a characteristic face, and so on, all due to a single dominant gene. Other syndromes may arise from a disease, whether acquired prenatally or postnatally. A familiar example is the syndrome of deafness, cataracts, mental retardation, neuromotor dysfunction, and cardiac problems that arises from prenatal rubella.

The essence of syndrome is twofold: the multiplicity of symptoms and the singularity of origin, whether viral, bacterial, genetic, chromosomal, teratogenic, or traumatic. Many communicative disorders, however, are nonsyndromal; that is, they may have many causes and/or few signs. This distinction is important for prevention, as it may permit the clinician to predict the probability of recurrence of a given disorder in a given family. It may also assist treatment to know if a given set of symptoms has a common origin.

A *sequence,* on the other hand, is just what it says it is: One thing leads to another. It is important, however, to note that there is still a multiplicity of symptoms and a singularity of cause. Persaud (1985) said that sequence "is a pathogenetic and not a causal concept. . . . " According to Siegel-Sadewitz and Shprintzen (1982), "A sequence of defects are [sic] causally related to a single anomaly. . . . " Hence, there is a "single localized malformation or disruption" that "may lead to single or multiple secondary defects. . . . " Siegel-Sadewitz and Shprintzen, like virtually everyone else, used the example of the Robin sequence.[1] This is a malformation that arises prenatally and is known to accompany a number of syndromes; it is marked by its three features of *micrognathia,* cleft palate, and *glossoptosis.* The point is that, developmentally, the micrognathia (severe under-development of the mandible) occurs first. This causes the tongue to remain high in the nasopharyngeal space, which, in turn, prevents the palatal shelves from closing. At birth, these infants have respiratory distress from glossoptosis (the "falling back" of the tongue) producing an airway obstruction. Many things might have been responsible for the micrognathia, but the sequence is micrognathia which causes the tongue to stay high, which, in turn, causes the cleft palate.

When a pattern of anomalies appears across individuals, whether or not they are in the same family, and this pattern has not been identified as a particular syndrome or sequence, it is known as an *association.* Persaud (1985) observed that this is a statistical, not a pathogenetic, notion. Recently, dysmorphologists and communicative disorders specialists have been interested in the CHARGE association:

---

[1] *Caution:* The terms Pierre Robin syndrome, Robin syndrome, Pierre Robin anomalad, and the like, are incorrect and are not currently in use.

FIGURE 1–2. CHARGE syndrome facial features

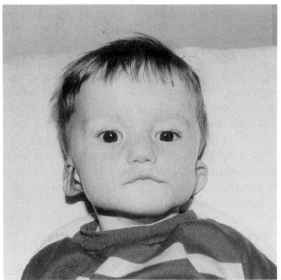

SOURCE: *CHARGE Syndrome: A Booklet for Families*, p. 33. Courtesy of Quota Club, Columbia, Mo. Copyright 1987.

*c*oloboma, *h*eart problems, *a*tresia of choanae, *r*etarded development, *g*enital hypoplasia, and *e*ar anomalies (Figure 1–2). What makes this assortment of symptoms an association is that they appear together nonrandomly. It is not a *mutation;* and, furthermore, more contemporary writings have called it the CHARGE syndrome (Davenport, Hefner, and Mitchell 1986).

Finally, the distinction between malformation and deformation is extremely important for diagnosis, treatment, and prevention. The term *malformation* is to be taken literally as "poor formation" (Smith 1981). It is "any morphologic defect caused by an error in the developmental process beginning at its most elementary level" (Siegel-Sadewitz and Shprintzen 1982). A *deformation,* however, is due to mechanical constraints that might be imposed by such things as abdominal tumors, small uterine space, or an unusual fetal position. It is essential to observe that deformations are usually much more easily repaired than malformations. Perhaps more important is the fact that they are not due to some genetic, chromosomal, or endocrine problem in the family. Smith remarked (italics his) that "the prognosis is *much* more favorable if the problem is deformation rather than malformation." Deformations appear in about 2 percent of all live births.

CONCLUSION

One might assume from the foregoing, then, that any discussion of prevention is perforce a discussion of etiology. Consequently, the organization of this book is according to etiology of communicative disorders. Although that is the case, in every instance the discussion of specific or suggested means for prevention is included, so that, for example, in a section on the learning disabilities and craniofacial anomaly that seem to result from fetal alcohol syndrome, we also include a review of the kind of primary and secondary prevention that might inhibit the incidence and reduce the prevalence of fetal alcohol syndrome.

It would be desirable if this book could incorporate all kinds of communicative disorders. It doesn't. The emphasis is on children. This is not because we are unconcerned with adults; all of our readers are adults. It is important to remember that some communicative disorders that arise in children might wait until after puberty to appear. We comment on some of them expressly, for example, otosclerosis. Another example that does not respect age is head injury. Adults as well as children suffer from the results of accidents, but relatively few children suffer from the effects of a stroke. Similarly, cancer of the larynx is relatively uncommon in children, but progressive sensory-neural hearing loss following cytomegalovirus is never encountered in adults. There is not a clear line.

The organization of the book is somewhat arbitrary but, I believe, reasonable. We begin with those inborn phenomena that may lead to communicative disorders at any time of life. We talk about chromosomes and genes. The reader's attention is then directed to teratogens; that is, those things that are not inborn but that could cause birth defects. Disorders of iatrogenic origin may arise in prenatal, perinatal, or postnatal life; the example of most frequent concern to us is ototoxicity. Traumas occur at any time of life, but particular traumas occur with greater incidence in early life (e.g., child abuse) and some in later life. Burns and chemical traumas are less common in infancy than they are later in childhood, but closed head injuries do not respect age.

Finally, this book addresses what can be done. We look at programs and procedures whereby communicative disorders specialists might institute and insist upon primary and secondary prevention. In other words, we want to put ourselves largely out of the business of tertiary prevention.

At the end of each chapter is a glossary of important terms in the text and a list of references. The book ends with sources of information and advice and a long bibliography.

GLOSSARY

association: a union or connection of things.
deformation: any change of form from that which is normal.
endemic: a condition or a disease found in a given community or among a certain group of people that prevails continually in a region, thereby distinguished from epidemic.
epidemic: a condition or a disease that attacks many people in a community simultaneously but is not continually present, thereby distinguished from endemic.
epidemiology: the study of epidemic diseases and epidemics.
glossoptosis: the "falling back" (ptosis) of the tongue (glosso-) into the oropharynx; hence, a downward displacement of the tongue.
incidence: the frequency of occurrence of a condition or a disease, or the rate at which it occurs, thereby distinguished from prevalence.
malformation: a failure of normal, correct, or complete development.
micrognathia: a malformation of the mandible characterized by extremely small size.
morbidity: any disease state.
mortality: the death rate; a state of being destined to die.
mutation: an alteration of form; genetically, a permanent, transmissible change that produces an individual unlike its parents.
prevalence: the frequency of occurrence of a given condition or disease in a group at any one time.
sequence: multiple anomalies resulting from a single defect or mechanical event.
syndrome: multiple anomalies resulting from a single pathogenetic process.

REFERENCES

AMERICAN SPEECH–LANGUAGE–HEARING ASSOCIATION. 1982. "Report of Committee on Prevention," *Asha*, 24, 425–26.
———1984. "Report of Committee on Prevention," *Asha*, 26, 35–37.
———1987. "Prevention of Communication Disorders: A Position Statement," *Asha*, 29, 51–52.
ANASTASIOW, NICHOLAS J. 1982. "Model Training Programs for Parents of Handicapped Infants and Children," in *Infant Communication: Development, Assessment, and Intervention*, ed. Dan P. McClowry, Arthur M. Guilford, and Sylvia O. Richardson. New York: Grune & Stratton.
BARR, BENGT. 1982. "Teratogenic Hearing Loss," *Audiol.*, 21, 111–27.
BELL, ALEXANDER GRAHAM. 1916. *The Mechanism of Speech*, 8th ed. New York: Funk & Wagnalls.
BERRY, MILDRED F., AND JON EISENSON. 1956. *Speech Disorders*. New York: Appleton-Century-Crofts.
BORDLEY, JOHN E., PATRICK E. BROOKHOUSER, JANET HARDY, AND WILLIAM G. HARDY. 1967. "Observations on the Effect of Prenatal Rubella in Hearing," in *Deafness in Childhood*, ed. Freeman McConnell and Paul H. Ward. Nashville, TN: Vanderbilt University Press.
DAVENPORT, SANDRA L. H., MARGARET A. HEFNER, AND JOYCE A. MITCHELL. 1986. "The Spectrum of Clinical Features in CHARGE Syndrome," *Clin. Genetics*, 29, 298–310.
GEISMAR, L. L. 1969. *Preventive Intervention in Social Work*. Metuchen, NJ: Scarecrow Press.
GERBER, SANFORD E., AND GEORGE T. MENCHER. 1983. "Is There an Increased Incidence of Congenital Deafness?" Mini-seminar presented to the annual convention of the American Speech–Language–Hearing Association.
JOHNSON, WENDELL. 1967. "Speech Disorders and Remedial Speech Services," in *Speech Handicapped School Children*, 3rd ed., ed. Wendell Johnson and Dorothy Moeller. New York: Harper & Row.

MARGE, MICHAEL M. 1984. "The Prevention of Communication Disorders," *Asha,* 26, 29–33.

McCABE, BRIAN F. 1963. "The Etiology of Deafness," *Volta Review,* 65, 471–77.

MILISEN, ROBERT. 1957. "The Incidence of Speech Disorders," in *Handbook of Speech Pathology,* ed. Lee E. Travis. New York: Appleton-Century-Crofts.

PERSAUD, T. V. N. 1985. "Classification and Epidemiology of Developmental Defects," in *Basic Concepts in Teratology,* ed. T. V. N. Persaud, A. E. Chudley, and R. G. Skalko. New York: Alan R. Liss.

SHAPIRO, SAM, MARIE C. MCCORMICK, BARBARA H. STARFIELD, AND BARBARA CRAWLEY. 1983. "Changes in Infant Morbidity Associated with Decreases in Neonatal Mortality," *Peds.,* 72, 408–14.

SIEGEL-SADEWITZ, VICKI, AND ROBERT J. SHPRINTZEN. 1982. "The Relationship of Communication Disorders to Syndrome Identification," *J. Speech Hear. Dis.,* 47, 338–54.

SMITH, DAVID W. 1981. *Recognizable Patterns of Human Deformation.* Philadelphia: Saunders.

UNITED STATES DEPARTMENT OF EDUCATION. 1984. *Annual Report on Public Law 94-142.* Washington, DC: Department of Education.

UNITED STATES NATIONAL INSTITUTE OF CHILD HEALTH AND HUMAN DEVELOPMENT. 1979. *Antenatal Diagnosis: Report of a Consensus Development Conference.* Washington, DC: Department of Health, Education, and Welfare.

VAN HATTUM, ROLLAND J. 1980. "Research Priorities in Speech," *Ann. Otol., Rhinol., Laryngol.,* 89, Suppl. 74, 161–64.

VAN RIPER, CHARLES. 1963. *Speech Correction,* 4th ed., Englewood Cliffs, NJ: Prentice Hall.

VENKATESAN, M. 1978. "Preventive Health: Positive Aspects," in *Marketing in Preventative Health Care: Interdisciplinary and Interorganizational Perspectives.* ed. P. D. Copper, W. J. Kehoe, and P. E. Murphy. Chicago: American Marketing Association.

WEGMAN, MYRON E. 1988. "Annual Summary of Vital Statistics—1987," *Peds.,* 82, 817–27.

WEST, ROBERT, MERLE ANSBERRY, AND ANNA CARR. 1957. *The Rehabilitation of Speech* 3rd ed. New York: Harper & Row.

WILSON, JOHN. 1984. "Prevention of Deafness in Developing Countries." Paper presented to the 17th International Congress of Audiology, Santa Barbara, CA.

WILSON, RICHARD, AND E. A. C. CROUCH. 1987. "Risk Assessment and Comparisons: An Introduction," *Science,* 236, 267–70.

2

Disorders
of Chromosomal Origin

Disorders of chromosomal origin are very common. In fact, about 7 in every 1,000 births will be affected by a chromosomal disorder. Furthermore, chromosomal disorders account for about half of all spontaneous abortions that occur in the first trimester of pregnancy. Consequently, dysfunction of the chromosomal system is etiologically very important for disorders of all kinds and especially those that exhibit disturbances of communication. As we discuss later, chromosomal disorders are amenable to primary, secondary, and tertiary prevention.

A chromosomal abnormality is something that can be seen under a microscope; consequently, in recent years, our understanding of chromosomes and what can go wrong with them has greatly improved and expanded. Moreover, each chromosomal disorder will present with a characteristic *phenotype*—the expression of the trait in some physiological, biochemical, or morphological manner that is unique and identifiable. The most frequently occurring abnormal phenotype is that of Down syndrome, or trisomy 21.

THE CHROMOSOMAL SYSTEM

What Is a Chromosome?

In the narrowest, most literal sense, a chromosome is a "colored body" from *chroma,* meaning "color" and *soma,* meaning "body." The reason these materials are called this is that certain stains are taken up by the chromosomes very deeply, permitting the microscopist to see these rod-shaped structures called chromosomes.

Although it used to be said that a human being was worth about $1.25 in minerals and was composed mainly of water, the fact is that the "stuff" of which humans are made is *deoxyribonucleic acid,* or DNA. It is this DNA of the chromosomes in which genetic information is encoded in what we call *genes.* DNA, then, is the genetic material found in the nucleus of each cell that constitutes the program or blueprint for the synthesis of protein molecules. These protein molecules, in turn, are the basis of all cellular functions and reactions. Each molecule of DNA has the structure of a double helix (Figure 2–1)

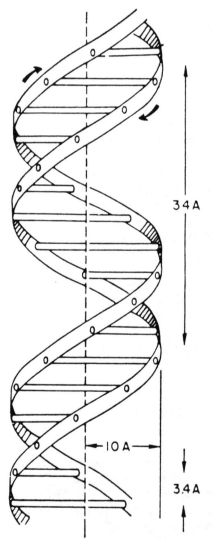

34 A

10 A

3.4 A

FIGURE 2–1.
The double helix
SOURCE: J. D. Watson, "Molecular Structure of Nucleic Acids," *Nature,* 171 (1953), 737. Reprinted by permission. Copyright © 1953 Macmillan Magazines Limited.

that uncoils to transmit genetic information (Figure 2–2) via synthesis to RNA, *ribonucleic acid.* This process may be thought of as a template for the formation of proteins (Figure 2–3). If a part of a DNA molecule that is essential to protein formation is damaged, and if cellular repair processes cannot correct this error, then it is very probable that the cell will not function as well as it should. Changes of DNA molecules are called *mutations.*

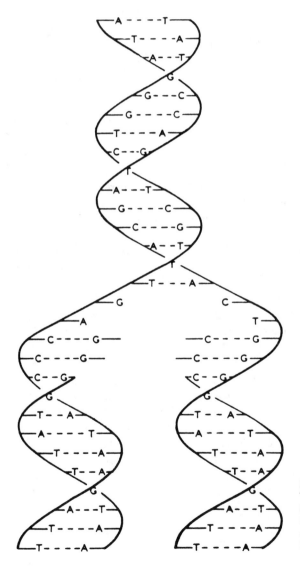

FIGURE 2–2.
The double helix uncoiled
SOURCE: H. Eldon Sutton, *Genes, Enzymes, and Inherited Diseases* (Orlando, Fla.: CBS Publishing, 1961), p. 38.

FIGURE 2–3. The genetic template

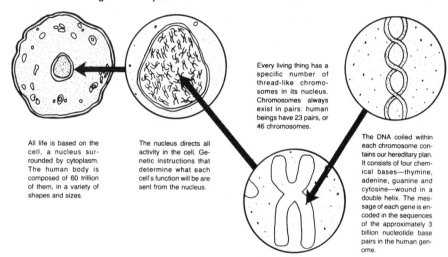

Every living thing has a specific number of thread-like chromosomes in its nucleus. Chromosomes always exist in pairs: human beings have 23 pairs, or 46 chromosomes.

All life is based on the cell, a nucleus surrounded by cytoplasm. The human body is composed of 60 trillion of them, in a variety of shapes and sizes.

The nucleus directs all activity in the cell. Genetic instructions that determine what each cell's function will be are sent from the nucleus.

The DNA coiled within each chromosome contains our hereditary plan. It consists of four chemical bases—thymine, adenine, guanine and cytosine—wound in a double helix. The message of each gene is encoded in the sequences of the approximately 3 billion nucleotide base pairs in the human genome.

SOURCE: *UC Focus,* October 1987, p.2. Reprinted by permission of the University of California.

Each living species has its own *karyotype*—that is, its own characteristic chromosome constitution, morphology, and number. Not only that, each karyotype has a particular gene map that refers to the specific locations of the genes on each chromosome. Hence, each gene has a unique locus. Again, each living species has a unique karotype, and each individual member of that species has its unique *genotype,* its own genetic constitution. Hence, the phenotype is the expression of the genotype. And the *genome* is the totality of the DNA content in that individual set of chromosomes.

Karyotyping of a cell's chromosomes makes them available for examination with respect to their number and structure. This is critical for our purposes because chromosomal disorders are, indeed, disorders of the number and/or structure of the chromosomes. Although it may be easy enough to count the numbers of chromosomes, it takes a great deal more expertise to examine their structures. Each chromosome is essentially X-shaped. The place where the arms of the X meet, the *centromere,* leads to the classification of chromosomes into three categories as shown in Figure 2–4: *metacentric, submetacentric,* and *acrocentric.* Familiarity with these three forms is one factor that permits us to identify structural abnormalities of chromosomes. Also, the arms of each of these chromosomes are labeled p for the short arm and q for the long arm; a ring-shaped chromosome is labeled r. Thus, for example, if the short arm of

FIGURE 2–4.   Forms of chromosomes

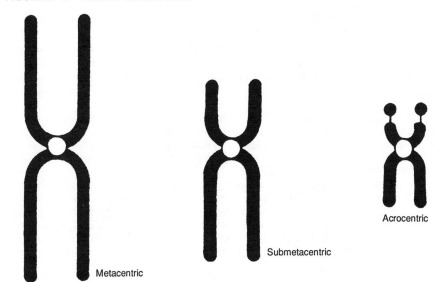

Metacentric

Submetacentric

Acrocentric

SOURCE: James S. Thompson and Margaret W. Thompson, *Genetics in Medicine,* 3rd ed. (Philadelphia: W. B. Saunders Co., 1980), p. 23. Reprinted by permission.

a given chromosome is missing, it is called "p-"; if it is the long arm, "q-". A later section of this chapter deals with what these structural abnormalities are and how they are described.

The transmission of genetic information from parent to child to succeeding generations is the central role of DNA. Remember,it is DNA that determines protein structure. In the process of doing this, DNA gets transcribed into RNA and, in turn, RNA gets translated into protein. Actually, this is not news: In 1928, Griffith performed an experiment that demonstrated that DNA is the genetic material.

But what are these acids, DNA and RNA? They are actually rather simple macromolecules composed of three types of units: a sugar, a base that contains nitrogen, and phosphate. In the RNA, which becomes protein, there are only four bases: *adenine, guanine, cytosine,* and *uracil.* Although the names of these particular substances are not essential for our purpose, it is important to observe that only 64 combinations are possible. Any triplet of three bases will constitute a *codon,* which is a unit of the genetic code. This is important because the number is amazingly small; because there are only four bases, the maximum number is $4^3 = 64$. Thus, the genetic code consists of 64, and only 64, codons. An example is the essential amino acid *serine,* which is made of the mRNA codon UCG (uracil, cytosine, and guanine). The sequence is also important: UCG produces serine, but CUG produces *leucine,* and GUC produces *valine.* Again, the names are not important; the important thing is that the number of combinations is both small and unique.

The situation has been brilliantly and succinctly stated by Wenthold (1980):

> The information contained in a gene is determined by the sequence of purine (adenine and guanine) and pyrimidine (cystosine and thymine) bases of the DNA . . . the basic amino acid backbone of the protein is formed at translation. Therefore, a change in the DNA sequence may result in an abnormal amino acid sequence in the protein product. Even a single nucleotide substitution may affect the growing polypeptides by insertion of an incorrect amino acid or by termination of the polypeptide's synthesis. Insertion of a single incorrect amino acid into the polypeptide may alter the properties of the protein so severely that it may be totally inactive, may function with limited efficiency, may function normally but have altered physical properties, or, . . . may cause little or no functional or physical change.

How Many Chromosomes Are There?
Where Are They?

Because we know that the number of combinations is small, it is conceptually simple (if mathematically difficult) to multiply the number of combinations by the number of cells. Thompson and Thompson (1980) estimated that the human genome contains about 2.79×10^9 nucleotide pairs, which is enough for about 3 million genes. The fact is, though, that only a small percentage of the total genome actually gets transcribed and translated. These are the so-called structural genes of which humans have about 30,000.

The total number of different chromosomes in humans is only 46. Each person has received 23 chromosomes from each parent. One of the 23 chromosomes is the sex chromosome, the one from the father that determines whether we are male or female. In the human animal, the female is said to be *homogametic* because she carries only X chromosomes. Human males are *heterogametic* because the male carries an X chromosome and a Y chromosome and produces both X and Y bearing sperm. All of us who are female, then, have received an X chromosome from each parent; those of us who are male received an X from our mother and a Y from our father. (By the way, this is not necessarily true of all higher species; in birds, for example, the female is heterogametic.) The remaining 22 chromosomes from each parent are called *autosomes.* Consequently, all somatic cells carry double the number of chromosomes, that is, 46, said to be the *diploid* number. On the other hand, the sex cells or gametes carry only 23 chromosomes, including the X or Y, or the *haploid* number.

The number of chromosomes is clinically very important. A person born with an incorrect number (i.e., other than 46) will display a chromosomal aberration, an abnormal phenotype. Any number that is not an exact multiple of 23 is called *aneuploid*. But remember that we are supposed to get 46 chromosomes; hence, we can have too many and still have that number be an exact multiple of 23. In such a case, it is said to be *polyploid*. Aneuploid and polyploid aberrations have different consequences.

Where are all these chromosomes? Virtually everywhere. Red blood cells have no nuclei and, hence, have no chromosomes; they may be the only exception. In other words, every single cell of the body, except for the red blood cells, carries a complete complement of 46 chromosomes. This is clinically useful because it permits one to take a small sample of tissue (usually blood or skin) for chromosomal analysis. One white blood cell will have the exact number of chromosomes in the exact structure as any other cell or any other tissue. Hence, by a process known as amniocentesis (discussed later in this chapter), it is possible to withdraw a very small sample of fluid from the intrauterine space and analyze that fluid to determine the chromosomal structure of a living fetus. In this way, prenatal diagnosis of chromosomal aberrations can be made. More than 250 disorders can be diagnosed via amniocentesis. Furthermore, because the amniotic fluid contains all the chromosomes, the sex of the fetus can also be determined.

THE MAJOR CHROMOSOMAL DISORDERS

Hypothetically, chromosomal disorders can occur on any one or more of the 23 chromosomes, but apparently this is not the usual case. It seems that some of the chromosome locations are more susceptible than others to aberrations; and the larger the chromosome (smaller number as they are ranked from large to small), the more likely it is that the aberration is lethal. Furthermore, there are only 64 codons, but most proteins are coded by hundreds or thousands of codons. Nevertheless, only certain aberrations are possible; aberrations, like all of life, are rule-governed.

The abnormalities of chromosomes may be either numerical or structural and may appear on the autosomes or on the sex chromosomes. It is important that we understand what is possible. Smith (1976) cautioned that genetic counseling should not be offered until the counselor or the medical geneticist actually has determined whether either parent is a carrier of a chromosomal abnormality. If there is no evidence of abnormality or if there is no history in the family, Smith pointed out that it is impossible to state the risk of recurrence. Therefore, he reminded us that it is presumptuous to suggest to parents that it may not recur. Is this really a problem? It certainly is. Smith continued that "roughly half the individuals with multiple defects have conditions which have not yet been recognized as a specific syndrome." Furthermore, only a small percentage of these has a true abnormality of chromosomal structure. Also, there is the problem of incomplete penetrance, as discussed in Chapter 3.

Disorders of Number or Structure

At one stage in development, chromosomes will disjoin. This may occur during *mitosis* or *meiosis*. When a pair of chromosomes fails to disjoin, aberrations of nondisjunction occur; this, in turn, may result in an aberrant number of daughter chromosomes. Remember that, in *homo sapiens,* the number of chromosomes is equal to 23. Each of us should carry $2n = 46$ chromosomes; hence, $2n$ is normal. Any other multiple, $3n$ or $4n$, for example, is polyploid and is not normal. When $3n$ occurs, it results in a condition known as *triploidy,* which is grossly deforming and lethal (Figure 2–5). It is more likely, however, that nondisjunction results in a number that is not a factorial multiple of n, an aneuploid. Some aneuploids are *trisomic,* meaning $2n + 1$. When trisomy occurs, three members of a given chromosome will arise. The most common example is trisomy 21, Down syndrome, where the extra chromosome appears at position 21 (Figure 2–6). Of course, trisomy can occur at other chromosome locations, notably 13 and 18, which are discussed below. Moreover, trisomy for two different chromosomes simultaneously occurs, but this happens only rarely.

Some chromosomal aberrations are abnormalities of structure rather than of number. Structural aberrations are due to chromosome breakage. In fact, a major issue for primary prevention is to identify and control those things that could cause chromosomes to break. These would include certain chemical *teratogens,* certain viruses, and ionizing radiation. (In fact, it is for this reason that X rays are rarely used today to visualize a fetus; ultrasonic images are preferred.) Thompson (1986) listed four kinds of causes of aberrations—late maternal age, genes predisposing to nondisjunction, autoimmune disease, and radiation—but observed that "there seems to be no evidence that viruses or teratogenic agents . . . cause nondisjunction in the offspring of exposed parents."

Chromosome abnormalities can lead to additional aberrations, all of which have relevance for communicative disorders and are amenable

FIGURE 2–5.   Triploidy

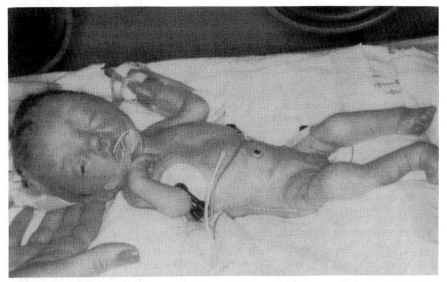

SOURCE: Photo courtesy of Roger G. Faix, M.D. Reproduced by permission from *Pediatrics,* 74, no. 2 (1984), 297. Copyright 1984.

FIGURE 2–6.   Down syndrome karyotype

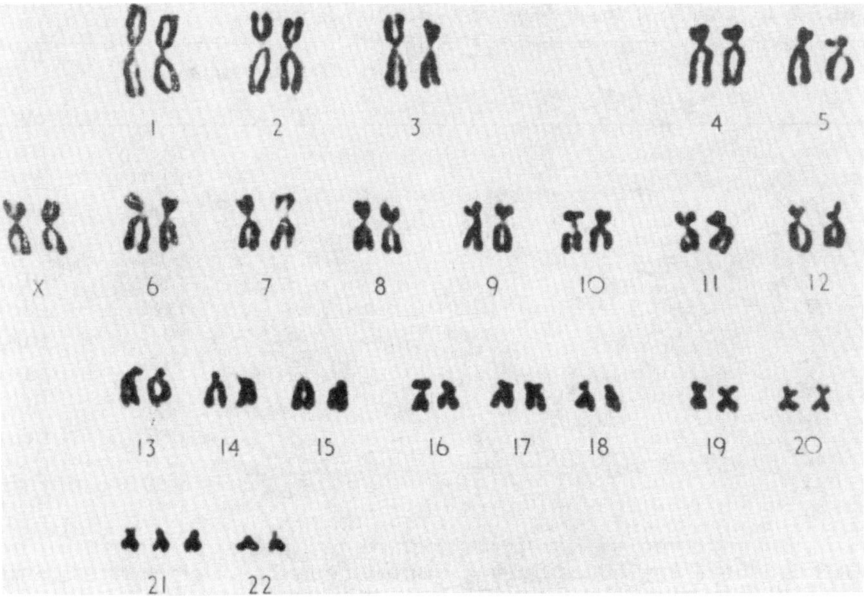

1	2	3		4	5
X	6	7	8	9	10	11	12
13	14	15	16	17	18	19	20
21	22						

(or potentially amenable) to primary or secondary prevention. For example, the trisomies, especially Down syndrome, are known to have late maternal age as a major etiological factor. Table 2–1 clearly shows the relationship between maternal age and the risk of Down syndrome. Good education should lead to pregnancies occurring at optimum ages. Early maternal age is also a problem; the incidence of birth defects appearing in children born to mothers under the age of 16 is four times what it is in the general population (Litch 1984). In 1981, girls aged 14 years and younger gave birth to 10,000 babies in the United States (Seessel 1985).

Autoimmune disease often appears in the form of high thyroid levels, and these are treatable. X-radiation during pregnancy has largely given way to ultrasonic radiation, and many viral diseases have been brought under immunologic control.

Trisomy 21, Down Syndrome   The most frequently occurring, and well-known, disorder of chromosomal number is Down syndrome. The classic paper, the one which gave the syndrome its name, was the 1866 lecture of J. L. H. Down, "Observations of an Ethnic Classification of Idiots." In the ensuing many years, literally volumes have been written on the subject of Down syndrome. Although Down correctly described the disorder, he was unaware of its chromosomal origin. It was Waardenburg (who has a syndrome named after him too) who first observed the chromosomal anomaly in 1932. Specifically, it was not until 1959 that the extra acrocentric chromosome was discovered at location 21 by Lejeune,

TABLE 2–1.   Maternal Age and Frequency of Down Syndrome

Maternal Age	Frequency of Down Syndrome	
	Fetuses	*Live Births*
<20	—	1/1,550
20–24	—	1/1,550
25–29	—	1/1,050
30–34	—	1/700
35	1/350	1/350
36	1/260	1/300
37	1/200	1/225
38	1/160	1/175
39	1/125	1/150
40	1/70	1/100
41	1/35	1/85
42	1/30	1/65
43	1/20	1/50
44	1/13	1/40
45	1/25	1/25

SOURCE: Data adapted from Margaret W. Thompson, *Genetics in Medicine*, 4th ed. (Philadelphia: W. B. Saunders Co., 1986), p. 121. Reprinted by permission.

Gautier, and Turpin. Figure 2–6 is a karotype of a female with Down syndrome; the extra chromosome at position 21 is obvious. The fact is that 95 percent of patients with Down syndrome have a trisomy 21 karyotype; 4 percent have *translocation,* and 1 percent are products of *mosaicism.*

Down syndrome is so familiar that a simple listing of its characteristics should be sufficient for its discussion:

Generalized hypotonia that extends through the oral cavity, resulting in a mouth-open posture with a protruding tongue (Figure 2–7)

Hyperflexibility of joints

A universal mental retardation that is rarely severe

A characteristic face with *brachycephaly*

FIGURE 2–7. Down syndrome

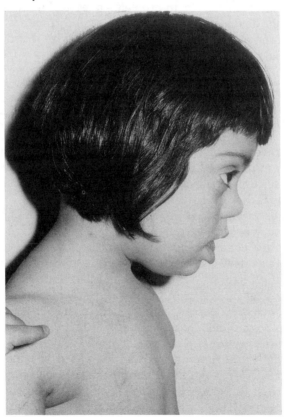

SOURCE: Sanford E. Gerber and George T. Mencher, *Auditory Dysfunction* (San Diego, Calif.: College-Hill Press, 1980), p. 93. Copyright 1980.

Occasional eye discoloration

Characteristic pinnae

Characteristic hands with *hypoplasia* of the fifth finger in about 60 percent of cases and a simian crease in about 45 percent

Anomaly of the heart in about 40 percent

Dry skin in about 75 percent accompanied by fine soft hair that is often sparse

Universal hypogonadism

Other abnormalities occur, but rarely, including seizures, strabismus, and cataracts.

The consequences for communication are manifold and appear in speech and language and hearing. The characteristic shape of the head (brachycephaly) results in a short anterior-posterior length of the oral cavity with a consequent protrusion of the tongue. The shortened vocal tract leads, almost inevitably, to problems of articulation. Clearly, disorders of language development and behavior will correlate with the mental retardation of the patient, so that some patients with Down syndrome are truly nonverbal. Furthermore, the anomalies of the upper respiratory system and the external (and probably middle) ear lead to recurrent otitis media. In fact, otitis media is endemic in the Down syndrome population.

The correlation of advanced maternal age with the incidence of Down syndrome is striking. Mothers under the age of 30 years will produce only one Down syndrome infant in 1,000 to 1,500 births. Mothers who are 45 years of age or older have the risk of delivering one Down syndrome infant in every 25 births. However, it appears that in some 24 percent of cases of Down syndrome, the extra twenty-first chromosome came from the father (Magenis et al. 1977).

Overall estimates have reported the incidence of Down syndrome in newborns to average about 1 in every 800 births. This incidence has remained rather constant over the years, even though the average maternal age has declined in the last decade or so. Perhaps this is due to two opposing factors: As more women are postponing a first pregnancy, the number of births in teenagers is simultaneously increasing. In the 1960s, about 10 percent of all births in the United States were to mothers aged 35 or older; by the mid-70s, it had dropped to 4.5 percent. These statistics may explain why the overall incidence has not changed.

Additionally, the prevalence has increased because many Down syndrome patients with cardiac anomalies have undergone heart surgery and thereby their lives have been prolonged. With more and more Down syndrome patients living longer, it has been observed that there is a high incidence of Alzheimer disease among them (Kelly 1980; Sinex and Merrill 1982). This raises questions of common etiology and considerations for prevention of both Down syndrome and Alzheimer disease. Barnes (1987) has reported that "the genetic defect in Alzheimer's disease is located on the same region of chromosome 21 that contains the gene for amyloid, a protein that accumulates abnormally in the brains of both Alzheimer's and Down's patients."

Prevention can be effected at the primary, secondary, and tertiary levels. The principle for primary prevention is in the area of education: we need to continue to instruct the childbearing public that there is increased risk in postponing pregnancies for a prolonged period (see Figure 2–8). Down syndrome has also become the prime example of a certain kind of secondary (or, for some people, primary) prevention: amniocentesis. Whether amniocentesis is primary or secondary prevention depends on the gestational age at which it is done and what the parents decide to do. In other words, if amniocentesis reveals a fetus with Down syndrome at a time sufficiently early for clinical abortion to be an option, then many people believe that it is up to the parents to make that choice. However, amniocentesis becomes secondary preven-

FIGURE 2–8. Prevalence of Down syndrome for mothers aged 30 to 40

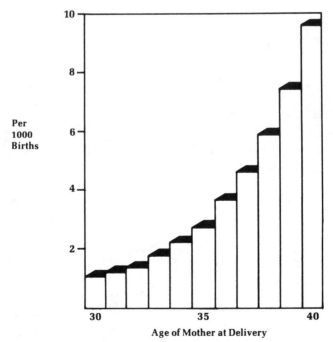

SOURCE: The President's Commission for the Study of Ethical Problems in Medicine and Biomedical and Behavioral Research, *Screening and Counseling for Genetic Conditions* (Washington, D.C.: Government Printing Office, 1983), p. 79.

tion (i.e., early identification) if it is done too late for clinical abortion to be an option or if the parents elect to continue the pregnancy. Tertiary prevention is, and must always be, available to the Down syndrome patient, or, for that matter, any patient with the consequences of chromosomal aberration.

Trisomy 13, Patau Syndrome   In 1960, Patau et al. described a trisomic syndrome characterized by multiple handicaps of the craniofacial area, hands, heart, and gonads. It is extremely rare, appearing with an incidence of only about 1 in 6,000 births, because 95 percent of trisomy 13 *conceptuses* abort spontaneously. Infants suffering the sequelae of Patau syndrome rarely come to the attention of the communicative disorders specialist even though they are frequently deaf and have clefts of lip and palate (Figure 2–9), again because of their greatly shortened life expectancy. Kelly (1980) stated that only 15 percent survive the first year; Konigsmark and Gorlin (1976) reported that the life span is "nearly always less than three months"; and Thompson and Thompson (1980) claimed that trisomy 13 is fatal within the first month of life in about half the infants with the disorder; no more than 5 percent survive past the third year. The result is that such infants don't come for tertiary preven-

FIGURE 2–9.   Trisomy 13 (Patau syndrome)

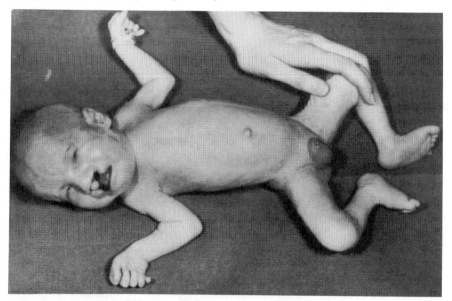

SOURCE: James S. Thompson and Margaret W. Thompson, *Genetics in Medicine,* 3rd ed. (Philadelphia: W. B. Saunders Co., 1980), p. 154. Reprinted by permission.

tion, habilitation, even though evidence suggests that they would be profoundly hearing impaired.

An extensive study by Sando et al. (1975) revealed a large number and variety of pathologies of the cochlea as well as of the vestibular system. These consisted of a shortened cochlear length with a widened aqueduct, anomalies of the modiolus, and a variety of other problems of the bony labyrinth. Interestingly, Sando et al. found no pathology of the organ of Corti and other parts of the membranous labyrinth. Paparella and Capps (1973) listed a variety of craniofacial anomalies appearing in this syndrome, some of which may suggest the presence of conductive hearing impairments. These include "low set ear, undifferentiated pinnae, absence of the external canal or the middle ear," and other *stigmata* of the midface. They, too, reported that these infants die within a short time.

Trisomy 13, then, is another example where primary prevention is in order. If a family has already produced a child with this syndrome, genetic counseling is highly appropriate. Although amniocentesis could reveal the extra chromosome, it is not likely to be done unless it is routine in pregnancies of older women.

Trisomy 18, Edwards Syndrome   Simultaneous with the first description of trisomy 13 by Patau et al. in 1960, Edwards et al. described trisomy 18 (Figure 2–10). It is the second most common autosomal trisomy, although 90% of conceptuses result in fetal wastage (Kelly 1980). Khoury et al. (1988) reported that 83.7 percent of cases of trisomy 18 are associated with intrauterine growth retardation. The incidence of live born infants with Edwards syndrome is about 1 in 8,000 births. Postnatal survival is poor; Thompson and Thompson (1980) reported the mean life expectancy to be only two months although some have lived as long as 15 years. The short life expectancy may be due to the severe heart malformations that occur in virtually all such patients.

The few studies of temporal bones that have been done on trisomy 18 infants indicate many middle ear anomalies and some inner ear anomalies as well. Among those have been malformed ossicles, absence of semicircular canals, and defective cochlear partition. Evidently there are no reports of clefts of the lip or palate in trisomy 18 as is the case in trisomy 13.

Obviously, tertiary prevention does not apply in the case of a trisomy 18 child who doesn't survive; however, primary and secondary prevention may be available. Maternal age is a factor in trisomy 18, as it is in trisomy 21 and other trisomies; hence, counseling for the older mother and amniocentesis are in order. Given that some trisomy 18 patients do survive, however, secondary prevention may also be available. Early identification is certainly possible, and it may be reasonable

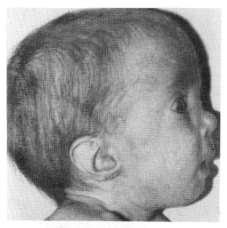

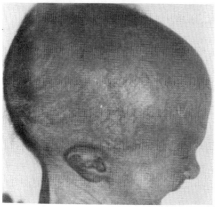

FIGURE 2–10.
Trisomy 18 (Edwards syndrome)
SOURCE: David W. Smith, *Recognizable Patterns in Human Malformation,* 3rd ed. (Philadelphia: W. B. Saunders Co., 1982), p. 17. Reprinted by permission.

in a given (even though rare) case to attempt therapeutic intervention for hearing impairment and mental retardation. It is important to state the case, as we have done elsewhere, that "the patient should receive appropriate amplification and rehabilitation for as long as possible" (Gerber and Mencher 1980). That is to say, although the patient's life expectancy may be short, there is no reason to deny treatment where it is indicated.

The eighteenth chromosome is vulnerable to deletion problems as well. These are 18p-, 18q-, and 18r, and each has a characteristic phenotype (Kelly 1980). Konigsmark and Gorlin (1976) referred to both 18r and 18q- syndromes indicating that 65 percent of these patients are reported to be deaf. Evidently, the hearing impairment associated with anomalies of the 18th chromosome is conductive. Some studies have reported stenosis of the external auditory meatus, for example, where others have revealed malformations of the ossicles and/or the tympanic membrane. Furthermore, these patients tend to be retarded, microcephalic, and to have facial anomalies which may on occasion interfere with their ability to produce intelligible speech. It seems that fewer than 100 cases of chromosome 18 arm deletions (18q-) have been reported, and these reports do not suggest a diminished life expectancy. There has also been a report of three children with 18p- syndrome (Thompson, Peters, and Smith 1986). These children were found to be less retarded than earlier literature would have caused one to expect; however, two of the three had severe linguistic deficits, and all three demonstrated articulatory difficulties.

Hence, programs of primary, secondary, and tertiary prevention should be made available. Primary prevention, again, takes the form of parent counseling for the reasons stated above, namely that chromosomal disorders appear with increased frequency in older mothers. Secondary prevention would arise probably from the observation that the child has an anomaly of the midface, which should lead the diagnostician to make chromosomal studies. Having acquired the evidence that this is, indeed, a deletion syndrome of the eighteenth chromosome, then the appropriate habilitative measures can be taken for hearing, speech, and language.

5p-, Cri du Chat Syndrome Deletion of the short arm of the fifth chromosome (5p-) results in a syndrome most uniquely named by the sound of the infant's cry. It is said that the cry of such an infant sounds like the cry of a cat, and hence is called Cri du chat syndrome. Presumably, this distinctive cry results from hypoplasia of the larynx. Figure 2–11 compares the spectrum of the cry of such an infant with the cry of a normal term newborn.

The patient with Cri du chat syndrome is mentally retarded and has a characteristic face (Figure 2–12). Evidently, there is no literature which suggests an increased risk of hearing impairment among 5p- patients, although they do have low-set pinnae. However, obviously, language disability at least concomitant with the amount of mental retardation should be expected. The narrow oral cavity may lead to additional problems with articulation. There is no known etiology, including advanced maternal age, for the Cri du chat syndrome.

Other Disorders of Structure Other deletion syndromes have been reported. For example, a few cases of 9p- have appeared (Figure 2–13). These children seem to be mentally retarded and language delayed, but little else is known about the consequences of this deletion. Abnormalities of chromosomes 4 and 12 have also been described (e.g.,

FIGURE 2-11. (a) Sonogram of a normal cry. (b) Sonogram of a Cri-du-chat (5p-) cry

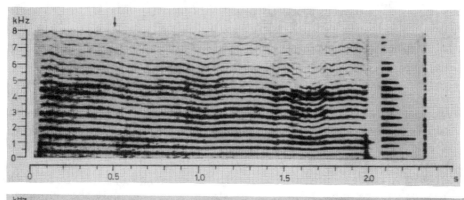

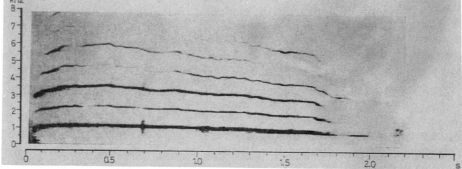

Courtesy of J. Hirschberg.

Kelly 1980; Nyhan and Sakati 1976). One supposes that deletion syndromes, whether of the short or long arm of any chromosome, probably arise from the same kinds of things that produce aneuploidy or polyplody: maternal age, ionizing radiation, environmental toxins, and so on. A case of arm addition has now come to our attention; 16q+ has been identified in a young man described as unintelligible, severely retarded, and sometimes aggressive toward himself and others (Figure 2-14).

Disorders of Sex Chromosomes

Remember that mammals, including *homo sapiens,* have their gender determined by the presence or absence of a Y chromosome. In humans, the Y is carried only by males; therefore, only a father can create a son. The mother gives only X chromosomes to her offspring. Hence, a child who receives the X chromosome from each parent will be female, and a child who receives a Y chromosome from the father will be male. Although that seems to be simple enough, things don't always work out

FIGURE 2–12. 5p- (Cri-du-chat syndrome)

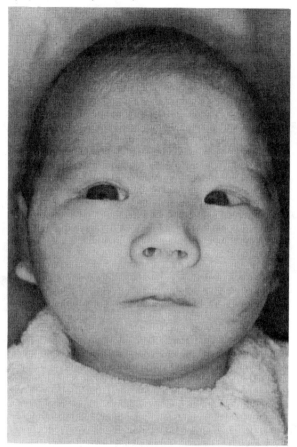

SOURCE: James S. Thompson and Margaret W. Thompson, *Genetics in Medicine,* 3rd ed. (Philadelphia: W. B. Saunders Co., 1980), p. 154. Reprinted by permission.

that way. For example, if the offspring has only one sex chromosome, and that one is X, the child will frequently appear to be male, although, 45X usually results in a female (see discussion below). Sometimes an offspring may end up with the wrong number of sex chromosomes. This results in, for example, XYY or XXX, when the number is too many, or X0 (i.e., 45X) when the number is too few.

Sex chromosome abnormalities appear in about 1 in every 400 male births and 1 in every 650 female births. Sex linked chromosomal disorders are always due to a mutant X chromosome; there are no known Y-linked disorders.[1] The reason that all aberrations are X-linked is that

[1] Some writers have pointed out that the only Y-linked trait is the family name!

FIGURE 2–13. 9p- syndrome

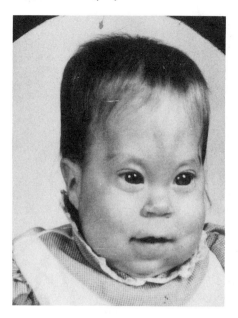

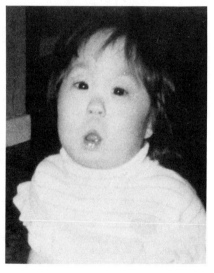

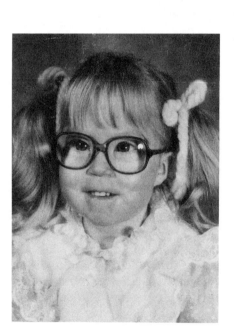

FIGURE 2–14. 16q+ syndrome

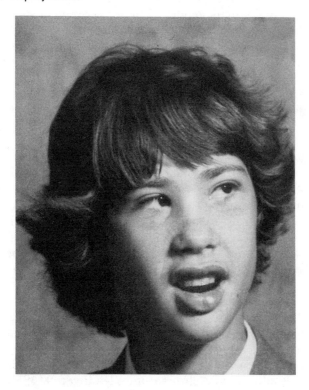

each pair of chromosomes has comparable gene determinates at the same position on each chromosome of each pair. So if one parent passes a normal X chromosome and the other an abnormal X chromosome to their daughter, the normal will dominate. But X dominates Y; hence, if the X chromosome is mutant and the father passes a Y, then the mutation will appear in the male offspring of such a mating and is called X-linked recessive. An X-linked recessive trait will be expressed in male offspring because there is no normal partner gene. The daughters of the male child, who receive his X, will all be carriers of the trait but will be normal; all of his sons, because they get his Y, will also be normal. On the other hand, an X-linked recessive trait will not be expressed in carrier females because the other X chromosome is normal. The risk for affected sons and carrier daughters of a normal and carrier female is 50 percent. A mutant X chromosome combined with a normal Y chromosome is what produces X-linked disorders; they pass from mother to son. Sex chromosome disorders occur more frequently in male than in female offspring because males are hemizygous.

Sometimes one of the sex chromosomes is not passed on at all, and this can lead to ambiguous gender. The most common such aberration is 45X, which means that the other sex chromosome is missing entirely. The description of normal, recall, is 46XX (a normal female) or 46XY (a normal male); the notation means that there are 46 chromosomes, including two sex chromosomes. Disorders with an extra sex chromosome are more common than those with a sex chromosome missing. In fact, the majority of sex chromosome disorders is found in the category 47XXX.

XYY Syndrome There has been a great deal of interest in males who have an extra Y chromosome (Jacobs et al. 1965). It seems almost a joke to suggest that the extra Y chromosome makes for extremes of supposedly masculine behavior. It turns out, however, that 20 percent of tall males studied in prisons display XYY syndrome. Hence, it has been suggested that this chromosomal disorder predisposes to criminal or psychopathic behavior. Statistics show, in fact, that the probability of imprisonment is six times greater for XYY males than for normal XY males.

The XYY syndrome does seem to be an example of a chromosomal disorder that is passed from father to son, as it apparently results from nondisjunction leading to YY sperm. Moreover, Grass et al. (1984) suggested that XYY males "may be at an increased risk of producing aneuploid progeny." Also, XYY sometimes is combined with syndromes where there are additional X chromosomes leading to XXYY and XXXYY variants.

Ethical questions having to do with prevention of XYY syndrome are difficult and unanswered. For one thing, it is improbable that one would know that a given patient had the XYY syndrome unless there were some reason to ask that specific question. Of course, there could be such reasons, that the patient had already demonstrated criminal behavior, for instance; but then it is too late for prevention of either the trait or the crime. An occasional infant may be identified as part of a newborn research survey or during some prenatal or perinatal studies for an apparently unrelated reason. Then what? One form of prevention would be clinical abortion, but this cannot possibly be justified. The vast majority of persons with the XYY syndrome are not criminal— even if they might turn out to be unpleasant persons. Should we suggest the early introduction of behavior modification procedures for patients in whom antisocial behavior has not appeared? How do we know that it will ever appear? Hence, although XYY may be subject to some forms of primary or secondary prevention, at the present state of knowledge, the only course available is tertiary prevention. It may be possible to prevent or control further antisocial behaviors in XYY patients.

FIGURE 2–15. 45X (Turner syndrome)

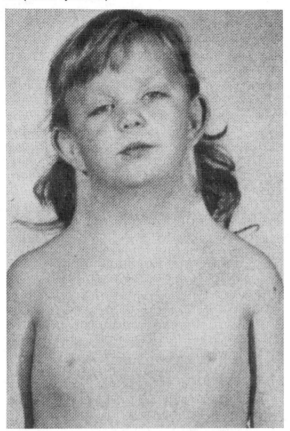

SOURCE: Jorge J. Yunis, ed., *Chromosomes in Biology and Medicine: New Chromosomal Syndromes* (Orlando, FL.: Academic Press, 1977), p. 94. Copyright 1977.

45X, Turner Syndrome Turner, in 1938, described a syndrome characterized by a reduced angle of the elbow, webbing of the neck, short stature, and sexual infantilism (Figure 2–15). The sexual infantilism is typically accompanied by hormone deficiency; estrogen replacement therapy is often indicated and a few individuals have been fertile. Ford et al. (1959) were the first to demonstrate that such patients lack a second sex chromosome. The karotype, then, is 45X; some literature identifies it as 45X0 to indicate that the other sex chromosome is missing. Thompson (1986) reported Turner syndrome to be the "only sex chromosome abnormality that appears in abortions with appreciable frequency . . . " In fact, she said that it is the most common cytogenetic abnormality and accounts for 18 percent of all abortions due to chromosomal aberrations, is present in 9 percent of all spontaneous abortions, and appears in 1.4 percent of all conceptions. In other words, Turner syndrome occurs fairly often.

Fraser (1976) reported that hearing losses are common in persons with sex chromosome disorders. Especially relevant for the immediate purpose, then, is the fact that patients with Turner syndrome frequently have conductive or mixed hearing impairments. Sensory-neural hearing loss has been reported in as many as 65 percent of Turner syndrome patients, and 10 percent of these patients demonstrate severe deafness. Furthermore, as many as one-third to one-half of these patients have been reported to have frequent, recurrent otitis media. Obviously, then, Turner syndrome is of concern to the communication disorders specialist.

This concern, however, need not usually extend beyond the consequences of the hearing impairment, although that is sufficient. Netley's (1983) review revealed that Turner syndrome females (obviously it does not appear in males) have deficits in nonverbal skills. Netley has also shown that 45X patients often do not show the normal right ear advantage in dichotic listening tests and that they are the ones with the most severe impairments of nonverbal abilities. Furthermore, Netley's patients had a mean WISC-R verbal IQ of 97.5 with a performance IQ of 84.4. In other words, the verbal cognitive function of these patients is normal and is about one standard deviation superior to their nonverbal function on this test. Curiously, Netley failed to distinguish between those Turner syndrome patients who do and those who do not have hearing impairments; one must suppose that his studies were limited to those with normal hearing.

There is a certain element of natural primary prevention, namely the large number of *abortuses* (more than 90 percent) with 45X. Nevertheless, it must be stressed to the parents that the recurrence rate is low. In one family that has come to our attention there is one 45X child among eight siblings, and she is not the youngest. Also, in the case of 45X, it may be the father's X chromosome that is missing. Of course, prenatal diagnosis can be available. The Turner syndrome phenotype is usually identifiable at birth, although it has sometimes been confused with Noonan syndrome (see Chapter 3). Early diagnosis should lead to early intervention. Because even in the case of hearing impairment, Turner syndrome patients have normal verbal abilities, auditory habilitation can be instituted at an early age both in the form of hearing aids and of frequent monitoring of the risk for recurrent otitis.

XXY, Klinefelter Syndrome Klinefelter syndrome (Klinefelter, Reifenstein, and Albright 1942) is another sex chromosome disorder that is not likely to be identified early unless there is reason to ask about it in a given patient, for example, if it had already occurred in that family. Usually it is discovered at puberty because it is characterized by the

FIGURE 2–16. 47 XXY (Klinefelter syndrome)

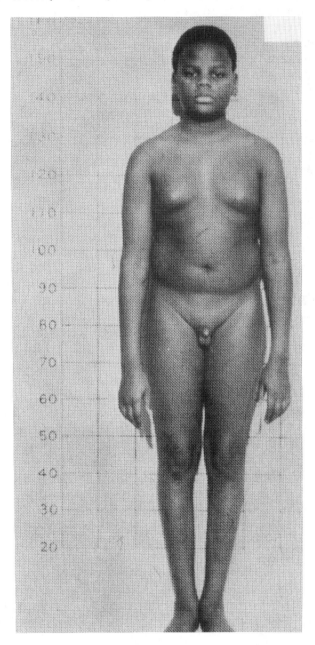

SOURCE: Courtesy of Dr. David L. Remoin.

stigmata of the additional X chromosome (hence, 47XXY). Because all patients with Klinefelter syndrome carry a Y chromosome,[2] they are all male; similarly, all patients with Turner syndrome are female because they never have a Y chromosome. The stigmata of Klinefelter syndrome appear at puberty because the secondary sex characteristics fail to arise; the patients tend to be eunuchoid. The typical patient will be rather tall, have poor development of male genitalia, and display the breasts of a small female (Figure 2–16).

Patients with Klinefelter syndrome suffer a progressive mental retardation, 20 percent have progressive hearing impairments, and Ludlow and Cooper (1983) reported that as many as 75 percent of cases studied display delays of language and phonological acquisition. As one would expect, therefore, verbal IQ scores have been lower than performance IQ—the opposite of Turner syndrome—but not always (Graham et al. 1988).

There are variants of Klinefelter syndrome, but common to all is the presence of a Y chromosome and more than one X chromosome. The literature has reported XXXY, XXXXY, and others. The addition of still more X chromosomes seems to increase the severity of the abnormality of the phenotype in sexual, intellectual, and communication development.

Treatment for Klinefelter syndrome patients who have developmental language problems is not inherently or necessarily different from that offered to other patients with language delays. Again, the issues of primary and secondary prevention are like those for other chromosomal disorders. Maternal age is a factor. Furthermore, prenatal diagnosis and genetic counseling should be offered to the family of such a patient. According to Smith (1976), the recurrence risk is not known but is expected to be rather low. This fact alone is a kind of primary prevention. Secondary prevention could be available to such a family in the case where they already have one child with Klinefelter syndrome. Amniocentesis may be done prenatally and/or chromosomal studies may be done in the early neonatal period. Bear in mind that the signs of Klinefelter syndrome do not usually appear until puberty; therefore, a family that already has a child with the syndrome would probably want to have another conceptus studied.

Fragile X Syndrome   The fact that there are sites of fragility on human chromosomes is not news. Hecht and Hecht (1984) claimed that this has been known for some 20 years or more. When fragility appears on an X chromosome—the best known and well understood of such

---

[2] However, Andersson, Page, and de la Chapelle (1986) reported that the Y-chromosomal DNA in XX males is found on the short arm of one of the X chromosomes. This was determined by the presence of a substance called Y-encoded testis-determining factor.

conditions—it results in a relatively common form of X-linked mental retardation. According to Carmi et al. (1984), this type of mental retardation affects at least 1 in every 1,000 live born males, and Wolf-Schein et al. (1987) added 1 in 2,000 females. Nielsen (1983) reported the fragile X syndrome to account for 2 to 6 percent of mentally retarded males.

There is a characteristic appearance including a large head, prominent forehead, long, narrow face, prominent chin, and large ears; however, there is an absence of clearly dysmorphic features; and these traits are not recognizable in infancy. Hockey and Crowhurst (1988) listed the syndromal features that appeared in more than half of the children they studied: big ears, big hands and feet, blond hair, hypotonia, light and soft skin, long face, macrocephaly, multiple pigmented nevi, narrow bifrontal diameter, photosensitivity, and strabismus. The single finding most commonly associated with fragile X syndrome is *macro-orchidism,* a remarkable enlargement of the testicles. This finding is rarely reported in prepubescent males, but it seems to be universal among those who have passed the age of puberty. No endocrinologic or histologic mechanism responsible for this enlargement has been identified. Furthermore, macro-orchidism is not specific to this syndrome.

According to Sparks (1984), expression of the mental retardation would arise in all males who inherit a fragile X chromosome. She, as well as Wolf-Schein et al. (1987), claimed that fragile X syndrome is second in frequency of occurrence only to Down syndrome as a cause of mental retardation. Families of patients who are known to have the fragile X syndrome have been investigated for speech and language function. Howard-Peebles, Stoddard, and Mims (1979) reported finding a general language disability in adults related to fragile X syndrome patients, and that none of these subjects had normal articulation. Moreover, Wolf-Schein et al. (1987) found that the language deviance observed in their male subjects "cannot be attributable to level of mental retardation." They were different from matched males with Down syndrome.

Brown et al. (1982) claimed to have seen four cases of fragile X syndrome with autism. Similarly, Levitas et al. (1983) diagnosed autism in six of their ten patients with fragile X syndrome. More recently, Brown et al. (1986) reported 13.1 percent of autistic males to be positive for fragile X. Nielsen (1983) found 20 of her 27 patients (74 percent) exhibited "severe psychiatric/behavioral" problems. Wolf-Schein et al. (1987) also found a similarity in the specific language characteristics of their patients and those with autism. However, one should not leap to a cause-and-effect conclusion, but only assume that there could be some frequency of association between these two syndromes which is larger than otherwise expected. Moreover, it is possible that some of the later appearing signs of fragile X are suggestive of Rett syndrome (Chapter 3). Nevertheless, the fragile X phenotype has been described as including self-mutilation, outbursts of violence, autistic behavior, and psychosis (Ho, Glahn, and Ho 1988).

However, as Hecht and Hecht (1984) pointed out, everyone has fragile sites and they are not always on the X chromosome. For example, Smeets, Scheers, and Hostinx (1984) reported fragility of the third chromosome; it was shown in 48 of 50 suspected subjects, meaning that it must be a rather common form of chromosome fragility. Nevertheless, they failed to report the consequences of this phenomenon. One would suppose from their observations that its consequences are not clinically significant since they stated "that everybody or almost everybody will express it under appropriate culture conditions."

What, then, about prevention? Carmi et al. (1984) claimed that children with fragile X syndrome can be detected in infancy with careful measurement of testes. However, they were careful to observe that macro-orchidism is not specific to fragile X, nor does it always occur with the fragile X syndrome. Furthermore, karyotyping would not necessarily reveal fragile X syndrome because it requires a particular kind of analysis that is not usually done. On the other hand, they urged "meticulous measurement of newborn and infant testes." They argued that this early detection would enable appropriate and timely counseling for the family and treatment for the infant, that is, secondary prevention. Indeed, their patient had "no speech" at the age of four years; hence, early identification could have been beneficial.

To introduce universal *orchidometry,* however, is to raise the fear suggested by Hecht and Hecht to frighten the family "that this is abnormal and warrants prenatal diagnosis." In other words, the fact that the patient may be both mentally and language retarded is in itself sufficient cause for diagnostic and therapeutic intervention. The detection of the fragile X chromosome is obviously irrelevant to that particular patient. Furthermore, there is no strong evidence that parents who have produced a child with fragile X syndrome would necessarily or ever produce another.

According to Cantu and Jacobs (1984), there is considerable variation in the expression of the fragile X syndrome even in the same family. What may be still more significant, in fact, is that they reported a variability of expression among different cells of the same individual, and they claimed that the fragile X chromosome is rarely seen in more than 50 percent of cells of patients who have the syndrome. Cantu and Jacobs concluded, therefore, that "the biologic basis . . . is not obvious . . . " Hence, one may conclude that primary prevention may be difficult if not impossible.

Clearly, the question does arise if such a patient has not been previously diagnosed in the same family. Furthermore, even if such a patient had been diagnosed, again note the observation of considerable variation within the same family (Varley, Holm, and Eren 1985) or even the same individual (Cantu and Jacobs 1984). Secondary prevention by universally applied orchidometry, it seems to us, is not warranted; this is an excessive attempt at secondary prevention. The fact remains, however, that if a child presents with intellectual and/or language delay, then that child should be treated accordingly. One cannot suggest that children who have developmental language problems and have fragile X syndrome are somehow therapeutically different from other children with developmental problems.

AMNIOCENTESIS AND PRENATAL DIAGNOSIS

In the preceding sections of this chapter it has been mentioned that amniocentesis could be available and prenatal diagnosis possible. Generally, there are three approaches whereby prenatal diagnosis may be made: amniocentesis, radiographic or ultrasonic visualization, and fetoscopy.

Amniocentesis

In 1961, Liley developed the technique now known as amniocentesis, and Steele and Breg reported the first chromosomal studies on amniotic fluid obtained in this way in 1966. By this procedure, the *amnion*—the fluid-filled sac that contains the fetus—is tapped through the abdomen and amniotic fluid is withdrawn. Amniocentesis permits the acquisition of two kinds of information: the karyotype of the fetus and the biochemical status of the fetus. The amniotic fluid contains the same constitution and distribution of chromosomes as the fetus who lives in that fluid. Hence, if a fetus is carrying a chromosomal disorder, that disorder can be discovered by analysis of the amniotic fluid.

The procedure for performing amniocentesis is conceptually relatively simple and is done commonly in the hands of a competent obstetrician. Modern amniocentesis is typically done under visual control using the ultrasonic imaging technique (discussed below). With the ultrasonic imager, the amniotic cavity may be seen on a television screen and the cannula required to withdraw the fluid is visualized. The needle carrying the cannula is introduced above the symphysis and is pushed toward the amniotic cavity (Figure 2–17). The cannula, as described by Jonatha (1974), is 1.24 mm thick. When the obstetrician is able to see the needle in the amniotic space, a small amount of fluid is withdrawn.

FIGURE 2–17. Amniocentesis under ultrasonic visual control

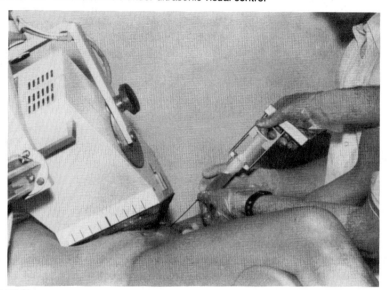

SOURCE: Courtesy of Dr. W. Jonatha.

This is a virtually no-risk procedure, and can be performed in the office in about five minutes; however, the ultrasonic equipment is not always available in the office. In addition, under ultrasonic visualization, it is possible to guide instruments to sample tissue from the forming placenta. This tissue is composed of chorionic villi which are produced by the embryo and therefore carry its chromosomes and genes.

Some years ago, the U.S. Department of Health, Education, and Welfare approved amniocentesis as a procedure by which genetic disorders may be detected (Culliton 1975). In 1980, the American Academy of Pediatrics' Committee on Genetics published a statement again endorsing the use of amniocentesis. The committee described the procedure as "a safe method for antenatal diagnosis." Epstein and Golbus (1977) pointed out that, in principle, all chromosomal aberrations can be detected by prenatal diagnosis. Of course, fetal karyotyping is not a general procedure, nor should it be; amniocentesis is performed only when there is reason to do so. In other words, it would be done when there is some question of the pregnancy leading to an abnormal birth. This applies particularly to Down syndrome because it does occur so frequently. In fact, Epstein and Golbus reported that the risk of having a child with Down syndrome is as great as 7.5 percent among mothers who have achieved the age of 45 years. Clearly, then, in such a case, amniocentesis is indicated. However, it happens that fewer than half of pregnant women who should have amniocentesis actually get it (Sepe et al. 1982).

Given that amniocentesis is performed, any karyotype may be observed. Consequently, a piece of fortuitous information that necessarily accompanies karyotyping is identification of the sex of the fetus. Obviously, though, amniocentesis would not be performed solely so that the parents might plan according to gender. Smith (1976) listed five conditions that should lead a clinician to consider amniocentesis. First is the often repeated fact of late maternal age. A second condition is that amniocentesis should be done for women under the age of 30 years who already have had a child with Down syndrome. Third, Smith recommended amniocentesis for a potential parent who has a known significant risk of producing a genetically abnormal offspring. This extends, fourth, to the case of a pregnant woman who is a known carrier of a serious X-linked disorder. And, finally, amniocentesis is obviously indicated for women who already have had children with serious chromosomal disorders, especially trisomy 13, trisomy 18, and XXY Syndrome. These are listed because the recurrence risk is unknown. Smith wisely observed, also, that there is a potential psychological benefit to mothers if they can know that they will not have a repetition of the problem of a serious chromosomal disorder.

Are there counterindications to the use of amniocentesis? There are none that are medically related; the risk of complications is less than 0.5 percent (National Institute of Child Health and Human Development 1979). However, misinformation can lead to psychological and social difficulties for parents who are carriers of some trait but who do not express it.

Karyotyping is not the only potential result of amniocentesis. Epstein and Golbus (1977) noted that cultured amniotic cells may be used to determine the biochemical status of a fetus. They also observed that biochemical disorders are of low incidence but are still very serious. At the time of their writing, 40 different biochemical disorders had been diagnosed by the technique of amniocentesis and another 35 were capable of diagnosis. By 1983, Starke reported that more than 190 disorders and defects could be diagnosed prenatally.

Again, the clinician doesn't ask every possible question but only those for which there is a reason. Significant among these would be tests for Tay-Sachs disease, glycogen storage diseases, and the *mucopolysaccharidoses*. Furthermore, the alpha fetoprotein test for neural tube defects can now be done via amniocentesis. The mucopolysaccharidoses are of concern to the communicative disorders specialist because we know that patients with *Hunter* or *Hurler* syndromes suffer progressive hearing impairment and progressive language disorders (see Chapter 8). Elevated alpha fetoprotein levels are associated with neural tube defects (e.g., spina bifida and anencephaly), hydrocephalus, congenital nephrosis, and several other disorders. Lowered alpha fetoprotein levels are associated with Down syndrome.

Ultrasonography

Earlier reference was made to the possibility that prenatal diagnosis may be made by radiographic or ultrasonic studies. The fact is that radiographic studies are done very rarely, due to the risk of chromosomal damage to the developing fetus. We know that ionizing radiation (e.g., X ray) can be harmful to a fetus. In fact, earlier in this chapter it was mentioned that ionizing radiation has been one of the principal sources of chromosomal disorders. Consequently, the use of X ray for prenatal diagnosis has been largely abandoned and this has been even truer since the development of diagnostic ultrasound for the purpose. An excellent review article with respect to this technique and its consequences is by Birnholz and Farrell (1984).

The use of ultrasonic imaging requires that acoustic pulses be transmitted into the body from a probe applied to the skin (Figure 2–18). Striking tissues of various density as they move through the body, these pulses are reflected with correspondingly proportional amplitude. The amplitude of the reflection, then, depends on the properties of the structure from which the pulses are being reflected. Thus, the amplitude of the reflection varies with composition, compressibility, and density of the structures (Birnholz and Farrell 1984). These reflections can be computerized, analyzed, and displayed on what is called a tissue reflectivity map. In this case, the images are synthesized line by line such that each line of the image represents the echo of an individual pulse. Consequently, one gets what Birnholz and Farrell called a "spatial map of echogenic centers within the tissues." A fetus is an ideal system with which to create such a map.

Because scientists know a great deal about fetal development, the ultrasonic map permits a rather careful determination of fetal age. This can be very important knowledge particularly if it is essential to delay or hasten the time of delivery due to some intrauterine upset. In fact, while much remains to be learned about fetal growth patterns, the ultrasonic image gives a better estimation of fetal development than any other calculation of the date of conception based on menstrual cycle. A common error in the determination of fetal age arises from inaccurate dating based on the time of the last menstrual cycle. Sonographic evaluation gives a more accurate estimate of fetal age, especially in cases where the fetus may be suspected of being large-for-dates (McGahan and Osborn 1985). Also, rapid uterine growth may be caused by events that could be harmful to the fetus such as *hydramnios* or an intrauterine mass.

FIGURE 2–18.   Patient undergoing sonography

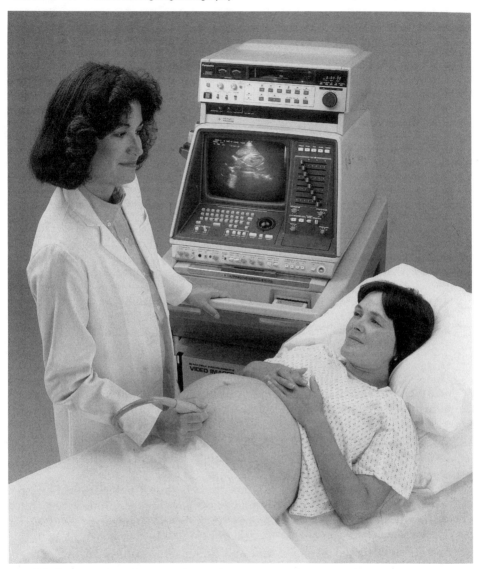

SOURCE: Courtesy of Hewlett-Packard Medical Products Group.

Importantly, moreover, the fetal anatomy is revealed as well as the fetal growth (Figure 2–19). Hence, it is possible to detect a number of anatomical abnormalities within roughly the first half of a pregnancy. These would include assorted structural anomalies such as those that occur in limbs, congenital heart defects, and neural tube defects. For

FIGURE 2–19. Sonogram of a fetus

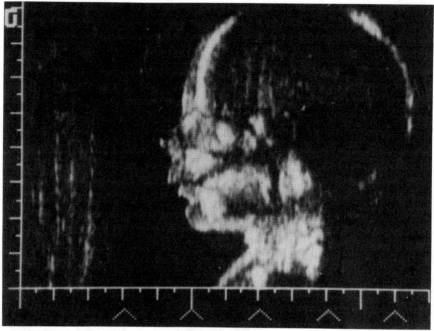

SOURCE: Courtesy of Dr. Jason Cordell Birnholz.

example, certainly the most profound birth defect is *anencephaly,* a severe deficiency of cerebral tissue that is always fatal. It can be identified by the ultrasonic imaging technique around the ninth week of gestation. Even Down syndrome can be visualized late in the pregnancy; but, of course, karyotyping of the amniotic fluid would provide an earlier diagnosis.

Of special relevance is the fact that the aural palpebral reflex (the eye blink) to sound has been demonstrated by this technique in the third trimester of prenatal development (Birnholz and Benacerraf 1983). It is well established that the APR—the aural palpebral or eye blink reflex— is reliably elicited in newborns and is a useful crude test of hearing. Because this response is present immediately after birth, it is reasonable to assume that it is present before birth as well. Using the ultrasonic imaging technique, Birnholz and Benacerraf have demonstrated that this is the case.

Finally, there is considerable promise for a great range of disorders to be diagnosed by this technique. In 1984, the American Academy of Pediatrics' Committee on Research reported that "modern ultrasound has brought another dimension to the early diagnosis of major malformations." The committee added that this technique could eventually lead to surgical correction in utero, an excellent form of primary prevention. Harrison, Golbus, and Filly (1984) observed that "It was not until the last half of this century that the prying eye of the ultra-sonographer rendered the once opaque womb transparent, letting the light of scientific observation fall on the shy and secretive fetus."

Fetoscopy

Fetoscopy permits direct visualization of the fetus *in utero*. One would suppose, therefore, that fetoscopy would be preferable to ultrasonography. However, over the past decades, the ultrasound technology has advanced much farther and more rapidly than that of fetoscopy. In his 1978 review, Omenn stated that there was "considerable enthusiasm" for fetoscopy until 1974. In fact, this enthusiasm was directed especially toward neural tube defects (e.g., spina bifida) as well as other major nervous system anomalies leading to mental retardation or poor organ function. And, he continued, there was progress in finer use of fiber optics and multiple lens systems. However, one needs to bear in mind that fetoscopy is invasive and ultrasonography is not. There is a 3 to 5 percent miscarriage rate with this procedure, and the narrow field of view limits utility (Starle 1983). Perhaps for such reasons, among others, the ultrasonic methods developed much more rapidly while, simultaneously, the biochemical methods that became possible under amniocentesis also developed. So, for example, while the fetoscope could indeed identify a neural tube defect, the alpha fetoprotein test of amniotic fluid turned out to be much less troublesome and equally or more sensitively diagnostic.

Fetoscopy is not in wide use today, at least not anywhere near as wide as ultrasonography. The 1980 statement of the American Academy of Pediatrics described fetoscopy and some other methods "as an adjunct to other forms of prenatal screening and diagnosis."

CONCLUSION

A large and varied content has been covered in this chapter. The point for the speech-language pathologist and the audiologist is that the disorders that arise from chromosomal aberrations should concern them. It is essential to know about chromosomes, about what happens to them, and what the consequences are. We are not medical geneticists or genetic counselors, but we must see their patients with understanding. We must also participate fully as professionals in prevention of all chromosomal disorders, not just those appearing in our patients.

GLOSSARY

abortus: the product of a conception (i.e., an embryo or fetus) that is lost in an abortion, whether spontaneous or induced.

acrocentric: a chromosome with very small short arms due to the centromere being close to one end.

adenine: one of the two major purines found in DNA and RNA.

amniocentesis: the process whereby the uterine wall is punctured to withdraw amniotic fluid by syringe.

amnion: the fluid-filled sac that contains a fetus or embryo.

amniotic fluid: the fluid that fills the uterus during pregnancy; the fluid in which the fetus is bathed.

anencephaly: markedly defective development of brain and cranial tissue.

aneuploid: an abnormal number of chromosomes; that is, a number of chromosomes not an exact multiple of the haploid.

autosomes: any and all chromosomes that are not sex chromosomes.

brachycephaly: a disproportionate shortening of the head; a reduction of the anterior-posterior dimension.

centromere: the primary constriction of a chromosome that divides the chromosome into two pairs of arms.

codon: a sequence of three bases in any strand of DNA and which specifies a single amino acid.

conceptus: produced by conception; an embryo.

cytosine: a pyrimidine found in DNA and RNA.

deoxyribonucleic acid (dna): a nucleic acid that is thought to be the component that produces chromosomes and many viruses and is considered to be the repository of hereditary characteristics.

diploid: the normal number of chromosomes (2 x 23=46); therefore, the state of a cell that contains 46 chromosomes.

genes: the functional units of heredity occupying a specific place on a chromosome and capable of directing the formation of proteins.

genome: the complete set of genes.

genotype: the variations of a gene at any given locus; hence, the genetic constitution of an individual.

guanine: one of the two major purines.

haploid: the normal number (23) of chromosomes in a gamete, i.e., an ovum or sperm.

heterogametic: capable of producing both X and Y chromosomes; in humans only the male is heterogametic.

homogametic: capable of producing only one type of sex chromosome; in humans the female is homogametic and produces only X chromosomes.

hydramnios: a condition of excessive amniotic fluid.

hypoplasia: defective or incomplete development of a body part.

karyotype: the complete set of chromosomes of an individual; therefore, a photograph of a karyotype.

leucine: one of the essential amino acids.

macro-orchidism: testicular enlargement.

meiosis: the process of cell division which results in gametes.

metacentric: a chromosome with the centromere placed such that the two sets of arms are of approximately the same length.

mitosis: the usual cell division process which results in two daughter cells with exactly the same DNA as the original.

mosaicism: an individual or cell with two different karyotypes; it results from somatic mutation.

mucopolysaccharidoses: a set of diseases characterized by a disorder of mucopolysaccharide metabolism and defects of bone, cartilage, and connective tissue.

mutation: a change of DNA that is revealed in change of both the phenotype and the genotype.

orchidometry: measurement of testes.

phenotype: the total nature of an individual in biochemical, physical, and physiological terms; the result of the genotype.

polyploid: any multiple of the haploid other than diploid; therefore, 3*n*, 4*n*, etc.

purine: a substance said to be the parent of certain amino acids such as adenine and guanine; it is not known to exist as such in the human body.

ribonucleic acid (rna): a nucleic acid found in all cells in both nuclei and cytoplasm.

serine: hexacosanoic acid; an amino acid.

stigmata: the evidence of a disease or condition.

submetacentric: a chromosome with its centromere placed such that the arms are of unequal length.

teratogen: any external agent causing congenital malformations.

translocation: the transfer of a segment of one chromosome to another.

triploidy: three times the haploid number; that is, 3 x 23=69.

trisomy: the state of there being an extra chromosome; for example, (2 x 23) + 1=47.

urasil: a base found in RNA.

valine: a constituent of most proteins.

REFERENCES

AMERICAN ACADEMY OF PEDIATRICS, COMMITTEE ON GENETICS. 1980. "Prenatal Diagnosis for Pediatricians," *Peds.*, 65, 1185–86.

AMERICAN ACADEMY OF PEDIATRICS, COMMITTEE ON RESEARCH. 1984. "Fetal Research," *Peds.*, 74, 440–41.

ANDERSSON, MEA, DAVID C. PAGE, AND ALBERT DE LA CHAPELLE. 1986. "Chromosome Y–Specific DNA Is Transferred to the Short Arm of X Chromosome in Human XX Males," *Science*, 233, 786–88.

BARNES, DEBORAH M. 1987. "Defect in Alzheimer's Is on Chromosome 21," *Science*, 235, 846–47.

BIRNHOLZ, JASON C., AND BERYL R. BENACERRAF. 1983. "The Development of Human Fetal Hearing," *Science*, 222, 516–18.

BIRNHOLZ, JASON C., AND E. E. FARRELL. 1984. "Ultrasound Image of Human Development," *Amer. Scientist*, 72, 608–13.

BROWN, W. T.,.et al. 1982. "Association of Fragile X Syndrome with Autism," *Lancet*, 1, 100.

————1986. "Fragile X and Autism: A Multicenter Survey," *Amer. J. Med. Gen.*, 23, 341–52.

CANTU, E. S., AND PATRICIA A. JACOBS. 1984. "Fragile (X) Expression: Relationship to the Cell Cycle," *Human Genetics*, 67, 99–102.

CARMI, RIVKA et al. 1984. "Fragile-X Syndrome Ascertained by the Presence of Macro-Orchidism in a 5-Month-Old Infant," *J. Peds.*, 74, 883–86.

CULLITON, BARBARA J. 1975. "Amniocentesis: HEW Backs Test for Prenatal Diagnosis of Disease," *Science*, 190, 537–40.

DOWN, J. L. H. 1866. "Observations on an Ethnic Classification of Idiots," *London Hospital Reports*, 3, 259–62.

EDWARDS, J. H., et al. 1960. "A New Trisomic Syndrome," *Lancet*, 1, 787–90.

EPSTEIN, CHARLES J., AND MITCHELL S. GOLBUS. 1977. "Prenatal Diagnosis of Genetic Diseases," *Amer. Scientist*, 65, 703–11.

FORD, C. E. et al. 1959. "A Sex-Chromosome Anomaly in a Case of Gonadal Dysgenesis (Turner's syndrome)," *Lancet*, 1, 711–13.

FRASER, GEORGE R. 1976. *The Causes of Profound Deafness in Childhood*. Baltimore, MD: Johns Hopkins University Press.

GERBER, SANFORD E., AND GEORGE T. MENCHER. 1980. *Auditory Dysfunction*. Houston: College-Hill Press.

GRAHAM, JOHN M., JR., et al. 1988. "Oral and Written Language Abilities of XXY Boys: Implications for Anticipatory Guidance," *Peds.*, 81, 795–806.

GRASS, F., et al. 1984. "Reproduction in XYY Males: Two New Cases and Implications for Genetic Counseling," *Amer. J. Med. Genetics*, 19, 553–60.

GRIFFITH, F. 1928. "The Significance of Pneumococcal Types," *J. Hygiene*, 27, 113–59.

HARRISON, MICHAEL R., MITCHELL S. GOLBUS, AND ROY A. FILLY. 1984. *The Unborn Patient.* Orlando, FL: Grune & Stratton.

HECHT, FREDERICK, AND BARBARA KAISER HECHT. 1984. "Autosomal Fragile Sites Not a Current Indication for Prenatal Diagnosis," *Human Genetics,* 67, 352–53.

HO, HSIU-ZU, T. J. GLAHN, AND JU-CHANG HO. 1988. "The Fragile-X Syndrome," *Dev. Med. Child Neurol.,* 30, 257–61.

HOCKEY, A., AND J. CROWHURST. 1988. "Early Manifestations of the Martin-Bell Syndrome Based on a Series of Both Sexes from Infancy," *Amer. J. Med. Gen.,* 30, 61–71.

HOWARD-PEEBLES, PATRICIA N., GAYLE R. STODDARD, AND MILDRED G. MIMS. 1979. "Familial X-Linked Mental Retardation, Verbal Disability, and Marker X Chromosomes," *Amer. J. Human Genetics,* 31, 214–22.

JACOBS, PATRICIA A., et al. 1965. "Aggressive Behaviour, Mental Subnormality and the XYY Male," *Nature,* 208, 1351–52.

JONATHA, W. 1974. "Amniocentesis in Early Pregnancy Under Ultrasonic Visual Control," *Electromedica,* 42, 94–96.

KELLEY, THADDEUS E. 1980. *Clinical Genetics and Genetic Counseling.* Chicago: Year Book Medical Publishers.

KHOURY, MUIN J., et al. 1988. "Congenital Malformations and Intrauterine Growth Retardation: A Population Study," *Peds.,* 82, 83–89.

KLINEFELTER, H. F., E. C. REIFENSTEIN, AND F. ALBRIGHT. 1942. "Gynecomastia, Aspermatogenesis Without Aleydigism and Increased Excretion of Follicle-Stimulating Hormone," *J. Clin. Endocrinol.,* 2, 615–27.

KONIGSMARK, BRUCE W., AND ROBERT J. GORLIN. 1976. *Genetic and Metabolic Deafness* Philadelphia: Saunders.

LEJEUNE, JEROME, MARTHE GAUTIER, AND RAYMOND TURPIN. 1959. "Etude des Chromosomes Somatiques de Neuf Enfants Mongoliens," *C.R. Acad. Sci.,* 248, 1721–22.

LEVITAS, ANDREW, et al. 1983. "Autism and the Fragile X Syndrome," *J. Dev. Beh. Peds.,* 4, 151–58.

LILEY, A. W. 1961. "Liquour Amnii Analysis in the Management of the Pregnancy Complicated by Rhesus Sensitization," *Amer. J. Obs. Gyn.,* 82, 1359–70.

LITCH, SUZANNE. 1984. "Prevention Curriculum in the Public Schools." Unpublished paper presented at the *Conference on Tomorrow's Child,* Irvine, CA, 1984.

LUDLOW, CHRISTY L., AND JUDITH A. COOPER, eds. 1983. *Genetic Aspects of Speech and Language Disorders.* New York: Academic Press.

McGAHAN, JOHN P., AND ALAN R. OSBORN. 1985. "Sonographic Evaluation of the Large-for-Dates Pregnancy," *Perinatology-Neonatology,* 9(4), 45–52.

MAGENIS, R. E., et al. 1977. "Parental Origin of the Extra Chromosome in Down's Syndrome," *Human Genetics,* 37, 7–16.

NATIONAL INSTITUTE OF CHILD HEALTH AND HUMAN DEVELOPMENT. 1979. *Antenatal Diagnosis,* NIH Publ.No. 79—1973. Bethesda, MD: National Institutes of Health.

NETLEY, C. 1983. "Sex Chromosome Abnormalities and the Development of Verbal and Nonverbal Abilities," in *Genetic Aspects of Speech and Language Disorders,* ed. Christy L. Ludlow and Judith A. Cooper. New York: Academic Press.

NIELSEN, KAREN BRONDUM. 1983. "Diagnosis of the Fragile X Syndrome (Martin-Bell Syndrome). Clinical Findings in 27 Males with the Fragile Site at Xq28," *J. Ment. Defic. Res.,* 27, 211–26.

NYHAN, WILLIAM L. AND NADIA O. SAKATI. 1976. *Genetic and Malformation Syndromes in Clinical Medicine.* Chicago: Year Book Medical Publishers.

OMENN, GILBERT S. 1978. "Prenatal Diagnosis of Genetic Disorders," *Science,* 200, 952–58.

PAPARELLA, MICHAEL M., AND MARY JAYNE CAPPS. 1973. "Sensorineural Deafness in Children—Genetic," in *Otolaryngology* vol. 2, ed. Michael M. Paparella and Donald A. Shumrick. Philadelphia: Saunders.

PATAU, K., et al. "Multiple Congenital Anomaly Caused by an Extra Autosome," *Lancet,* 1 (1960), 790–93.

SANDO, ISAMU, et al. 1975. "Temporal Bone Histopathologic Findings in Trisomy 13 Syndrome," *Ann. Otol., Rhinol., Laryngol.,* 84, Suppl. 21, 1–20.

SEESEL, THOMAS V., ed. 1985. *National School Health Services Program.* Princeton, NJ: Robert Wood Johnson Foundation.

SEPE, STEPHEN J., et al. 1982. "Genetic Services in the United States 1979–80," *Amer. Med. Assn. J.,* 248, 1733–35.

SINEX, F. MAROTT, AND CARL R. MERRILL, eds. 1982. *Alzheimer's Disease, Down's Syndrome, and Aging* New York: The New York Academy of Sciences.

SMEETS, D. F. C. M., J. M. J. C. SCHERES, AND T. W. J. HUSTINX. 1984. "The Fragile Site on Chromosome 3," *Human Genetics,* 67, 351.

SMITH, DAVID W. 1976. *Recognizable Patterns of Human Malformation: Genetic, Embryologic, and Clinical Aspects,* 2nd ed. Philadelphia: Saunders.

SPARKS, SHIRLEY N. 1984. *Birth Defects and Speech-Language Disorders,* San Diego, CA: College-Hill Press.

STARKE, LINDA, ed. 1983. *Screening and Counseling for Genetic Conditions.* Washington, DC : President's Commission for the Study of Ethical Problems in Medicine and Biomedical and Behavioral Research.

STEELE, MARK W., AND W. ROY BREG, JR. 1966. "Chromosome Analysis of Human Amniotic Fluid Cells," *Lancet,* 1, 383.

THOMPSON, JAMES S., AND MARGARET W. THOMPSON. 1980. *Genetics in Medicine,* 3rd ed. Philadelphia: Saunders.

THOMPSON, MARGARET W. 1986. *Genetics in Medicine,* 4th ed. Philadelphia: Saunders.

THOMPSON, RONALD W., JO E. PETERS, AND SHELLEY D. SMITH. 1986. "Intellectual, Behavioral, and Linguistic Characteristics of Three Children with 18p- Syndrome," *J. Dev. Beh. Peds.,* 71–7.

TURNER, HENRY H. 1938. "A Syndrome of Infantilism, Congenital Webbed Neck, and Cubitus Valgus," *Endocrinol.,* 23, 566–74.

VARLEY, CHRISTOPHER K., VANJA A. HOLM, AND MUAZZEZ O. EREN. 1985. "Cognitive and Psychiatric Variability in Three Brothers with Fragile X Syndrome," *J. Dev. Beh. Peds.,* 6, 87–90.

WAARDENBURG, P. J. 1932. *Das Menschliche Auge und Seine Erbanlagen.* The Hague: Nijoff.

WENTHOLD, ROBERT J. 1980. "Neurochemistry of the Auditory System," *Ann. Otol., Rhinol., Laryngol.,* 89, Suppl. 74, 121–31.

WOLF-SCHEIN, ENID G. et al. 1987. "Speech-language and the Fragile X Syndrome: Initial Findings," *Asha,* 29, 35–8.

3

Disorders of Genetic Origin

A large proportion, probably the majority, of the incidence of hearing impairment is of genetic origin. At least one-third of all cases of congenital deafness is of genetic origin, and it is likely that figure is closer to one-half. If we exclude disorders that arise from disease or injury, it is probable that many (if not most) speech and language disorders are genetically based, including stuttering. In fact, probably 75 percent of cases of stuttering are genetic (Ingham 1987). Certainly there are numerous instances of genetically based multiple handicaps that include disorders of speech, language, and/or hearing among their stigmata, as, for example, Noonan syndrome, the second most frequently occurring multiple handicap. With this awareness, it has become essential for the communicative disorders specialist to have more than a mere acquaintance with rules of inheritance and the means to prevent genetic disorders.

Until the twentieth century, our understanding of genetics was more mystical than biological. Aristotle—from whose ideas we suffered for so many centuries—proposed that organisms were formed through sexual production in a manner by which the female egg provides the substance and the male seminal fluid provides the form. He apparently believed, though, "Nothing . . . can be produced contrary to . . . nature." A belief in the mystical influence of the semen persisted into the sixteenth century when the great biologist William Harvey named it the *aura seminalis*. In fact, during the seventeenth and eighteenth centuries, our understanding of inheritance did not improve substantially. There were those who claimed the existence of a homunculus that was preformed in both parents and was waiting to be nourished so that it might grow into an adult form. Obviously, then, the number of children a couple might have was determined by the number of homunculi already in place. Still in the eighteenth century, biologists believed that tissues and organs that appeared during the development of an organism arrived de novo, that is, from nothing at all. They ascribed this process to mysterious vital forces. Even Charles Darwin believed that each body organ and component was preexistent in so-called invisible copies to be transported by the bloodstream to sex organs and there assembled into gametes.

This notion of preformation was finally rejected by the parent of modern embryology, Kaspar Wolff, in the latter half of the eighteenth century. Wolff knew about differentiation and growth of embryonic cells (see Persaud 1985). The classic experiment in genetics was the work of the monk Gregor Mendel. Interestingly, Mendel's data were published in 1866, but no one seems to have noticed or cared until 1900. Hence, genetics is literally a twentieth-century science.

WHAT ARE GENES? WHERE ARE THEY?

The dictionary tells us that a gene is a functional unit of heredity that occupies a given place on a chromosome and is capable of every division of prenatal life. Genes are the germ tissue of living creatures, the irreducible structures appearing at the first primordial level of development.

Generally, this unit consists of a molecule of DNA that contains the appropriate numbers of *purine* and *pyrimidine* (which are bases) in a certain sequence such that they can code amino acids needed for protein synthesis (see Chapter 2). More simply, genes are pieces of DNA that find their homes (so to speak) on every chromosome. They are the units of genetic information encoded in the DNA of the chromosomes. All genes occur in pairs except those that appear on sex chromosomes. A gene located on any chromosome other than a sex chromosome is said to be *autosomal*. Conversely, genes located on sex chromosomes are called sex-linked genes, X-linked or Y-linked.

In essences, then, genes (like chromosomes) are everywhere. If a given gene is located at the same spot as another on a given chromosome, they are said to be *linked*. Sometimes, genes can appear in alternative forms; these are called *alleles*. However, one chromosome carries only a single allele at a given locus. There may be multiple alleles in any given population of genes, and any allele may occupy any given locus.

Chromosomes of the same number are said to be *homologous*. The alleles, then, are genes that appear at the same locus on any given pair of homologous chromosomes. If the alleles are identical on the two chromosomes, the individual who carries them is said to *homozygous.* If the alleles are not identical, the individual is *heterozygous.* In a genotype where both genes at a given location are mutants, the alleles are said to be compound.

Forms of Genetic Transmission

An allele that is expressed in a heterozygous individual is said to be *dominant.* Thus, a dominant genotype will be expressed in the phenotype. If homozygosity is required for the allele to be expressed, it is said to be *recessive.* Consequently, what we are talking about is actually the phenotype when we say that the genotype has been expressed. However, convention has it that we speak of dominant and recessive genes. The third form of genetic transmission arises when the alleles appear on the X or Y chromosomes, that is, they are sex-linked.

The relationship between the genotype and the phenotype is not always obvious or forthright. The fact that a given allele exists in a genotype does not necessarily mean that it will be expressed in the phenotype. McKusick (1978) estimated that there are 30,000 structural genes in the human animal. Furthermore, he calculated that these can be expressed in 2,786 abnormal conditions of which 1,473 are autosomal dominant, 1,108 autosomal recessive, and 205 X-linked. Indeed, there is a great deal of variability in phenotypic expression. Moreover, many phenotypes are determined by more than one gene; they are said to be *polygenic.* Additionally, some genetic traits are influenced by the environment and are therefore said to be products of *multifactorial inheritance.*

During development, the number of interactions between the genotype and its environment is literally innumerable, making it truly impossible to draw a direct line from genotype to phenotype. Therefore, we must be aware of two notions important to the geneticist: penetrance and expressivity (or expression). *Penetrance* refers to the proportion of genotypes producing or leading to a given phenotype; *expressivity* is the degree to which a particular effect is expressed by individuals.

Consider the following: Not all the children of deaf parents will be deaf themselves because the penetrance varies; furthermore, even among deaf siblings, expressivity varies such that one child may have a greater hearing impairment than another. Moreover, there are interactions between genes and the environment that are sometimes beneficial; for instance, congenital deafness does not always result from prenatal rubella. Why not? It may be that some of us are genetically predisposed to environmental effects more than others, or some of us are more resistant. These phenomena, penetrance and expressivity, serve to make the life of the genetic counselor or medical geneticist still more difficult.

Nevertheless, it is essential to understand them in dealing with parents, patients, and families.

Consider an example from our clinic. Both Mr. and Mrs. H were congenitally deaf. They had two children, and both children were congenitally deaf. One might easily conclude that a homozygous dominant gene is at work here and is being passed phenotypically to the children through one or both parents. In this case, that would have been a wrong conclusion. Different genotypes may produce the same phenotype (variable penetrance), and the same genotype may produce different phenotypes (variable expression); that was the case in this family. Although both parents did have genetic forms of deafness, one of them was found to be dominant and the other recessive. It turned out, on further examination, that the children had inherited the dominant form of deafness from their father. They did not express the recessive form of deafness that was expressed in their mother. She had *Pendred syndrome;* they did not. On the other hand, note that 50 percent of deaf children have deaf parents, but only 10 percent of the children of the deaf are deaf themselves. Many instances do not have a genetic component.

Another example would be stuttering. Recall that 75 percent of cases of stuttering seem to be inherited, but the form of inheritance is not the same for all stutterers. Stuttering appears more frequently in the male children of female stutterers than in their female children. This suggests that some of these cases may be X-linked, especially as the children of male stutterers rarely show the disorder.

Dominant inheritance Among McKusick's 2,786 abnormal genetic conditions, the majority (1,473 = 53 percent) are dominantly inherited. The simplest definition of genetic dominance derives directly from Mendel's experiments. Suppose that one parent carries a given trait— say, blue eyes or left handedness—and the other does not. The process by which one trait would appear and the other would not is called dominance. In more specific language, if one parent is heterozygous for a given autosomal dominant gene and the other parent is homozygous for the normal allele, 50 percent of the products of that mating will express the trait.

In fact, this is the usual pattern of inheritance for autosomal dominant traits because it less frequently happens that both parents will carry the *same* dominant alleles or that either parent will be homozygous for the dominant allele. Such kinds of dominant transmission do occur, but they are rare. Examples would be when both parents are homozygous for the dominant trait, one parent is homozygous for the dominant trait and the other is heterozygous, one parent is homozygous for the dominant trait and the other is homozygous for the normal, or both parents are heterozygous for both the normal and abnormal alleles.

Normals occur, of course, when both parents are homozygous for the normal alleles. Figure 3–1 displays a case of dominant transmission.

Although we say that 50 percent of the offspring of the typical dominant mating will express the phenotype, penetrance just doesn't work that way. Take a familiar example: If you toss a perfectly balanced coin often enough, it will come up heads half the time and tails half the time. But the fact that it came up heads last time does not imply an increase in the probability that it will come up tails the next time. In other words, the 50–50 chance of the phenotype expressing the genotype reappears with each mating. Hence, it is conceivable that the penetrance would be such that a parent who expresses a trait could still produce no

FIGURE 3–1. Dominant inheritance

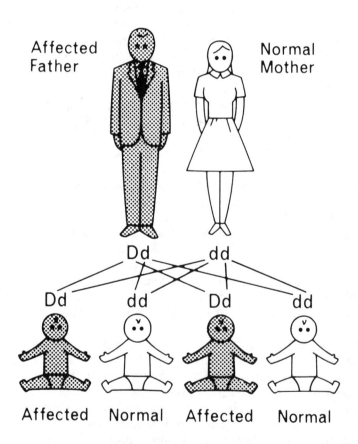

SOURCE: Marilyn J. Krajicek and Alice I. Tearney, eds., *Detection of Developmental Problems in Children* (Austin, TX.: PRO-ED, Inc., 1977), p. 66.

children with that phenotype, or it is possible that all of the children would have the trait.

The fact that the deaf H parents produced two deaf children does not necessarily tell us that either parent is homozygous for dominant deafness; we need more information. It turned out that Mr. H was dominantly homozygous for deafness; but the fact that his children were deaf was not a sufficient reason to suspect it. In their case, one parent was homozygous for that trait and the other was not, which necessarily leads us to consider penetrance in every mating product. Expressivity is a different issue; one of the H children was much more seriously impaired than the other.

As we should expect, a large number and variety of communicative disorders are genetically determined. Assuming (and we should) that McKusick's estimates of the relative proportions of dominant, recessive, and X-linked inheritance apply to communicative disorders as much as to other kinds of anomalies, we should conclude that somewhat more than half of all genetically determined communicative disorders are due to dominant inheritance. Furthermore, because both penetrance and expressivity vary in dominant disorders, it is probable that some proportion of patients whose communicative disorders are supposed to be of unknown origin are actually of genetic origin and more often dominantly inherited than inherited by either of the other two mechanisms. This could explain why deafness appears in a family where it is not known to have appeared before, why children with language problems sometimes have a parent who may have difficulty with spelling, why children with phonologic delays may have parents who were "late talkers", and so on. Furthermore, because there is not a one-to-one correspondence between genotype and phenotype, genotypes are expressed in many different phenotypes; the communicative disorders of the children need not match those of their parents to have been inherited.

Recessive inheritance An autosomal recessive trait can be expressed only in homozygotes. In other words, people who express a recessively inherited phenotype must have received the recessive gene from both parents (Figure 3–2). Again, because penetrance is variable, the phenotype may not appear at all. However, because both parents must be heterozygous in order for any offspring to be affected, all of the children will be carriers of the trait, whether or not they express it. In a typical family in which the parents are heterozygous for a recessive trait (Aa × Aa), one-quarter of the children will be AA and will be affected by the trait, one-quarter will be unaffected (aa), and one-half will be carriers (Aa).

There is an important, if rare, exception to this rule: when the same homozygous alleles are in both parents, that is, same locus. If two

FIGURE 3–2.   Recessive inheritance

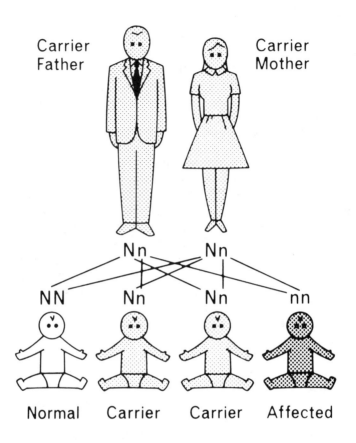

Carrier Father

Carrier Mother

Nn   Nn

NN   Nn   Nn   nn

Normal   Carrier   Carrier   Affected

SOURCE: Krajicek and Tearney (1977), p. 69. Courtesy of PRO-ED, Inc.

phenotypically normal individuals carry the autosomal recessive abnormal gene, as described above, their risk for producing a child with that genotype and that phenotype is 25 percent. However, whether or not both families have expressed the trait, if the trait was caused by the same autosomal recessive gene, their risk for producing the abnormal phenotype is 100 percent (Carrel 1977).

We had an interesting illustration of this exception in our clinic. Mr. and Mrs. J were healthy parents with normal hearing, but they had three sons all of whom were profoundly hearing impaired. What happened? The best guess in light of other information is that both parents were heterozygous for the deafness gene with the abnormal alleles at the same gene location. Therefore, although they did not express the trait, their children had to. This could have arisen simply from statistical probabilities, or from something else.

Consider another example. It appeared to be a case similar to the one above in which normal parents had two deaf children and no knowledge of family history of deafness. It took some very good detective work on the part of a genetic counselor to discover that these parents were distant relatives. In other words, their deaf children were the products of *consanguinity*. It seems that these parents were descended by five generations from deaf brothers: the great-great-great grandfather of one was the brother of the great-great-great grandfather of the other. Evidently at work was a heterozygous recessive gene that was not expressed in five generations because, in all of those matings, the normal allele of the mate appeared. Five generations later, however, a male carrying a heterozygous deaf gene mated with a female carrying an identical heterozygous deaf gene, and all of their offspring expressed the trait. This is not at all a strange story.

Consanguinity, in fact, is a frequent cause for the expression of recessive traits, and is more nearly the norm in some parts of the world than in others. Generally, there are two reasons for this. One is that the geography of the region permits very little interchange outside of the community. Hence, for example, birth defects (including those with consequences for communication) are relatively very common in some of the remote areas of the Andes. Simply stated, no one comes or goes from those mountain valleys, and everyone is related. The other reason for the appearance of consanguinity, frequently seen in the Middle East, is cultural. Middle Eastern custom and tradition, and some religious mandates, have it that one would not marry outside the family. So it is typical for a man to marry his niece, for example. In other cultures, such as some communities of southern India, a man's niece is the daughter of his brother and he may not marry her. His sister's daughter, however, is not his niece; he can marry her.

If we examine parts of the world where consanguinity is the norm, we find that the incidence of genetic disorders is very high. The world's highest incidence of congenital deafness does appear in the Andes, in Bolivia and Peru. The incidence of congenital deafness in Israel had been nearly double what it is in North America because immigrants from Arab lands to that country have intermarried for many centuries as a matter of custom. Cleopatra was married to her brother because he was the only person in the world who was her equal. The final evidence of the effect of consanguinity is that the incidence of birth defects in Israel has decreased with the education of these immigrant families on the point. In some Muslim countries—Kuwait is one where the data are known—

the rate of consanguineous matings exceeds 90 percent due to ancient custom and to religious mandate. If the reader finds Kuwait, India, or Bolivia to be exotic, note that the incidence of birth defects in the Appalachian regions of the United States and among the so-called Pennsylvania Dutch is also very high and for the same reasons.

Consanguinity will increase the penetrance incidence of recessive traits. Hence, although McKusick's (1978) estimates would predict that about 40 percent of cases are due to autosomal recessive inheritance, there are places where the proportion is much greater. Fraser (1976), in his magnificent volume on the subject, concluded that "it is not to be expected that the distribution of the various mutant alleles causing deafness, whether dominant or recessive, autosomal or X-linked, is either qualitatively or quantitatively uniform; indeed marked differences are known to exist."

The forms of recessive inheritance are only one contribution to this lack of uniformity. Part of the problem is that the geneticist's art does not yet permit us to determine if a given autosomal recessive disorder is related to the same or to different loci. Some may be explained by a single major locus hypothesis; perhaps stuttering is an example. As Carrel (1977) pointed out, the risk for the offspring expressing the trait is 100 percent for parents who have the same mutant alleles; otherwise, it may be as low as 1 in 200 (0.5 percent) given the range of possible loci at which the same mutant alleles could appear.

X-linked inheritance   In reading a descriptive term "X-linked inheritance," we should ask about the absence of Y-linked inheritance. As it turns out, things don't happen that way; there are few known Y-linked traits in humans. Although we might suppose that mutant alleles could appear with equal likelihood on X or Y chromosomes, contemporary knowledge contains no Y-linked anomalies. A Y antigen necessary to male development is located on Y. Consequently, in Homo sapiens, the terms "sex-linked" and "X-linked" may be interpreted synonymously. Remember, though, that only males receive Y chromosomes; hence, the female off-spring get X chromosomes from both parents, but the males get the X only from their mothers. Therefore, in the case of X-linked recessive inheritance, it is only the mother's allele on the X chromosome that matters, and that is why X-linked disorders pass from mother to son (Figure 3–3). The son, who has only one X chromosome, will have the disorder which is carried on that chromosome penetrate. The daughter, who has two X chromosomes, one normal and one abnormal, will be a carrier for the trait but it will not penetrate. In other words: "The distribution of X-traits in families follows the course of the X chromosome carrying the abnormal gene" (Thompson 1986).

FIGURE 3–3. X-linked inheritance

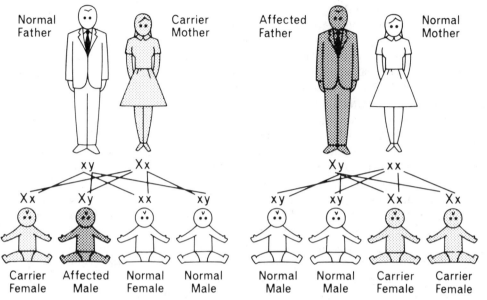

X-Linked Inheritance (Through Carrier Woman)	X-Linked Inheritance (From Affected Male)

Normal Father — Carrier Mother

x y   X x

Xx   Xy   xx   xy

Carrier Female   Affected Male   Normal Female   Normal Male

Affected Father — Normal Mother

X y   x x

xy   xy   Xx   Xx

Normal Male   Normal Male   Carrier Female   Carrier Female

SOURCE: Krajicek and Tearney (1977), pp. 72 and 73. Courtesy of PRO-ED, Inc.

Variations

In the preceding discussion, we have learned that genes are bunches of protein collected as pairs of alleles on each and every chromosome except for the sex chromosomes. The basic amino acids of the normal proteins are derived from the information contained in the genes such that they are formed at the time DNA transcribes into RNA. Thus, a change in the DNA sequence may result in an abnormal amino acid sequence. This is what causes abnormal inheritance—whether dominant, recessive, X-linked, or sporadic—but which may also be without effect. Wenthold (1980) observed that even a single incorrect amino acid "may alter the properties of the protein so severely that it may be totally inactive, may function with limited efficiency, may function normally but have altered physical properties, or, . . . may cause little or no functional or physical change." In fact, some gene mutations may even be beneficial.

All new heritable variations arise by mutation. Hence, it may be claimed that any genetic change is a mutation, but the custom is to define mutation as a change that does not depend on some normal combination of genes or rearrangement of chromosomes. Many mutations are lethal; they lead to the death of the fetus. On the other hand, geneticists have introduced the notion of *fitness*, which, in a restricted sense, means only the ability to transmit one's genes to one's heirs and for them to transmit in turn to their heirs.

A case in point is sickle cell anemia. Three different genotypes may result in this phenotype; hence, there can be two or more alleles at a given locus that occur fairly often. This is known as *polymorphism*. In the case of polymorphic sickle cell anemia, there is an advantage to the heterozygotic form. Heterozygotes are resistant to malaria, and malaria remains the world's leading cause of death (Grant 1981). Although the phenotype may eventually suffer from the sickle cell anemia disease, the patient is equally resistant to malaria. This is not true for the homozygotic form of sickle cell anemia. Homozygotes have a fitness of zero; that is, they do not pass on the risk for sickle cell anemia and the beneficial protection against malaria. Consequently, they do not produce ill offspring, but they are as susceptible to sickle cell anemia as are their heterozygotic neighbors and they are also susceptible to malaria.

Of course, the truth is not always easily discernible. Traits that are due to *sporadic inheritance*—that is, they appear in families where they have never appeared before—do not reproduce. So, although a new phenotype may have appeared, a new genotype has not. Mutations, on the other hand, produce new phenotypes and new genotypes for that family. There are situations, such as *achondroplasia*, in which at least 80 percent of the patients are due to new mutations. Because achondroplasia arises sporadically, there is no increase in the recurrence risk for parents of such a child of having any more. But the child has a 50 percent chance of reproducing this disorder because this mutation does produce a new genotype, resulting in an autosomal dominant phenotype. Achondroplastic dwarfs are typically hearing impaired. Another example is *mandibulofacial dysostosis*, or Treacher Collins syndrome. Perhaps as many as half of the incidents of this craniofacial disorder are new mutations, and the disorder is autosomal dominant.

This discussion excludes, for the time being (see Chapter 4), the issue of mutagens and genetic predispositions toward them. Moreover, we have introduced the concepts of penetrance and expressivity, meaning that the inherited trait may or may not appear and, if it does, it may appear with various degrees of severity. All of the preceding discussion, in fact, is based on single gene inheritance. There is another category of genetic disorder.

Multifactorial inheritance has also been called polygenic, meaning determined by many genes at different loci. This is an illustration of the rule that different phenotypes may result from the same genotype and that different genotypes may result in the same phenotype. Also, multifactorial genetic inheritance is frequently influenced by the environment, and that makes it even more difficult to be absolutely confident that it is truly multifactorial. Nevertheless, some disorders that are of consequence to the communicative disorders specialist are known to be inherited multifactorially, particularly cleft lip with or without a cleft of the palate. Kelly (1980) stated that the polygenetic or multifactorial forms of inheritance are continuous (for example, height) and are greatly influenced by environmental agents. Therefore, he preferred the term "multifactorial causation."

The rest of this chapter deals with some of the very many communicative disorders that are, in whole or in part, inherited. Keep in mind, however, that we often don't know with total confidence about a particular patient or a given disorder. Also remember the caution that the same genotype may have different phenotypes, the same phenotype can result from several genotypes, and many (most?) disorders are polygenic or multifactorial. So, although the following discussions indicate the form of inheritance, be alert to other possibilities and to unknowns. When reading, bear in mind the limitations that would be characterized by descriptors like "usually," "typically," and the like.

INHERITED COMMUNICATIVE DISORDERS

Autosomal dominant inheritance refers to the transmission of the trait expressed in the heterozygous state. What does that mean? It indicates that all heterozygous offspring will express the phenotype. Look at the idealized pedigree in Figure 3–1. Suppose that we have a family in which one parent demonstrates the phenotype (Dd) and the other parent is normal for that genotype (dd). Hypothetically, then, if they had four children, they could have two sons and two daughters, two children who are homozygous and unaffected, and two children who are heterozygous and do not express the phenotype but are carriers for the dominant allele. These two carriers, then, have a risk of producing the trait in their children that is still 50 percent. However, if both parents express the same autosomal dominant disorder (Dd), something that is very rare, the risk of reproducing it is 75 percent (Carrel 1977). In the real case, contrary to the ideal case, these risks remain the same with each succeeding pregnancy. Hence, it is possible that all or none of the offspring will express the trait, but they all could be carriers of that trait.

At this point in our discussion, remember that the terms "congenital" and "genetic" are not synonyms. The term *congenital* describes any condition, genetic or nongenetic, that exists at birth. The term *genetic,* on the other hand, refers to any condition which is transmitted through gene structure (as described earlier) that may or may not appear at birth.

The uninitiated student may have some difficulty with this second notion. It is easy enough to understand that congenital defects may be caused by things other than abnormal genes, but some of us don't appreciate that there are genes—even dominant ones—that have delayed or progressive effects on the phenotype. Yet such is the case, and, for the outstanding example, look at the later section on otosclerosis.

The majority of *monogenic* disorders—that is, those caused by a single defective gene—are of the autosomal dominant form. Kelly (1980) reported the incidence of autosomal dominant disorders to be 7 to 8 per 1,000 births, claiming, furthermore, that "the more common dominant disorders are those in which the major impact occurs later in life. . . ." Again, consider otosclerosis. Nevertheless, the proportion of genetic deafnesses without associated handicaps that are diagnosable at or soon after birth has been described by Konigsmark (1971) as "many."

Dominant Congenital Deafness

The most common form of hereditary deafness that is present at birth is dominant, severe, and sensory-neural and is not accompanied by vestibular disorders. All of these observations are important to the diagnostician, and perhaps the most important one is that the condition exists and is diagnosable at birth. Both behavioral and electrophysiologic diagnostic procedures may be applied in such cases, but they are not the topic of this book. The reader is advised to look elsewhere, for example,at Gerber (1977) and Northern and Downs (1984). The point is that these disorders are present at birth, they can be diagnosed at birth, they should be diagnosed as early in life as possible, and habilitation should be begun at the earliest feasible time. The time-worn adage "he will outgrow it" is just plain false; a practitioner's comment to "wait and see what happens" is bad advice.

Can dominant congenital deafness be prevented? Except in cases of sporadic appearance or new mutations, it has to be true that the trait has already appeared in one or both parents and/or elsewhere in the family or its history. In other words, it could be relatively simple for a medical geneticist to discover if this is a dominantly inherited trait given that the audiologist, the speech-language clinician, the pediatrician, and the otolaryngologist have collectively made the diagnosis. If the deafness is polygenic, then it is probable that it is also polymorphic, being expressed in more than one way. It is important to remember that dominant congenital deafness without associated handicaps is the single most frequently occurring category of congenital genetic deafness. Although many genetic deafnesses are not congenital and many congenital deafnesses are not genetic, among those that are both, this is the most common.

How, then, is it preventable? A kind of primary prevention is genetic counseling. Deaf parents may or may not choose to have deaf children or additional deaf children. Nevertheless, the family in which one or both mates is deaf can be counseled about the risks of producing deaf children; the decision to do so is theirs. If they choose not to reproduce, then primary prevention has occurred.

What we in the communicative disorders professions have been stressing for many years, however, is secondary prevention. Very early diagnosis and intervention are both possible and available. It may not be possible to prevent the child from being deaf, but early diagnosis and intervention should be expected to minimize the handicap that results from the deafness. We know from the work of many scientists (e.g., Greenough 1975; Webster and Webster 1979) that plasticity of the developing nervous system can be influenced in beneficial ways if only to inhibit further deterioration. The effects of early sensory deprivation and the release from deprivation have been documented repeatedly.

The child who is born with a severe hearing impairment that is dominantly inherited should be expected to benefit from early and adequate amplification, and such amplification should be provided unless there is some odd reason why it should not. For example, the youngest child in the nearly 50-year history of our clinic who has been fitted with hearing aids was seven weeks of age at the time. This is mentioned here not because it is remarkable, but because it is (or ought to be) unremarkable. The risk of acoustic trauma from excessive amplification, although it is real, is simply not very probable (Ross and Giolas 1978). In other words, the risks attendant upon not amplifying are greater than the risks that could accompany excessive amplification. This is secondary prevention.

There are those who have argued against this kind of secondary prevention on the ground that the danger of disrupting the parent-infant bond is great within the first few months of life, and hence that bond should not be disrupted by informing the parents of the handicap and taking remedial action. In our experience, we have never made a diagnosis of profound congenital deafness in an infant that was a surprise to the parents; indeed, it may have been very distressing, but not surprising. Obviously, the lack of surprise is to be expected with the patient whose deafness is dominantly inherited; it has probably already appeared elsewhere in the family, possibly in the parents themselves. Moreover, as Moses and Van Hecke-Wulatin (1981) observed, the risk to the child's educational and cognitive development from not treating exceeds the risk of the consequences of upsetting the parent-infant bond.

Finally, dominant congenital deafness cannot be prevented except insofar as a family that carries such a genotype elects to have no children. If they do decide to reproduce, such a family provides an ideal basis for secondary prevention. The first item on the high-risk register for congenital deafness developed by the national Joint Committee on Infant Hearing (1982) is family history. But it sometimes happens that deaf parents are not interested in primary or secondary prevention. Many deaf parents, although preferring to have hearing children, accept the risk of producing deaf children. And we have seen deaf parents delay the provision of amplification for their deaf babies on the grounds that, in their opinion, it isn't very important anyway. Find your friends who are deaf adults; typically they don't wear their hearing aids.

In summary, then, note that dominantly inherited disorders constitute the majority of genetic diseases. However, the majority of those are not congenital. That, then, leads to the next section.

Dominant hereditary degenerative deafness   Returning to the 1971 *nosology* of Konigsmark, we find that what he called "dominant progressive nerve deafness" was the second most frequently occurring hereditary deafness with an onset in childhood. This is not entirely consistent with the comment of Kelly (1980), mentioned earlier, that the dominant disorders commonly appear later in life. Perhaps deafness is an exception, or perhaps Kelly's notion of "impact" doesn't apply to things present at birth. On the other hand, Fraser (1976) suggested that the "formal demonstration" of the dominantly inherited phenotype is impossible because of reduced penetrance and variable expression. These don't occur in cases of recessively inherited deafness. Hence, it is entirely possible that the parents of a child whose deafness seemed to appear first at a few months of age and progressed from then on may be normal hearing themselves.

On the other hand, if the parents are deaf, then one can enjoy the luxury of being a talented diagnostician. In our clinic, for example, we observed the T family, one in which both parents and all four children were profoundly and bilaterally hearing impaired. The luxury was that we became involved with this family only at the birth of the fourth child; we already knew that both parents and all three siblings were deaf. However, the T's fourth child was obviously not deaf at one week of age, seemed to have lost some hearing by one month, much more by three years of age, and by seven years she was the only one of the four children who displayed absolutely no responses at all on customary air conduction audiometry. In such a case, then, one can be an astute diagnostician and make an educated guess of dominant degenerative deafness.

Fraser (1976) taught us that

> another even more substantial difficulty in the diagnosis of dominant forms of deafness is due to the undoubted fact that a certain proportion of cases is caused by fresh mutations, that is, transmission in a germ cell from one or the other parent of an abnormal allele which is not present in the somatic cells of the parent concerned.

In such a case, which is more common than any of us would like, the disorder did not appear in the parents or their ancestors but does appear in the children and in succeeding generations. Furthermore, in the case of hereditary progressive disorders, diagnosis may be confused by the fact that other *exogenous* events may have occurred by the time the impairment was first diagnosed.

Fraser found that 25 percent of the children he studied seemed to be products of a fresh mutation. In the 1976 encyclopedic work of Konigsmark and Gorlin, the comment is made that these early onset hearing losses appear in the first or second decade of life. But they also appear earlier. Of course, Konigsmark and Gorlin also suggested that "several disease entities have been included in this category" and pointed out that they should be distinguished by age of onset.

It appears that we do have children like those born deaf to Mr. and Mrs. T, and we also see patients who display a form of hearing impairment which is called by the paradoxical term "early presbyacusis." It seems evident, a priori, that a child who is born hearing and appears to be deaf by three months of age is probably not in quite the same category as a person who begins to lose hearing in the fifth decade of life, or perhaps the fourth, and reports that this was also true in one of the parents. This distinction is clearly important from the position of primary prevention; and, given the possibility of intervening events or instances of morbidity over a lifetime of any duration, it may be exceedingly difficult to distinguish between late onset deafness and auditory impairment due to exogenous factors. Hence, a careful and thorough pedigree is clearly essential for primary prevention in siblings and/or later generations.

Secondary prevention for the very young child with hereditary degenerative hearing impairment mandates that the child be seen repeatedly, as was the case with the fourth T child. The 1982 position statement of the Joint Committee on Infant Hearing insists that a child with a family history who passes an initial hearing screen must be rescreened periodically for some time. Probably, in fact, it should be done semiannually for at least the first three years of life. If it can be established, as it was in the T family, that a given patient clearly demonstrates a dominantly inherited and degenerative condition, then primary prevention can be offered. However, if we are dealing with the mysterious entity of early presbyacusis, then there is no prevention (in that patient) other than tertiary.

It is extremely difficult to be confident about a progressive hearing loss that appears in the fourth or fifth decade of life because such a patient has already been exposed to a variety of diseases, environmental hazards, noises, and so on. Take the example from our clinic of a father and son—both with moderate, severely sloping, sensory hearing impairments—who worked together in a lumberyard. What is the culprit: the father's genes or the noise in the lumberyard? The probable answer is both, but without an extensive family history we cannot be sure.

Dominant unilateral deafness The third item in Konigsmark's 1971 nosology is dominant unilateral deafness. His review of the literature at that time revealed only a few cases, but that may have been an underestimation. He found that this form of hearing impairment is dominantly transmitted, present at birth, does not progress, and is severe. He also reported normal vestibular findings. The more recent work of Bess (1984) and of Bess and Tharpe (1984) has drawn attention to the issue of unilateral deafness that the topic has deserved but not had.

There is actually very little literature on dominant unilateral deafness with no associated abnormalities. Even though we expect the variation of both penetrance and expressivity in dominantly inherited disorders, we also know that these unilateral impairments seem to appear much more frequently in patients who have other anomalies as well. Nevertheless, Konigsmark and Gorlin (1976) concluded that "this form of deafness is transmitted by an autosomal dominant gene that shows variable expressivity, sometimes causing bilateral congenital deafness and sometimes only unilateral deafness."

This conclusion, while undoubtedly correct, is based almost entirely on the family pedigree, shown in Figure 3–4 (Smith 1939). That pedigree shows deafness appearing in 12 of 30 family members over four generations. Of the 12, 9 had severe unilateral sensory deafness. Probably, dominant unilateral deafness, which appears in families that also have dominant bilateral deafness, is likely not a genetically different condition from that described for dominant congenital deafness. It is only the expression that is different. In other words, it is a somewhat different phenotype arising from the same genotype. Hence, the forms of prevention are the same as with children with bilateral hearing impairments.

That last comment is important in terms of tertiary prevention, habilitation, because we have ignored the fact that children with unilateral hearing impairments are indeed handicapped. We have already concluded that one ear is enough for most purposes, and it probably is. But the work of Bess shows that one ear is not enough for *all* purposes, and the statistics clearly indicate that young children with severe unilateral hearing impairments (of whatever cause) do exhibit problems not encountered with people who have two normal ears.

Noonan Syndrome

A major example wherein the family history is frequently unknown, and therefore suitable to illustrate that point, is Noonan syndrome. In 1963, Noonan and Ehmke described a number of children with cardiac,

FIGURE 3–4.   Pedigree of dominant unilateral deafness

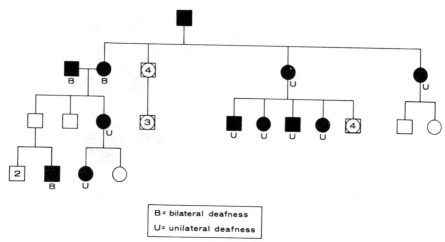

B= bilateral deafness
U= unilateral deafness

SOURCE: Bruce W. Konigsmark and Robert J. Gorlin, *Genetic and Metabolic Deafness* (Philadelphia: W. B. Saunders Co., 1976), reprinted by permission.

pulmonary, and craniofacial abnormalities. Although this phenotype, which we now know as Noonan syndrome, had been observed earlier, it was from this time that it was distinguished from other disorders. The patient with Noonan syndrome (Figure 3–5) presents with short stature, facial anomalies, congenital cardiac defects, skeletal abnormalities, genital malformations, and mild mental retardation. In fact, more than 50 different major and minor anomalies have been observed to occur in Noonan syndrome (Gorlin, Pindborg, and Cohen 1976).

Noonan syndrome is thought to be second only to Down syndrome in frequency of occurrence among conditions presenting with multiple congenital anomalies. Perhaps that is why it has sometimes been confused with other syndromes (Berman, Desjardins, and Fraser 1975). It has even been said to have a Turner phenotype, but Turner syndrome appears only in females. The incidence of Noonan syndrome has been reported to occur from 1 in 1,000 births (Summitt 1969) to as few as 1 in 2,500 births (Nora et al. 1974).

Virtually all writers on the subject of Noonan syndrome have included among its stigmata an observation of low set and/or abnormal auricles (Figures 3–6 and 3–7). This fact alone should lead one to consider the probability of congenital conductive hearing impairment; however, it has been described in detail only once (Gerber 1986). The patient did have a mild, low frequency hearing loss (down to 25 dB HL at 250 Hz) and a somewhat flattened tympanogram, and these were in the absence of ear disease.

FIGURE 3–5.   A child with Noonan syndrome

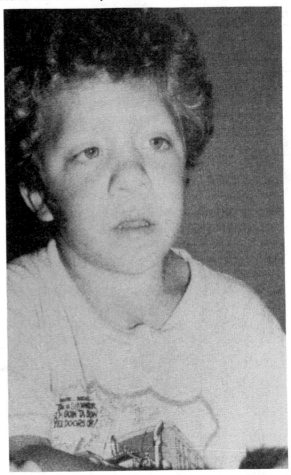

SOURCE: Courtesy of D. Elaine Pressman, ed., *Human Communication Canada.*

Curiously, also, the literature reveals only two studies of speech and language in Noonan syndrome (Hopkins-Acos and Bunker 1979; Wilson and Dyson 1982).   The patient of Hopkins-Acos and Bunker (who is the same child described by Gerber [1986]) had reasonably good receptive language at three and a half years of age, but his expressive language was limited to gestures and isolated vowel sounds.   One could not blame his relatively poor expressive language and his relatively good receptive language on his hearing impairment or on his mild mental retardation. In other words, his expressive language deficit seems to have been a property of the syndrome.

FIGURE 3–6. In Noonan syndrome, the pinnae are lowset

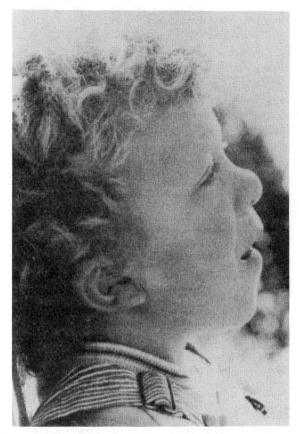

SOURCE: Courtesy of D. Elaine Pressman, ed., *Human Communication Canada.*

Although some writers have confused Noonan syndrome with other disorders, there does seem to be consensus that it is dominantly inherited but with variable penetrance and expression. For these reasons, perhaps, it may be misdiagnosed. Sparks (1984) claimed that Noonan syndrome arises sporadically, but that is apparently not true.

Noonan syndrome is a complex example of a dominantly inherited communicative disorder in which diagnosis may be incorrect or delayed because of the incomplete penetrance. Therefore, primary prevention is difficult at best, and there is a risk of postponing secondary prevention. The report by Hopkins-Acos and Bunker (1979) is an example of tertiary prevention in the form of habilitation of a particular child with Noonan syndrome. Also, the fact that this same child had surgery on both the

FIGURE 3–7.   An abnormally shaped auricle in Noonan syndrome

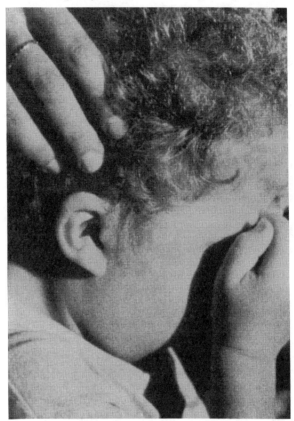

SOURCE: Courtesy of D. Elaine Pressman, ed., *Human Communication Canada.*

cardiac system and genitourinary system may be considered a form of secondary prevention. Finally, the conclusion of Konigsmark and Gorlin (1976) that Noonan syndrome is due to "possible autosomal dominant inheritance with incomplete penetrance" could sometimes lead families to genetic counseling.

Other Recessively Inherited Disorders

Recall that McKusick (1978) estimated that 40 percent of all heritable disorders are autosomal recessive. Also, Carrel (1977) supposed that there are five to ten different gene locations for deafness. Both parents must carry the gene, albeit probably at a different location, for the trait to appear; and then the risk is 25 percent. If the parents carry the gene at the same gene location, the risk is 100 percent; it will always be expressed. But remember that the figure of 25 percent is a risk factor;

that is, on the average the trait will appear in one of four births; but it could appear in all or none of a couple's children. For this reason, it is difficult to predict the occurrence of a trait, especially in a family where it has not appeared.

Consider the case of a firstborn child delivered in good health following a normal pregnancy to a family which honestly denies knowledge of any given trait in the family history. Primary prevention has certainly not occurred, and secondary prevention may be unlikely because no one knows that the child has a problem. Let us suppose that this child is severely hearing impaired and has no associated handicaps; in fact, this is the usual form of congenital deafness. This infant will not likely be on a high-risk register and is likely to go without identification for some months.

Let us consider, for example, mental retardation. Recall that we have posited mental retardation as the most common communicative disorder. Opitz (1969) calculated that 3 percent of all newborns will eventually be diagnosed as retarded, but only 2.5 percent of retarded persons have a family history. So we must conclude that mental retardation arises sporadically and/or from exogenous causes, or family history is simply unknown.

Another important example are the hemoglobinopathies, especially sickle cell disease and the thalassemias. Hemoglobin is that constituent of blood that carries oxygen from the lungs to the tissues. Recall the earlier observation that even a single protein substitution can be expressed in significant ways. In sickle cell disease, there is a single substitution in the second position of the code for glutamic acid such that it is altered to valine (Thompson, 1986). The normal (Hb A) sequence is val-his-leu-thr-pro-*glu*-glu-lys. The substitution produces val-his-leu-thr-pro-*val*-glu-lys. This causes the normal hemoglobin, Hb A, to be converted to Hb S, the hemoglobin that underlies sickle cell disease. In addition to the serious effects of this disease, including death, it has been shown that there is a high incidence of bilateral sensory-neural hearing loss (12 percent of patients) and of central nervous system involvement in those patients who have such a loss (Friedman et al. 1980).

Thalassemias are the most common single gene disorders in the world (Thompson 1986). There are many variants; but, for our purpose, thalassemia major (also called Cooley anemia) is especially relevant. This is a severe and progressive hemolytic anemia that typically appears in the latter half of the first year of life. Such patients have maxillary hypoplasia with associated dental abnormalities that, obviously, can affect articulatory ability. Additionally, endocrine abnormalities may prevent sexual maturation, and diabetes mellitus is common. The disorder is treated, or at least ameliorated, by transfusion; otherwise, it is usually fatal.

X-Linked Communicative Disorders

Disorders that are inherited by X-linked transmission are really rather rare. Sparks (1984) claimed that 109 disorders are known to be X-linked and another 98 are suspected. As Opitz observed in 1969: "There exist few well-documented X-linked malformation/retardation syndromes." One reason for this state, he observed, is that

> Occasionally it is impossible to determine from pedigree data whether the disorder affecting several siblings is due to X-linked or recessive autosomal inheritance; this is particularly true if the parents are normal and not consanguineous, if no other cases have been observed in the family, and if the affected individuals are all males.

Nevertheless, there are two classes of disorders which may be encountered by the communication disorders specialist. One is *Duchenne muscular dystrophy* and the other is one of the group of seven called collectively the *mucopolysaccharidoses* (see Chapter 8). Both of these disorders are eventually fatal, so the task for us is to improve the quality of life while it lasts.

Duchenne muscular dystrophy, by virtue of being X-linked, is found only in males. It appears around the age of 2 years, but sometimes not until as late as 6 years of age. It then spreads rapidly from the pelvic girdle up to the pectoral area, the trunk, and extremities. Typically, the child is wheel-chair-bound by the age of 10 and does not survive into the teens. Karagan and Zellweger (1978) found the full-scale WISC IQ of boys with this disorder to be significantly below normal and the verbal portion much lower than performance. Sparks concluded that "early verbal disability" is characteristic of this disease, and it thereby becomes our concern.

Primary prevention of Duchenne muscular dystrophy is subject to all the difficulties cited by Opitz and mentioned above. If, of course, the disease had already appeared in the family, then they are forewarned (one hopes) and genetic counseling should be made available. Secondary prevention is difficult as the symptoms don't appear very early in life. For tertiary prevention, Sparks recommends "very limited language goals with the flexibility to change them as the disease progresses."

The mucopolysaccharidoses are six to nine (depending on how they are described) clinically related diseases, all of them fatal and all of them with communicative implications. One of them, Hunter syndrome (MPS-II), is X-linked. The communicative consequences of all the mucopolysaccharidoses are essentially the same (see chapter 8).

The Unusual Audiogram

Audiometrists are accustomed to seeing abnormal audiograms that are flat (usually indicative of conductive impairments) or falling toward the high frequencies (usually indicative of sensory impairments). There are exceptions and some of those are diagnostic. What most auditory technicians are not accustomed to seeing are audiograms that show hearing that improves from low to high frequencies or, more peculiarly, audiograms that display the best hearing in the middle frequencies.

A number of cases (at least in excess of 100) have been identified indicating that these are dominantly inherited disorders. Konigsmark (1971) referred to dominant low frequency hearing loss and dominant midfrequency hearing loss with no associated abnormalities. Both of these, he claimed, appear in childhood, are slowly progressive, range from mild to severe, and have normal vestibular findings. Later (Konigsmark and Gorlin 1976), he suggested that this hearing impairment may be of early onset or may be congenital. Furthermore, the dominant low frequency hearing loss seems to progress to ever higher frequencies, which suggests that it may be the same kind of entity as early presbyacusis.

An important distinction between dominant low frequency and dominant midfrequency hearing losses is that it appears that the midfrequency hearing loss is stable, whereas the low frequency hearing loss progresses to higher frequencies. Clearly, this distinction is important for the planning of habilitation for such a patient. Is it going to get worse? If yes, then steps need to be taken that are different from those for a person in whom the hearing loss will not get worse. Again, however,we might be looking at many different entities, all of which are dominantly inherited and all of which show the complete range of penetrance and expression.

Hearing loss that seems to be limited to low or midfrequencies may be produced by a number of things other than inheritance. Consequently, prevention depends heavily on establishing that this is indeed a genetic condition. There are two ways to accomplish this: One, of course, is by making a pedigree of the family; the other is diagnosis by exclusion of such things as prenatal viral disease, ototoxicity, or noise. Given that is accomplished, the implications for prevention at all levels are the same as those for other dominantly inherited hearing impairments.

Otosclerosis

Otosclerosis is probably the most outstanding example of a progressive, dominantly inherited disorder. It is one of the most frequently occurring diseases among the human species, appearing in as many as one in eight Caucasian women, about half that number of white men, rarely among black people, and virtually never among orientals. Race aside, however, this is a considerable number of people. Studies of otosclerosis have appeared in literally hundreds of publications.

The summary of Konisgmark and Gorlin indicated that the characteristics of otosclerosis include autosomal dominant transmission with a penetrance of about 40 percent, gradual progression of hearing impairment occurring in the early decades of life, and normal vestibular responses, in the presence of conductive or mixed symmetrical hearing losses. Typically, otosclerosis is a disease that appears clinically in the third decade of life. Although an occasional case of otosclerosis has been reported in a child, such instances are relatively rare. It is probable, of course, that the progression of otosclerosis begins much earlier than the third decade, but it is so slow that the patient does not complain until after the age of 20. Furthermore, because the penetrance is only 40 percent, many people who actually do have the pathology associated with otosclerosis do not display the clinical signs, or at least do not display them with sufficient severity that they complain. In fact, it has been claimed that only 10 percent of people who have otosclerosis really have a hearing loss that is a problem for them (Goin 1976).

A question about the genetics of otosclerosis had been raised repeatedly in past years: why does it appear so much more frequently in women of childbearing age? If, in fact, the disease is dominantly inherited, it should not appear with greater penetrance or expression in females than in males. There are two ways out of this apparent paradox. One is for the medical geneticist to draw a complete and extensive pedigree, which should reveal that this disorder has appeared in males as well as females in the same family and that other forms of hereditary deafness have not appeared. The other solution is to examine the metabolic and biochemical status of the patient and/or the patient's disease. It appears that the kinds of metabolic changes that normally appear in women of child-bearing age aggravate the underlying pathology of otosclerosis. That is why it seems to appear more often in women and especially in women in the third decade of life. Extensive studies of the genetics and the pathology of otosclerosis have led to a firm conclusion that the disease is of genetic origin, is of late onset, is progressive, and is aggravated by metabolic changes accompanying pregnancy. There are numerous reports of women with known otosclerosis whose hearing deteriorates suddenly during pregnancy and in whom the deterioration stops following the birth of the child.

Otosclerosis, then, must be the outstanding example of inherited progressive deafness with no associated handicaps if only because it occurs so frequently. Fraser (1976) observed that there are no examples of clinically undifferentiated conductive losses that are passed on by an autosomal recessive trait. Hence, he concluded that a progressive conductive hearing loss is likely to be inherited in an autosomal dominant manner, although he suggested that X-linked recessive inheritance may be possible. Furthermore, he concluded that the most common type is otosclerosis. Differential diagnosis is not always easy, and that fact underlines the need for construction of a careful pedigree. In Fraser's extensive studies, he found cases of otosclerosis appearing with other genetically inherited hearing impairments (e.g., Usher syndrome) and cases of otosclerosis with profound hearing impairment from another cause. Again, because otosclerosis is so common, one might expect it to occur in patients who have other problems.

Prevention at all levels is indeed possible and available for otosclerosis. Primary prevention is to be found in the family history. Women who have otosclerosis are expected to produce daughters with otosclerosis and, with less frequency, sons with otosclerosis. The audiogram that accompanies otosclerosis is frequently distinguished by Carhart's notch (Figure 3–8), a notch in the bone conduction audiogram at 2,000 Hz that is not found with other conductive hearing impairments. Less often, but also signifi-

FIGURE 3–8. An audiogram showing Carhart's notch

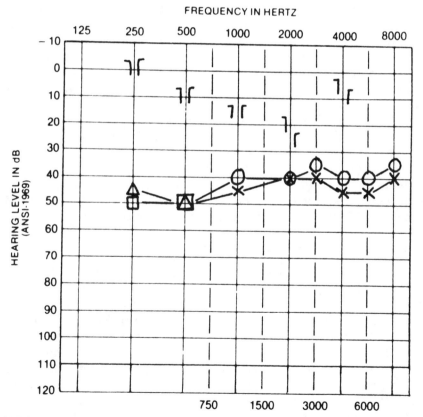

SOURCE: Frederick N. Martin, *Introduction to Audiology,* 3rd ed. (Englewood Cliffs, N.J.: Prentice-Hall, 1986), p. 253. Courtesy of Prentice-Hall, Inc. Copyright 1986.

cantly, the otologist may observe Schwarze's sign, an apparent reddish glow of the tympanic membrane peculiar to otosclerosis. Of course, what is most distinctive is the fact that the hearing impairment is familial, progressive, and conductive. Audiometric studies are a form of secondary prevention because the disease can sometimes be detected early. Tertiary prevention of otosclerosis is most commonly in the form of surgery. Stapedectomy or, occasionally, stapedolysis has a very high success rate. Paparella (1973) claimed no more than a 3 percent failure rate in the treatment of otosclerosis by stapedectomy. Those are quite good odds.

ANOMALIES OF THE NECK, HEAD, AND FACE

Many *morphogenic* alterations of facial appearance are dominantly inherited, some are recessively inherited, and all include a probability of dysfunction of both hearing and articulation. Although they are discussed in detail in Chapter 6, it is important to observe here that many of them have genetic origins. We must always consider the admonition of Stool and Houlihan (1977): "We assume that any child who has a marked facial deformity suffers from a hearing loss until we determine that he has adequate hearing."

Moreover, craniofacial alterations may signal nervous system problems as well. Wiznitzer, Rapin, and Van De Water (1987) examined 100 patients with complex ear anomalies some of whom did and some of whom did not have hearing impairment. They found that 85 of these patients had neurologic dysfunction: 56 with cranial nerve disorder, 64 with central nervous system problems, 11 with vestibular system difficulties, and 74 with anomalies in other organ systems.

External Ear Malformations

Jaffe (1978a, 1978b) has written on the significance of external ear malformations vis-a-vis other disorders. The fact is that the external ear in the human animal performs no important purpose as it does in some other higher animals. Observe, for example, your cat or dog. Notice that the external ear is mounted on the top of the head, unlike yours which you will find (I trust) on the sides of your head. You may also notice that your cat or dog is capable of moving the pinnae for the ostensible purpose of using them as localizing antennae. You and I can't do that. It seems that Homo sapiens has lost, or never acquired, the function of the external ear found in other higher animals.

The external ear does some important purposes: Facetiously, we can put earrings on the external ears, and they are useful for keeping our eyeglasses from falling off our heads. But they do serve two more important purposes. There is some reason to believe that the human pinnae do act as localizing antennae for high frequencies and as significant diagnostic clues. It has been amply demonstrated (for example, by van Gogh) that we don't need them for purposes of hearing. It has also been demonstrated, however, that malformations of the external ear (not deformations) are usually indicative of more serious malformations of the middle ear and/or other parts of the craniofacial complex. It is this point that Jaffe has discussed extensively. In a series of papers (1978a, 1978b), he has shown surgically confirmed middle ear anomalies that were signaled in the first instance by anomalies of the external ear. Also, Konigsmark (1971) listed four different dominant hereditary deafnesses that are characterized or signaled by external ear malformations. Of these four, he claimed that three of them present with conductive hearing loss (which one might expect) and one with what he called "neural hearing loss." According to Konigsmark, hearing loss occurs in about 90 percent of patients who have preauricular pits (Figure 3–9). Of these, he said, the hearing loss appears in 90 percent of the patients, the pits in 85 percent, and branchial fistulae in about 20 percent.

Again, this is a disorder that is dominantly inherited, is slowly progressive, and appears in the first or second decade of life. This particular disorder is especially significant and interesting for the following reasons. It has been our experience, in a handful of cases, that preauricular pits tend to go unnoticed or to be thought of as insignificant.

FIGURE 3–9. A pre-auricular pit

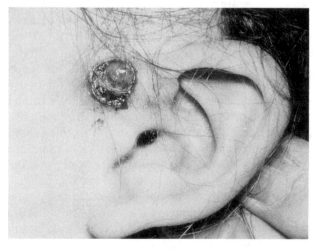

SOURCE: Sanford E. Gerber and George T. Mencher, *Auditory Dysfunction* (San Diego, Calif.: College-Hill Press, 1980), pp. 14–17. Courtesy of College-Hill Press. Copyright 1980.

Clearly, if this is a dominantly inherited disorder that includes among its stigmata a sensory hearing impairment, then it is important that the pits are not bypassed or misdiagnosed. For example, we once saw a grown woman who had been complimented all her life on the "cute dimples" that were found in the upper part of her face. These so-called "dimples" were preauricular pits; they were increasing in size and depth and migrating toward the middle ear cavity. The woman was hearing impaired.

Malformations of the external ear are generally of two kinds, which may or may not occur together. *Microtia* is the term that describes a significant reduction in the size or alteration of the shape of the external ear. *Atresia* refers to the failure of any body opening to open; hence, aural atresia refers to a primitive, incomplete, or missing ear canal. A moment's reflection about the embryology of the external ear suggests that it is reasonable to expect both to occur. However, that is not always the case, and when atresia appears without microtia, it often goes undiagnosed. It is obvious that aural atresia, in its own right, must lead to a conductive hearing impairment as there is no airborne pathway to the middle ear. Figure 3–10 shows the range of possibilities of microtia from a somewhat malformed pinna to virtually total absence of the pinna. Curiously, although this anomaly is typically dominantly inherited, it occurs more often in males than in females, twice as frequently unilaterally as bilaterally, and twice as common on the right side as it is on the left. Figure 3–11 is a photograph of a child with microtia and aural atresia.

Jaffe (1977) cited a number of patients in whom malformations of the external ear were associated with malformations of the middle ear and concomitant hearing impairments. Certainly, some of these anomalies are dominantly inherited and some inherited otherwise. He correctly observed that anomalies of the pinna are frequently overlooked or at least underregarded. It is probable that, more often than not, a primary care provider would not explore the situation further.

Jaffe stressed that hearing tests should be performed when a pinna anomaly is recognized. For example, he reported examining five children in whom the superior crus of the pinna was absent in one ear. Two of these children had a congenital fixation of the stapes footplate, and a third had an anomaly of the stapes such that only the footplate remained. It must be understood, further, that these are children in whom the external auditory meatus was present; there was no atresia of the ear canal. In one such family there were six children who had low set, cupped pinnae, congenital conductive hearing losses, but patent ear canals. Again, the pinna anomaly, in the absence of atresia, was a signal of a congenital conductive hearing impairment. Further, he reported a family in which a father and four

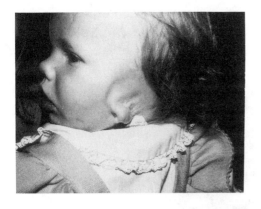
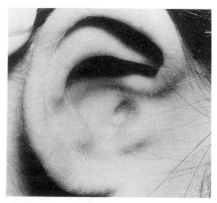

FIGURE 3–10.
Range of microtias

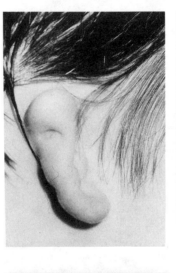
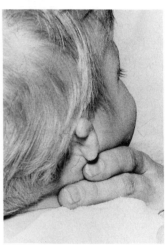

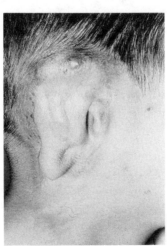
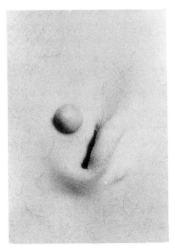

SOURCE: Sanford E. Gerber and George T. Mencher, *Auditory Dysfunction* (San Diego, Calif.: College-Hill Press, 1980), pp. 14–17. Courtesy of College-Hill Press. Copyright 1980.

FIGURE 3–11. Microtia and atresia

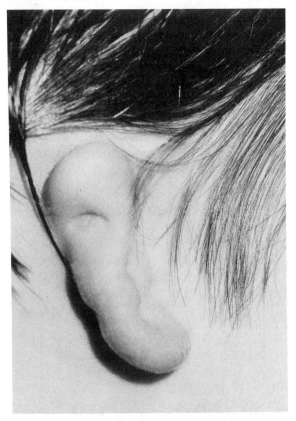

SOURCE: Sanford E. Gerber and George T. Mencher, *Auditory Dysfunction* (San Diego, Calif.: College-Hill Press, 1980), p. 18. Courtesy of College-Hill Press. Copyright 1980.

children had abnormal pinnae, preauricular fistulae, and bilateral conductive hearing losses. Again, this is a case of dominant inheritance.

External ear malformations accompanied by stenosis or atresia of the external auditory meatus also occur. Cremers (1985) reported on families in which both autosomal dominant and autosomal recessive patterns of inheritance occurred. As Cremers pointed out, congenital aural atresia is frequently associated with syndromes of the head and neck, as we discuss them below. Here we are talking about atresia of the ear canal in which there is no other immediately obvious anomalies of the craniofacial system. This is not to say, however, that there are no such anomalies; as we mentioned earlier, they may not be immediately visible.

The Cremers patients included a transmission of unilateral meatal atresia from father to son—hence, the conclusion of a dominant form of inheritance. Cremers observed, moreover, that bilateral meatal atresia in the absence of frank anomalies of the head and neck has been reported only once. Thus, we should expect external ear malformations to occur unilaterally, rarely, and genetically. Specifically, Cremers reported that 5 of his 33 patients had atresia of genetic origin. Interestingly, he was unable to determine the etiology of the atresia in the other patients, but "environmental causes are still expected."

Given Cremers's observations that there can be environmental causes, it appears that primary prevention might be difficult indeed. Of course, in that minority of cases where genetic factors are clear, the same kinds of primary prevention that apply to other genetic disorders would apply here. Environmental factors are a different problem, and are reviewed in some length later in this volume.

Secondary prevention, however, is clearly possible as has been repeatedly stressed by Jaffe (1977, 1978a, 1978b). Examination of the external ear should lead one to suspect accompanying anomalies of the middle ear. Jaffe's experience has been that that certainly is the case; hence, early identification both by cursory examination and, when necessary, by tympanostomy can be carried out. Furthermore, both Jaffe and Cremers (as well as many others) have reported that these problems are usually amenable to surgical correction. For example, Jaffe reported one patient with a 49 dB hearing loss who came to surgery and who recovered 30 dB of that conductive impairment.

One would suppose that surgery is a kind of tertiary prevention, but it is the secondary level that brought such a patient to this state. It needs to be stressed, furthermore, that pinna anomalies (with or without atresia) should not be surgically corrected for purely cosmetic reasons. Remember that they are almost always unilateral in the absence of other craniofacial problems or sensory hearing impairments, are not particularly handicapping, and the child need not be unduly subjected to surgical intervention. However, this is a condition that requires very careful evaluation by a pediatric otologist. It needs to be determined if a given patient is suffering a progressive hearing impairment and/or anomaly (such as a preauricular cyst) that could lead to problems more serious than a simple microtia. In other words, cosmetic surgery, for purely cosmetic reasons, should not usually be considered. Cosmetic surgery for valid medical and communicative reasons should be considered.

Finally, we are reminded again that anomalies of the external ear rarely occur in isolation; usually they are part of a complex of anomalies of the head and neck. These are discussed in Chapter 6 on craniofacial anomalies, a very broad topic.

Disorders of the Integument

An in-depth study of embryology is probably not required to recognize the developmental association between the auditory system and the *integument* (i.e., hair, teeth, nails, and skin). The Latin root of the word "integument" refers to a covering; hence, the body's covering is known as the integumentary system.

Genetic hearing impairment appearing with alterations of the integumentary system is so common that it merits fully 50 pages in the encyclopedia of Konigsmark and Gorlin (1976). However, as they pointed out, virtually all cases of hearing loss with integumentary disease are found in the Waardenburg syndrome. Other cases of integumentary system disease with genetic hearing loss have occurred very, very rarely. It was the opinion of Konisgmark and Gorlin that the syndromes "can be diagnosed rather easily because of skin, nail, or hair changes that occur along with the generally severe hearing loss." Most of these syndromes, although easily identified and diagnosed, have been described in only one or two families. On the other hand, Waardenburg syndrome may be far more common than is either known or knowable.

Table 3–1 is a list of genetic hearing losses that accompany integumentary system disease. It is included to show the range of possibilities. However, they are not discussed here because they occur so rarely and because Waardenburg syndrome is such an outstanding model for all of them. The interested reader should consult the work of Konisgmark and Gorlin for the details of a particular disease or to find information about a particular patient.

In 1951, P. J. Waardenburg described what he called "a new syndrome combining developmental anomalies of the eyelid, eyebrows, and nose root with pigmentary defect of the iris and headhair and congenital deafness." Actually, he had suggested the same phenomenon in a 1948 publication written in Dutch and published in the Netherlands. Although not the first to note this particular association—a paper written in German in 1916 by van der Hoeve may have been the first to describe this syndrome—Waardenburg was the first to recognize it as an inheritable disorder.

Waardenburg syndrome is a particular favorite illustration for geneticists because, as it is dominantly inherited, it is an outstanding model of variable expression. The syndrome is delineated (as Waardenburg described it) by a characteristic face with a wide separation of the medial canthi which causes the patient to appear to have widely spaced eyes, heterochromia irides (different colored eyes), a white forelock in the hair, and sensory hearing impairment (Figure 3–12). What is interesting and important about this disorder is the variable expression such that some or all of these symptoms may appear with various degrees of severity, or none at all.

TABLE 3–1. Genetic Hearing Losses with Integumentary System Disease

---

Waardenburg Syndrome
Oculocutaneous Albinism and Congenital Sensory-Neural Deafness
Multiple Lentigines (Leopard) Syndrome
Recessive Piebaldness and Congenital Sensory-Neural Deafness
X-Linked Pigmentary Abnormalities and Congenital Sensory-Neural Deafness
Dominant Piebald Trait, Ataxia, and Sensory-Neural Hearing Loss
Vitiligo, Muscle Wasting, Achalasia, and Congenital Sensory-Neural Deafness
Atypical Erythrokeratoderma, Somatic Retardation, Peripheral Neuropathy, and Congenital Sensory-Neural Deafness
Generalized Spiny Hyperkeratosis, Universal Alopecia, and Congenital Sensory-Neural Deafness
Keratopachydermia, Digital Constrictions, and Sensory-Neural Deafness
Anhidrosis and Progressive Sensory-Neural Hearing Loss
Generalized Alopecia, Hypogonadism, and Sensory-Neural Deafness
Knuckle Pads, Leukonychia, and Mixed Hearing Loss
Dominant Onychodystrophy, Coniform Teeth, and Sensory-Neural Hearing Loss
Dominant Onychodystrophy, Triphalangeal Thumbs, and Congenital Sensory-Neural Deafness
Recessive Onychodystrophy, Triphalangeal Thumbs and Halluces, Mental Retardation, Seizures, and Congenital Sensory-Neural Deafness
Recessive Onychodystrophy and Congenital Sensory-Neural Deafness
Pili Torti and Sensory-Neural Hearing Loss
Scanty Hair, Camptodactyly, and Sensory-Neural Hearing Loss
Atopic Dermatitis and Sensory-Neural Hearing Loss

SOURCE: Bruce W. Konigsmark and Robert J. Gorlin, *Genetic and Metabolic Deafness* (Philadelphia: W. B. Saunders Co., 1976).

DiGeorge, Olsted, and Harley (1960) estimated that Waardenburg syndrome would account for about 2.3 percent of the congenitally deaf population. Konigsmark and Gorlin suggested that the number could easily be twice that due to the variability. For example, in our clinic, we have seen two very interesting families both of which are highly illustrative of this variable expression. The first to come to my attention all looked like they had walked out of a textbook on Waardenburg syndrome. However, only the infant who was brought to our clinic had a severe bilateral sensory hearing loss. Her mother had a severe unilateral hearing loss; the mother's aunt had normal hearing, but her daughter was also quite deaf. All of them exhibited all of the other features of Waardenburg syndrome. A year or so later, the J family appeared. Mr. J had all the stigmata of Waardenburg syndrome except for deafness. In fact, he reported that the deafness had never appeared in his family until the birth of his first daughter. He was fully aware of the consequences of Waardenburg syndrome; he knew its name, he knew what caused it, and he knew that they had it. Yet Mr. J had two daughters; one was deaf and the other had essentially none of the signs of Waardenburg syndrome.

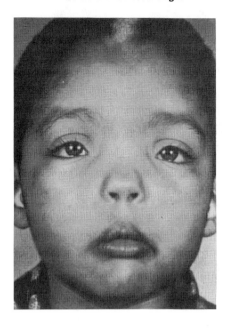

FIGURE 3–12.
Waardenburg syndrome
SOURCE: Robert J. Ruben, "Deafness of
the Inner Ear and Sensorineural Deafness," in
Charles D. Bluestone and Sylvan E. Stool,
eds., *Pediatric Otolaryngology,* vol. I (Philadel-
phia: W. B. Saunders Co., 1983), p. 581.
Reprinted by permission.

In the absence of sensory hearing impairment, and in the absence
of a clearly established pedigree of the family, it may be impossible to
determine if Waardenburg syndrome really does exist in a given case.
Different colored eyes do occur otherwise; some people have been known
to have a white streak in the hair produced by the local beautician;
characteristic shapes of eyes and mouth can occur in syndromes other
than that of Waardenburg. Hence, the true prevalence of Waardenburg
syndrome may not be knowable. None of these signs of Waardenburg
syndrome would cause a patient to appear before an audiologist or
otologist. Only about 20 percent of patients with Waardenburg syndrome
have hearing impairment of sufficient severity to be clinically significant.
Furthermore, many of the signs associated with Waardenburg syndrome
result in a particularly attractive patient rather than one who is singu-
larly unattractive as would be expected with most craniofacial disorders.

If Konigsmark and Gorlin were correct—and they undoubtedly
were—Waardenburg syndrome would account for at least 2 percent of the
incidence of congenital deafness. Furthermore, since only about 50 percent of patients with Waardenburg syndrome have severe hearing impairment, the risk for genetic transmission may be greater than expected. It
is indeed a dominantly inherited disorder with variable expression; consequently, deafness can appear in an isolated case within a family knowing that it has Waardenburg syndrome, the J family, for example.

Clearly, primary prevention is possible in families like the two
described. However, because the expression is so highly variable and

because the deafness often does not appear, the risk of producing a handicapped child in a given family cannot be predicted. Secondary prevention, though, is always and immediately available. On the one hand, there are families like the ones just described who know they have Waardenburg syndrome; on the other hand, a child born with the stigmata of this syndrome is typically easily identifiable. Secondary prevention, then, takes the usual form of early identification and early intervention. Proper procedures of habilitative audiology and, where indicated, special education for the hearing impaired can and should be brought to such children. Hearing aids almost always will be of benefit.

The many forms of deafness with alterations of skin pigment come under the general category of genetic hearing loss with integumentary system disease (Konigsmark and Gorlin 1976). With the exception of Waardenburg syndrome, they are rather uncommon taken one at a time. However, there have been reports of a few of these and a few of those in the literature over the years amounting to a rather goodly number of cases. They tend, as a group, to be rather easily diagnosed because they are characterized by obvious changes of skin accompanied by usually severe hearing impairments. Moreover, the pigmentary disorders are of great interest for research because many animals (e.g., white angora cats) are genetically deaf and serve as models for our understanding of such disorders in humans.

The pathology in these animals, and presumably in depigmented humans as well, is entirely limited to cochlear structures. Wever and Lawrence (1954) found that "these animals have normal middle ears, but their inner ears are malformed. There is a complete absence of hair cells and varying atrophy of the supporting cells. The nerve supply of the cochlea, however, is often only moderately affected and sometimes both nerve fibers and ganglion cells are present in nearly normal amounts."

Apparently, there has been only one study of human temporal bones of a patient who had deafness and integumentary system disease. Myers, Stool, and Koblenzer (1971) reported the Scheibe type of cochleosaccular abnormality in this case. However, the appearance of a Scheibe anomaly is consistent with the description of the animals. Our own (appropriately little noticed) paper on the subject revealed a dalmatian dog that made no obvious responses to sound up to 19,000 Hz and at levels as high as 110 dB SPL (Gerber 1968). Wever and Lawrence included dalmatians in their discussion of albinotic cats. Thus, the pathology in the case of the deaf dalmatians is assumed to be identical to that of the albinotic animals. More importantly, however, the pathology in the case of albinotic people is probably the same also.

The 1971 nosology of Konigsmark lists, in addition to Waardenburg syndrome, six dominantly inherited deafnesses that accompany integumentary system disease. None of them comes anywhere near the frequency of occurrence of Waardenburg syndrome; all of them had amounted to 70 patients (Konigsmark 1971).

One might ask why we should care about a group of rather peculiar disorders that cumulatively have appeared fewer than 100 times in the medical literature. There are two answers to that question. The first is that patients who have alterations of skin, hair, or nails may appear at a dermatology clinic where the relationship of these symptoms to progressive sensory deafness could be unknown. Therefore, it is incumbent upon our colleagues in dermatology to ensure that such patients are referred to audiology and otolaryngology. The other reason is that, as communicative disorders clinicians, it is important that we be alert to the possibility of degenerative disorders and to the understanding that these phenomena may be inherited. It then becomes incumbent upon us to make referrals to genetic counselors.

There is a still more general, and potentially more important, need to understand such phenomena. Study of dalmatian dogs, angora cats, albino (waltzing) guinea pigs, the Kreisler mouse, and so on, eventually leads to the ability to understand the mechanism of congenital inherited deafness. Ruben and Van De Water (1983) proposed that "the prevalence of genetic disease as the etiological factor of hearing loss in the elderly is approximately 50 percent." Consequently, they insisted that "genetic disease, although becoming manifest in later life, is fundamentally congenital." There are, they continued, "no preventative or cure interventions for sensorineural hearing loss of genetic origin with the exception of genetic counseling." They insisted, quite properly, that our clinical mission is to prevent or cure such disorders and that to do this "there must be an acquisition of knowledge of the embryologic mechanisms which control the expression of normal inner ear development and the mechanisms by which mutated genes disrupt these developmental mechanisms and cause hearing loss."

What Ruben and Van De Water have to say about hearing impairment applies also to speech and language impairments whether or not they are accompanied by auditory dysfunction. In fact, we know substantially less about the genetics of speech and language dysfunction than we do about congenital and/or progressive sensory hearing impairments. As a clinical scientist, I may be unable to prevent the birth of a child with an inherited communicative disorder, but my only ethical act is to do everything I can to minimize the handicap that results from that disorder. That is secondary prevention. The study of these biochemical and/or mutagenic disorders may eventually lead to primary prevention. Still, as clinicians, we need to be able to confront questions of the probability of a disorder becoming increasingly severe and eventually disabling, to know when and where to refer patients with these disorders, to understand the distinctions between those that are dominantly inherited and those that are recessively inherited, and the like.

The 1976 survey by Fraser concluded that "these alleles show a 100 percent penetrance and complete expressivity with regard to bilateral profound hearing loss . . . " He did point out that complete expression is not universal even though he found it among his patients. Nevertheless, in light of the comments of the preceding paragraph, we need to be especially sensitive to the very high probability that these dominant disorders will penetrate and will be expressed in future generations. Fraser also believed that heterochromia of the irides "may be of causal significance . . . ". The phenomenon of different colored eyes is not unique to the syndrome of Waardenburg. Fraser's data indicate a prevalence of pigmentary disorder syndromes with deafness to range from 1.17 per 100,000 persons in the general population to as many as 6.10 per 100,000. In either case, the number is not large but is illustrative of the fact that progressive sensory-neural hearing impairments do occur often with these pigmentary disorders. Hence, again, we must be sensitive to the probability of degenerative disorders.

Ocular and Oculomotor Disorders

A moment's reflection on the development of the fetal face should lead one to expect a conjunction of eye with ear anomalies. We have just discussed at some length the fact that discoloration of the eye is often a clue to progressive hearing impairment. There are known syndromes of deafness and blindness as well as hearing impairments with other visual handicaps; most of these are recessively inherited. Konigsmark's 1971 nosology listed only three dominantly inherited deafnesses associated with eye disease. Among them, he reported only 35 cases being known, with three syndromes: (1) dominant saddle nose, myopia, cataracts, with slowly progressing hearing loss; (2) dominant myopia, peripheral neuropathy, skeletal abnormalities, and slow to moderately progressing severe hearing loss appearing in the first or second decade of life; and (3) dominant corneal dystrophy with slowly progressing moderate hearing loss in adulthood. By 1976, Konigsmark and Gorlin were able to list the following dominantly inherited disorders characterized by deafness, visual handicaps, and usually with other handicaps:

1. A syndrome characterized by retinitis pigmentosa, nystagmus, hemiplegic migraine, and sensory-neural deafness
2. A syndrome characterized by myopia, cataract, saddle nose, and sensory-neural hearing loss which is sometimes called Marshall syndrome
3. A syndrome in which one finds myopia, blue sclerae, Marfanoid habitus, and sensory-neural deafness

4. Another syndrome characterized by myopia, peripheral neuropathy, skeletal abnormalities, and sensory-neural deafness
5. Konigsmark's description of progressive optic atrophy and congenital sensory-neural deafness
6. A similar condition with the addition of ataxia

All of these have been reported by several clinical studies; nevertheless, the total number of patients continues to be small.

The importance of our consideration of such patients is similar to the significance of those with integumentary system disorders. With this group, however, we must be even more alert to the probability of progressive hearing handicap accompanied by progressive visual handicap. It is irrelevant, in this instance, whether a given patient's disorder is dominantly or recessively inherited. Rather, it is important that we understand the probability of progression of the disorder.

It happens that those disorders in which deafness and blindness progress are usually dominantly inherited. The recessive disorders are characterized more frequently by nonprogressive deafness accompanied by progressive visual handicap. Also, it is to be noted that some of these dominantly inherited syndromes are characterized additionally by neuropathy and/or by musculoskeletal disorders. In other words, although the numbers are small, we will confront patients with multiple handicaps. And, most important, the patient who will become both deaf and blind requires a treatment quite different from the one who is either but not both. This is a place where a strong case must be made for secondary prevention. Obviously, it is critical to know if this is a dominantly inherited progressive disorder or one that is not going to progress whether dominantly or recessively inherited. What we do for a deaf child who is going to become blind is obviously different from what we do for the deaf child who will continue to have normal vision.

Dominantly inherited disorders of all kinds become ideal candidates for genetic counseling as primary prevention. Secondary prevention, as mentioned earlier, is truly essential for some of these disorders. Early identification is always indicated, but it is indispensable in the case of progressively degenerating disorders. Also, for some of these disorders, secondary prevention may take the form of correction of such things as cataracts or the provision of lenses for the severe myopia.

The neuropathy and musculoskeletal disorders, however, may not be correctable and may or may not lead to communicative disorders other than hearing impairment. Some of these patients do present with facial anomalies that might interfere with the acquisition of normal articulation. Again, sometimes surgery may help, sometimes not. The early introduction of amplification is always important, and is still more important for the patient who will become visually impaired. We must do our utmost to approach acoustic normality in such a patient. Still, to the extent that we know that both hearing and vision will deteriorate severely, then we must be prepared to introduce other forms of communication to these patients. This is our responsibility; that is, the rehabilitative audiologist and the speech-language pathologist are the essential care providers.

The primary example of all of the above is Usher syndrome (Usher 1914). It is the most common cause of deaf-blindness in every country that reports such a statistic. Usher syndrome is distinguished by profound congenital deafness accompanied by progressive blindness due to *retinitis pigmentosa*. It arises due to monogenic autosomal recessive inheritance, and may account for as many as 10 percent of children who are born deaf. Similarly, among patients who have retinitis pigmentosa, hearing loss appears in 4.3 to 6.3 percent (Vernon 1976).

Primary and secondary prevention efforts can be available to families or individuals with Usher syndrome. The genetic counselor should explain the risk of recessive inheritance to families with a history of Usher syndrome—primary prevention. The risk of recurrence is 25 percent in the patient's sibs and offspring (Bergsma 1973). Secondary prevention should always be available in the form of repeated visual examinations for all hearing impaired children. A fundoscopic examination is essential to the assessment of any child suspect for hearing loss (Gerber and Mencher, 1978).

INHERITED DISORDERS OF THE NERVOUS SYSTEM

In the 1971 nosology, Konigsmark listed three dominantly inherited forms of deafness associated with nervous system disease: (1) dominant neuroma (von Recklinghausen disease); (2) sensory radicular neuropathy; and (3) dominant photomyoclonus, diabetes, nephropathy, and sensory-neural hearing loss. All of these are progressive, all appear in the second or third decade of life, and all may become severe. In the 1976 nosology, Konigsmark and Gorlin added three more disorders to those three: (1) ataxia, hyperuricemia (abnormally high level of uric acid in the blood), renal insufficiency, and sensory-neural deafness; (2) ataxia, cataract, cytosis, and sensory-neural deafness; and (3) myoclonic epilepsy, ataxia, and sensory-neural deafness.

Tumors

Of special concern is the distinction between dominantly inherited bilateral acoustic neuromas and dominantly inherited von Recklinghausen disease. The gene for von Recklinghausen disease has been located on the seventeenth chromosome (Barker et al. 1987). Konigsmark and Gorlin (1976) did not use the expression von Recklinghausen disease but are more careful to describe it as von Recklinghausen *neurofibromatosis*. The reason this is important is that the pathology is different in the condition they described and in von Recklinghausen neurofibromatosis. A *neurofibroma* is a slowly growing tumor that originates in a nerve and is composed of Schwann cells, those that ensheathe the nerve's axon; frequently, such tumors are called *Schwannoma*. It has been found that the genetic defect in bilateral acoustic neurofibromatosis is loss of alleles on the twenty-second chromosome (Seizinger et al. 1987).

The Schwannomas that accompany von Recklinghausen neurofibromatosis are cutaneous as well as auditory and do not appear in the syndrome of acoustic neuromas and neural deafness. Furthermore, Konigsmark and Gorlin said that patients with neurofibromatosis "may occasionally have meningiomas, astrocytomas, or rarely bilateral acoustic neuromas." Although von Recklinghausen neurofibromatosis is inherited by autosomal dominant transmission, the consequences are different from the dominantly inherited bilateral tumors. These tumors, unlike those of von Recklinghausen "can reach remarkable size, affecting severe distortion of the brain stem, enlarging and eroding the bony walls of the internal meatus, and finally extending extradurally into the middle cranial fossa" (Konigsmark and Gorlin 1976).

Although the tumors do not appear until the second or third decade of life, life expectancy from then on is relatively short. The average life expectancy after the onset of symptoms is about 20 years, but some patients have been known to survive as long as 44 years. What may be most essential about the distinction between dominant neuromas and dominant neurofibromatoses is the rate of growth of the tumors. The neurofibromatoses grow much more slowly, and consequently life expectancy is correspondingly increased. Obviously, this is important to the patient, but also to the clinician as well. In either case, however, life expectancy is such that the patient will survive into adulthood and should be treated accordingly. Moreover, it has been established that children with neurofibromatoses are often retarded (14 percent), they have lower scores on the Peabody Picture Vocabulary Test than their unaffected siblings, and they have a high incidence (35 percent) of voice quality abnormalities (Levy et al. 1986). Eliason (1986) found 56 percent of the 23 children she studied to have a visual-perceptual disability and the majority of those also had language deficits. Clearly, these are issues for the speech-language pathologist.

Because these are dominantly inherited disorders, genetic counseling is in order. Neurofibromatosis is a common genetic disorder; Eliason claimed that it appears once in 3,000 live births. Secondary prevention is constituted of surgical removal of the tumors. However, removal of a neuroma or a neurofibroma of the auditory nerve or of the cerebellopont-ine angle frequently necessitates destruction of the cochlea. This is a sufficiently severe problem when it occurs unilaterally (which is not an inherited disorder), but if both cochleae need to be destroyed, the result is a profoundly deafened patient. Furthermore, surgical removal of the tumor associated with von Recklinghausen neurofibromatosis has not been encouraging. It is only a small proportion of cases in which the evidence indicates that life has been prolonged by the surgery. Death results in either case from these tumors encroaching upon adjacent cranial nerves. Obviously, if a tumor of the eighth nerve gets sufficiently large, it will affect not only the seventh nerve (the facial) but also the ninth and tenth. These latter two are critically involved in pulmonary and cardiac function.

The issue for both secondary and tertiary prevention, then, is to determine the rate of growth of the tumor. If the tumors are surgically removed, and if the patient is left with a profound (in fact, total) bilateral hearing impairment, the role of the rehabilitative audiologist is paramount. In such a case, the only treatment is instruction in alternative forms of communication. Obviously a hearing aid won't help, and it is extremely doubtful that a cochlear implant would be of benefit. The fact is, however, that it is unusual to remove both tumors. It is less unusual to remove one and to hope that the other will not grow larger to necessitate removal. Unfortunately, sometimes that is not the case.

Catlin (1981) warned about other lesions producing similar symptoms. These include meningiomas, cysts, aneurysms, arteriovenous malformations, congenital cholesteatomas, Ménière disease, and tumors of the fifth or seventh nerves. Again, the thing that sets apart the two neurofibromatosis disorders is the fact that they always occur in the family, no generations have been skipped (according to the published literature), and so autosomal dominant inheritance is obvious. This is a case, of course, where the diagnostic skills of the audiologist are essential.

This is secondary prevention: Are both ears deteriorating? Are they deteriorating at the same rate? Is the patient experiencing symptoms in addition to or instead of loss of acoustic sensitivity? Does the patient benefit from a hearing aid? The audiologist and radiologist are undoubtedly the strongest allies of the neurosurgeon in these cases. Catlin (1981) indicated that auditory and labyrinthine dysfunctions are the first cranial nerve signs to appear with tumors. Other signs of nervous system dysfunction appear later. Although this is not a book on diagnosis, it should be evident to the reader that the use of auditory evoked potentials is critical in mapping the progress of these disorders.

Other dominantly inherited impairments that have associated nervous system disease occur quite rarely. Apparently the most common of these rare disorders is the syndrome characterized by sensory radicular neuropathy and progressive sensory-neural deafness. These patients undergo a progressive loss of sensation in the extremities (feet, hands, and lower limbs) accompanied by a sensory-neural hearing impairment. These seem to begin simultaneously usually in the second or third decade of life. It is important to distinguish this disorder from similar ones. There are occasional reports of sensory neuropathy without deafness or with deafness that does not progress. There may also be some evidence of a recessive form of this disorder. This last distinction is an important one because, in the recessively inherited condition described by Hirschowitz, Groll, and Ceballos (1972), there is poor prognosis for survival because this form is characterized by gastrointestinal and cardiac difficulties as well.

All the nervous system disorders so far discussed incorporate hearing impairments. Communicative disorders of the nervous system that are inherited and that do not incorporate auditory symptoms are more difficult to describe. In fact, "It has yet to be demonstrated . . . that speech and/or language function can be directly and specifically affected by genetic mechanisms. Dyslexia and stuttering offer two disorders where this could be the case" (Darby, Kidd, and Cavalli-Sforza 1985).

It seems appropriate at this point for me to state a set of prejudices in these matters. First, there is no such thing as behavior; that is, there is no behavior disembodied from the organism doing the behaving. True, much of the time, even most of the time, it is the behavior that gets treated, and that is appropriate and desirable. But, as clinicians, we must be aware that treating the behavior is intended in some beneficial way to alter the organism. Second, everything is caused, even those things for which we cannot identify a cause. Again, it is not necessary to know the cause in order to treat, but it is frequently desirable for treatment and always essential for prevention. When our colleagues in the medical sciences describe a disease or process as being *idiopathic,* they mean that the cause is unknown, not that there is no cause. Dyslexia is an ideal example.

Dyslexia

Dyslexia is a family of disorders all of which are characterized by an inability to read or read well. It seems to appear in one or both of two forms. The first may be a problem of visual processing; that is, the patient is genuinely unable to identify and/or order correctly a sequence of written symbols. This results in, for example, reversals such that letters or even whole words get turned around as in reading "ward" as "draw" or "eat" as "tea." The second form is expressed in some kind of failure to make a visual to acoustic transformation. In this case, the patient seems to be constitutionally incapable of phonic concepts; this child is unable to learn which symbols represent which sounds. Regehr (1987) considered these two subtypes to be reading disability with verbal/language problems and reading disability with visual/spatial problems. The first of these is known to be inherited. Furthermore, Regehr and Kaplan (1988) have distinguished yet another inherited form of dyslexia, namely, reading disability with motor problems. In fact, they hypothesized "that the reading and motor problems are related, perhaps as part of one genetic disorder characterized by underlying cerebellovestibular dysfunction."

Kinsbourne and Caplan (1979) called these disorders "constitutional dyslexia" in order to distinguish them from an even more mysterious entity, minimal brain dysfunction (now more often called attention deficit disorder). They considered constitutional dyslexia to be "a hereditary cognitive deficit selective for reading. . . . " The case for heritable dyslexia was put just as strongly by Darby, Kidd, and Cavalli-Sforza (1985): "It is a familial disorder and in some cases is possibly transmitted through an autosomal-dominant mode of inheritance." Galaburda (1983) apparently believes that dyslexia is a monogenic disorder expressed in bilateral thalamic lesions.

The problem with making a diagnosis of dyslexia is that an inability to read is not demonstrated until the children are 5 or 6 years old and someone tries to teach them to read. But these children did not suddenly become dyslexic at that time; it just had not been a problem before. Consequently, our ability to predict—and therefore prevent—dyslexia depends upon our knowledge of family history.

Cooper and Ludlow (1985) suggest the basis for making such a judgment: (1) that there is a strong family history; (2) that disabilities are similar among affected family members; and (3) documentation of transmission of the dyslexia from one generation to another. There are data to show that dyslexia often meets these criteria. In fact, one might argue that a reading disability in a given patient *must* meet these criteria for a diagnosis of dyslexia to be made. Again, Kinsbourne and Caplan (1979) make the case that it is the genetic nature of the disorder which distinguishes it from other reading problems. Smith et al. (1983) conclude:

> A gene playing a major role in this type of specific reading disability has tentatively been localized to chromosome 15, and the disorder appears to be inherited as an autosomal dominant trait . . . . These children had only reading and writing disabilities and no other evidence of intellectual or motor problems.

In other words, they fit the definition of a genetically based disorder with no associated handicaps.

Finally, given that there is a set of children whose reading problems arise from a particular genotype, the issue of primary prevention again appears. Again, the resolution is in the form of genetic counseling for a family who is sufficiently concerned about this particular problem to seek it. Secondary prevention, however, seems more difficult. To my knowledge, there is no diagnostic procedure available which would predict dyslexia in a child who has yet to demonstrate the symptoms and whose family has been unaware of a difficulty. Nevertheless, it is my belief that such secondary prevention could become possible when we have clear methods and reasons that distinguish dyslexic children from other children before they fail to learn to read.

Stuttering

Stuttering continues to be one of the great mysteries of human communication, indeed, of human life. Over the years there have been diverse ideas about what it is, such as Van Riper's (1939) conceptualizations of primary and secondary stuttering, Johnson's (1944) "diagnosogenic" view that stuttering arises in the ear of the listener when normal nonfluency exceeds some statistical expectation, and West's (1958) hypothesis that "spasmophemia" is some underlying biochemical cause. Actually, all of these notions are valid in some way or to some extent, but none explains the origin of stuttering. Van Riper was certainly correct that young children do display dysfluencies that are merely part of development, whereas some older children demonstrate what he called secondary symptoms of behavioral accretions to the act of stuttering. Johnson was right in supposing that families' reactions to normal nonfluency (or to Van Riper's primary stuttering) may aggravate the disorder. And West had to be correct in his assumption that there is something that underlies this particular verbal behavior, and he confessed that he didn't know either what "spasmophemia" means.

It is now many years since Severina Nelson first gathered the data that show that stuttering runs in families (1939). A review of the current literature would show support for hypotheses of genetic causation of stuttering. Indeed, Nelson and her colleagues (Nelson, Hunter, and Walter 1945) did show that stuttering was concordant in twins; that is, it appears in both of them. More recently, it has been shown that 83 percent of monozygotic twins were concordant for stuttering (Godai, Tatarelli, and Bonanni 1976). What does this signify? Monozygotic twins, recall, are genetically identical; they arose from the same germ cell, one zygote. Therefore, any genetic trait that appears in one *must* appear in the other. On the other hand, dyzogotic (i.e., fraternal) twins are not genetically identical, and have no more and no less in common than siblings who are not twins. The ideal question to be answered, then, would require the separation of monozygotic twins at birth so that they would never be raised in the same family environment. If, in such a case, a given trait appears, then it must be inherited. Moreover, in the case of similarly separated dizygotic twins, it could appear in one and not the other.

Although Godai, Tatarelli, and Bonanni (1976) found concordance in 83 percent of 12 pairs of monozygotic twins, they found only 10.5 percent in 19 dizygotic pairs. In other words, the percentage of monozygotic twins who stutter greatly exceeds the proportion of dizygotic twins who stutter. And this finding is convincing evidence that stuttering is inherited. However, because the proportion is not 100 percent, there must be nongenetic factors operating as well, at least in some cases.

The Yale Family Study of Stuttering (Kidd 1984) began in 1973 to collect data on the hypothesis of a genetic basis for stuttering. By 1984, it included information on more than 600 persons who, at some time, had been diagnosed as stutterers but who had no history of neurologic impairments such as epilepsy, cerebral palsy, or mental retardation. Additional data were collected on several thousand first degree relatives of these stutterers so that family pedigrees could be prepared. It is not necessary here to recount all the findings of this massive study, but a summary of its results is informative.

Most important is the conclusion that the person at highest risk of becoming a stutterer is a male relative of a female stutterer, and the one at least risk is a female relative of a male stutterer. This is not news: The White House Conference on Child Health and Protection of 1931 found a preponderance of stuttering in males under the age of ten years as compared to older males or females of any age. Thus, West, Ansberry, and Carr (1957) concluded that "maleness, or something associated with it, is a factor in stuttering." Kidd (1984) concluded that female stutterers have more of the factors that promote stuttering than males, as they have more affected family members. He posited, then, that there is an inherited neurologic susceptibility to stuttering.

The point is, though, that the probability that the gene will penetrate is greater for males than for females; in fact, stuttering appears in five times as many males as females (Records, Kidd, and Kidd 1977). The explanation offered by several experts is that males have a lower threshold for inheriting the trait; hence, stuttering appears more often in the male offspring of stutterers than in female offspring. But that doesn't explain why the risk is greater for those males whose mothers stutter than for those whose fathers do, except for Kidd's hypothesis that, in females, there is a preponderance of factors that promote stuttering in their offspring.

It isn't simple. Kidd (1983) observed that "stuttering does not show a simple pattern of inheritance in families." Nevertheless, it is clear that stuttering is usually an inherited trait, given the high concentration in families. Kidd concluded that stuttering—although it is usually *endogenous*—fails to demonstrate a single-gene pattern; that is, it is probably not monogenic. On the other hand, he proposed a single-major-locus model with three different genotypes:

> Both the male and female penetrances are virtually zero for homozygotes for the normal genotype; both are one (or 100%) for homozygotes for the stuttering allele. A striking sex difference is found for heterozygotes: Penetrance is about 40% for a heterozygous male but only 11% for a heterozygous female . . . . Especially noteworthy is that the model does not require that the interaction of genetic and nongenetic factors be confined to heterozygotes and yet biological principles would suggest that interaction is most likely to be significant in heterozygotes.

Thus, some incidents are inherited by a multifactorial mode, perhaps some by an X-linked mode, and some not at all. One wants to suppose an X-linked mode of transmission, given that male children of female stutterers have a much higher risk of stuttering than any other combination, such as female children of female stutterers, female children of male stutterers, and male children of male stutterers. In fact, 17 percent of the daughters and 36 percent of the sons of female stutterers do stutter (Sparks 1984). One rejects a hypothesis of X-linked inheritance because there are many instances of father to son transmission—22 percent of their sons but only 9 percent of their daughters—and an X-linked trait could not have appeared in the mother of a stutterer.

Where does this lead? One must conclude that stuttering is not a single or unique inherited disorder. It is apparently a multifactorial inheritance characterized by an increased susceptibility in males and increased preponderance of factors that lead to stuttering in their mothers.

Then what about prevention? The statistics render an a priori risk for the children of stutterers, but one cannot imagine a family deciding to have no children on that basis. Thus, that form of primary prevention is not likely. It is especially unlikely given West's old idea of spasmophemia rendering stutterers who never stutter. Maybe those are the female children of female stutterers. Secondary prevention, early intervention, continues to be controversial. For one thing, there is no simple or direct metric that separates normal nonfluency from Van Riper's primary stuttering. Indeed, it may be diagnosogenic, to use Johnson's term, insofar as the stuttering child is one whose parents say he is.

What to do? Happily, this is not a book on stuttering, so this writer can avoid answering the question. But a general answer does exist: There are programs of early intervention. Gregory (1984), for example, has suggested "modifications of the environment" in early intervention. And Costello has written often on management of the young chronic stutterer (e.g., 1984). It suffices for our purpose to indicate that early intervention strategies do exist, have been employed, and do succeed. Stuttering is a disorder of childhood, as evidenced, among other data, by Andrews' (1984) finding that 1.6 percent of eight-year-old children stutter but that rate drops to 1.2 percent by 15 years of age. Furthermore, 79 percent of the children he studied stopped stuttering before the age of 16. Finally, remember Ingham's (1987) finding that 75 percent of cases of stuttering are inherited.

Other Inherited Nervous System Disorders

What else is possible? Certainly, delayed development of expressive language is possibly heritable. Ludlow and Cooper (1983b) have edited an entire book on the subject. It is not appropriate to rewrite it here, but note that with respect to delayed development of speech and language, they report that interpretation of published studies is difficult. It is their view that the data are questionable in light of methodological problems. One of the problems is that the incidence of delayed language associated with any given genetic trait is very small. For example, Garvey and Mutton (1973) studied all of nine children with language problems and found sex chromosome abnormalities in five of them. One might suppose that five of nine is significant, except that the nine came from a pool of 450. One ought not to underestimate the importance of this association in the five children, but one must also be aware that the two clinical phenomena could be unrelated.

Number problems persist. These are small sample studies, so it is difficult to make generalizations. On the other hand, the study of chromosomal abnormalities that are relatively common and rather well understood—Klinefelter syndrome or Turner syndrome, for example—does reveal language difficulties in those groups. Another problem is that children who have chromosome anomalies that are expressed have a variety of difficulties. Fragile X syndrome, for example, is recognized as one of the most common causes of mental retardation; and, mentally retarded people by definition are developmentally delayed in language as in all other areas. The nature of this subproblem in Fragile X patients has been called "characteristic speech delay" (Ho, Glahn, and Ho 1988). To resolve the problem, it would be necessary to find children who are not otherwise delayed, have no difficulties with receptive language, and do have problems with expressive language and karyotype them. That is just what Garvey and Mutton (1973) did, and they found five children from a pool of 450.

Another possibility may be Rett syndrome. Hagberg et al. (1983) described this progressive disorder as characterized by ataxia, autism, dementia, mental retardation, and "loss of purposeful hand use . . . ". What is curious is that it seems to appear only in females and yet is a genetic disorder. Moreover, Hagberg (1985) suggested that Rett syndrome may be more common than PKU in female infants (about 1 in 15,000). Unfortunately, too little is known to introduce primary prevention, and symptoms usually appear too late for secondary prevention. At this point, only a pedigree may be used as a means of prevention of future incidences. One needs to be concerned, however, as Witt-Engerstrom and Gillberg (1987) found that 37 of their 50 cases (78 percent) of Rett syndrome had earlier been diagnosed as autistic. In fact, Moeschler et al. (1988) noted that previous diagnoses of their patients had "included Prader-Willi syndrome, Angleman syndrome, toxic reaction to pertussis vaccine, CNS dysgenesis, and encephalitis."

As any speech-language clinician can report, the most common problem is one of delayed or distorted phonological development. Ludlow and Cooper (1983a) reported finding no studies "on the genetic bases of developmental speech misarticulations." Again, one can find phonological difficulties appearing in children who have other problems; for example, developmental dyspraxia accompanying X-linked mental retardation. In summary, then, we really don't know about the genetic basis of language delay or disability. It is reasonable to suppose that there is one and that it is very common, probably the most common etiology. We have yet to learn that, however.

CONCLUSION

What have we learned? Ultimately, not much, as demonstrated especially by the section immediately above. As specialists in the study, diagnosis, and treatment of disorders of communication, we are relative newcomers to understanding genetics and the genetically based disorders we encounter. We must come to a state where we can answer the question put by Ludlow and Cooper (1983b):

> The recent emergence of the discipline of behavioral genetics has altered the study of the hereditary bases of many behavioral traits, including specific cognitive abilities, psychopathology, and intelligence. The question naturally arises, does this discipline have the potential for improving our understanding and treatment of speech and language disorders?

Clearly, the answer is affirmative, but effecting the answer in our practice is still ahead of us.

GLOSSARY

achondroplasia: a hereditary, congenital disturbance that results in a form of dwarfism characterized by short limbs and normal trunk, small face, anomalies of spine and hands, and occasionally sensory-neural deafness.

allele: alternative form of any given gene found at the same locus on *homologous* chromosomes. Only two alleles can exist in any one individual; however, if more than two alleles exist in the population, they are called multiple alleles.

atresia: congenital absence or closure of any bodily orifice; especially, for our purpose, aural atresia, congenital absence of the external auditory meatus.

autosomal: pertaining to an autosome, that is, any chromosome that is not a sex chromosome or gamete.

congenital: present at birth for any reason, but not necessarily genetic.

consanguinity: relationship by descent from a common ancestor.

dominant inheritance: the expression of any trait even if it is *heterozygous.*

Duchenne muscular dystrophy: a heritable disorder usually appearing in boys.

endogenous: growing from within the organism; hence, arising from causes internal to the organism rather than imposed from the environment.

exogenous: something that develops or originates outside the organism.

expressivity: the extent to which a genetic trait demonstrates its effect; a trait with variable expression, or expressivity, may appear from mild to severe and/or in different forms among individuals.

fitness: the ability to transmit genes that survive from one generation to the next.

genetic: anything that depends upon genes.

heterozygous: heterozygote is an individual having two different alleles at the same locus on a pair of *homologous* chromosomes.

homologous: chromosomes that correspond in structure, position, origin, and so on—hence, allogenic.

homozygous: a homozygote is an individual who has a pair of identical alleles at a given locus on homologous chromosomes.

idiopathic: a condition that appears without evident cause.

integument: any bodily covering: skin, hair, teeth, nails, and so on.

linkage: the property of genes with loci within a measurable distance.

mandibulofacial dysostosis (Treacher Collins syndrome): an autosomal dominant disorder with high penetrance and variable expressivity distinguished by characteristic facies.

microtia: extreme hypoplasia or aplasia of the pinna usually accompanied by aural *atresia.*

monogenic: produced by a single gene.

morphogenic: arising from early differentiation of cells and tissues.

mucopolysaccharidoses: a group of heritable diseases characterized by a disorder of metabolism of mucopolysaccharide, a protein found in blood groups.

multifactorial inheritance: also called *polygenic* inheritance; refers to many genes at different loci that have small additive effects.

mutation: a change in the genotype that is perpetuated in the phenotype.

neurofibroma: a tumor of peripheral nerves due to an abnormal proliferation of Schwann cells—hence, schwannoma.

neurofibromatosis: a familial (i.e., inherited) condition characterized by the formation of *neurofibromas* that may be distributed over the entire body.

nosology: the science of disease classification; hence, any system of classification of diseases.

Pendred syndrome: an autosomal recessive disorder that is distinguished by congenital sensory-neural deafness and goiter; the goiter is usually not detectable at birth.

penetrance: the frequency of phenotypical expression of a genotype; if the trait appears less than 100 percent of the time, it is said to have reduced penetrance.

polygenic: multifactorial inheritance, that is, inherited due to many genes at different loci; sometimes called quantitative inheritance.

polymorphic, polymorphism: the appearance of two or more genetically determined alternative phenotypes in a population at a rate greater than may be explained by *mutation.*

purine: a colorless, crystalline substance that participates in the creation of metabolic end products; the purine bases include adenine and guanine, which are constituents of nucleic acids (see Chapter 2).

pyrimidine: another organic compound that is a fundamental form of the pyrimidine bases.

recessive inheritance: a trait that is expressed only in individuals homozygous for the gene involved.

retinitis pigmentosa: a group of diseases, usually genetic (transmitted as dominant, recessive, or X-linked), marked by progressive blindness due to retinal atrophy, attenuation of the retinal vessels, and contraction of the field of vision.

Rett syndrome: a genetic disorder that appears only in females and is often misdiagnosed as autism.

sporadic inheritance: a trait that appears in a single individual in a family with no evident genetic basis.

X-linked inheritance: inherited from genes located on the X chromosome; X-linked traits pass only from mother to son.

REFERENCES

ANDREWS, GAVIN. 1984. "The Epidemiology of Stuttering," in *Nature and Treatment of Stuttering: New Directions,* ed. Richard F. Curlee and William H. Perkins. San Diego: College-Hill Press.

BARKER, D., et al. 1987. "Gene for von Recklinghausen Neurofibromatosis Is in the Pericentromeric Region of Chromosome 17," *Science,* 236, 1100–102.

BERGSMA, DANIEL, ed. 1973. *Birth Defects Atlas and Compendium.* Baltimore: Williams & Wilkins.

BERMAN, PAIGE, CLAUDE DESJARDINS, AND F. CLARKE FRASER. 1975. "The Inheritance of the Aarskog Facial-Digital-Genital Syndrome," *J. Peds.,* 86, 885–91.

BESS, FRED H. 1984. "The Minimally Hearing-Impaired Child," *Ear and Hearing,* 6, 43–47.

———AND ANNE MARIE THARPE. 1984. "Unilateral Hearing Impairment in Children," *Peds.,* 74, 206–16.

CARREL, ROBERT E. 1977. "Epidemiology of Hearing Loss," in *Audiometry in Infancy,* ed. Sanford E. Gerber. New York: Grune & Stratton.

CATLIN, FRANCIS I. 1981. "Otologic Diagnosis and Treatment of Disorders Affecting Hearing," in *Medical Audiology,* ed. Frederick N. Martin. Englewood Cliffs, NJ: Prentice-Hall.

COOPER, JUDITH A., AND CHRISTY L. LUDLOW. 1985. "The Genetics of Developmental Speech and Language Disorders," in *Speech and Language Evaluation in Neurology: Childhood Disorders,* ed. John K. Darby. Orlando, FL: Grune & Stratton.

COSTELLO, JANIS M. 1984. "Treatment of the Young Chronic Stutterer: Managing Fluency," in *Nature and Treatment of Stuttering: New Directions,* ed. Richard F. Curlee and William H. Perkins. San Diego: College-Hill Press.

CREMERS, COR W. R. J. 1985. "Meatal Atresia and Hearing Loss. Autosomal Dominant and Autosomal Recessive Inheritance," *Intl. J. Ped. Otorhinolaryngol.,* 8, 211–13.

DARBY, JOHN K., KENNETH K. KIDD, AND LUIGI LUCA CAVALLI-SFORZA. 1985. "Molecular Genetics in Speech and Language Disorders," in *Speech and Language Evaluation in Neurology: Childhood Disorders,* ed. John K.Darby. Orlando, FL: Grune & Stratton.

DIGEORGE, ANGELO M., RICHARD W. OLSTED, AND ROBISON D. HARLEY. 1960. "Waardenburg's Syndrome," *J. Peds.,* 57, 649–69.

ELIASON, MICHELLE J. 1986. "Neurofibromatosis: Implications for Learning and Behavior," *J. Dev. Beh. Peds.,* 7, 175–79.

FRASER, GEORGE R. 1976. *The Causes of Profound Deafness in Childhood.* Baltimore: Johns Hopkins University Press.

FRIEDMAN, ELLEN M., et al. 1980. "Sickle Cell Anemia and Hearing," *Ann. Otol.,* 89, 342–47.

GALABURDA, ALBERT M. 1983. "Definition of the Anatomical Phenotype," in *Genetic Aspects of Speech and Language Disorders,* ed. Christy L. Ludlow and Judith A. Cooper. New York: Academic Press.

GARVEY, MAUREEN, AND DAVID E. MUTTON. 1973. "Sex Chromosome Aberrations and Speech Development," *Arch. Dis. Childhood,* 48, 937–41.

GERBER, SANFORD E. 1968. "The Deaf Dalmatian," *The Voice,* 17, 12–14.

GERBER, SANFORD E., ed. 1977. *Audiometry in Infancy.* New York: Grune & Stratton.

GERBER, SANFORD E. 1986. "Congenital Conductive Hearing Impairment in Noonan Syndrome," *Human Communication Canada,* 10, 21–23.
———AND GEORGE T. MENCHER, eds. 1978. *Early Diagnosis of Hearing Loss.* New York: Grune & Stratton.
GODAI, U., R. TATARELLI, AND G. BONNANI. 1976. "Stuttering and Tics in Twins," *Acta Geneticae Medicae et Gomellologiae,* 25, 369–75.
GOIN, DONALD W. 1976. "Otospongiosis," in *Otolaryngology: A Textbook,* ed. Gerald M. English. New York: Harper & Row.
GORLIN, ROBERT, JENS J. PINDBORG, AND M. MICHAEL COHEN, JR. 1976. *Syndromes of the Head and Neck.* New York: McGraw-Hill.
GRANT, MURRAY. 1981. *Handbook of Community Health,* 3rd ed. Philadelphia: Lea & Febiger.
GREENOUGH, WILLIAM T. 1975. "Experiential Modification of the Developing Brain," *Amer. Scientist,* 63, 37–46.
GREGORY, HUGO H. 1984. "Prevention of Stuttering: Management of Early Stages," in *Nature and Treatment of Stuttering: New Directions,* ed. Richard F. Curlee and William H. Perkins. San Diego: College-Hill Press.
HAGBERG, BENGT. 1985. "Rett Syndrome: Swedish Approach to Analysis of Prevalence and Cause," *Brain and Development,* 7, 277–80.
———JEAN AICARDI, KARIN DIAS, AND OVIDIO RAMOS. 1983. "A Progressive Syndrome of Autism, Dementia, Ataxia, and Loss of Purposeful Hand Use in Girls: Rett's Syndrome: Report of 35 Cases," *Ann. Neurol.,* 14, 471–79.
HIRSCHOWITZ, BASIL I., A. GROLL, AND RICARDO CEBALLOS. 1972. "Hereditary Nerve Deafness in Three Sisters with Absent Gastric Motility, Small Bowel Diverticulitis and Ulceration, and Progressive Sensory Neuropathy," *Birth Defects,* 8, 27–41.
HO, HSIU-ZU, T. J. GLAHN, AND JU-CHANG HO. 1988. "The Fragile-X Syndrome," *Dev. Med. Child Neurol.,* 30, 252–65.
HOPKINS-ACOS, PATRICIA, AND KAREN BUNKER. 1979. "A Child with Noonan Syndrome," *J. Speech Hear. Dis.,* 4, 495–503.
INGHAM, ROGER J. 1987. "Stuttering: Recent Trends in Research and Therapy," in *Human Communication and Its Disorders,* ed. Harris Winitz. Norwood, NJ: Ablex.
JAFFE, BURTON F., ed. 1977. *Hearing Loss in Children.* Baltimore: University Park Press.
——— 1978a. "Topographical Signs Associated with Congenital Hearing Loss," in *Early Diagnosis of Hearing Loss,* ed. Sanford E. Gerber and George T. Mencher. New York: Grune & Stratton.
———1978b. "Deformities of the External Ear Associated with Middle Ear, Inner Ear, or Distant Malformations," *Clin. Plastic Surg.,* 5, 413–18.
JOHNSON, WENDELL. 1944. "The Indians Have No Word for It," *Quart. J. Speech,* 30, 330–37.
JOINT COMMITTEE ON INFANT HEARING. 1982. "Position Statement, 1982," *Peds.,* 70, 496–97.
KARAGAN, N. J., AND HANS U. ZELLWEGER. 1978. "Early Verbal Disability in Children with Duchenne Muscular Dystrophy," *Dev. Med. Child Neurol.,* 20, 435–41.
KELLY, THADDEUS E. 1980. *Clinical Genetics and Genetic Counseling.* Chicago: Yearbook Medical Publishers.
KIDD, KENNETH K. 1983. "Recent Progress on the Genetics of Stuttering," in *Genetic Aspects of Speech and Language Disorders,* ed. Christy L. Ludlow and Judith A. Cooper. New York: Academic Press.
———1984. "Stuttering as a Genetic Disorder," in *Nature and Treatment of Stuttering: New Directions,* ed. Richard F. Curlee and William H. Perkins. San Diego, CA: College-Hill Press.
KINSBOURNE, MARCEL, AND PAULA J. CAPLAN. 1979. *Children's Learning and Attention Problems.* Boston: Little, Brown.
KONIGSMARK, BRUCE W. 1971. "Hereditary Congenital Severe Deafness Syndromes," *Ann. Otol., Rhinol., Laryngol.,* 80, 269–88.
———AND ROBERT J. GORLIN. 1976. *Genetic and Metabolic Deafness.* Philadelphia: Saunders.
LEVY, S., et al. 1986. "Communication and Neuropsychologic Dysfunction in Children with Neurofibromatosis." Paper presented at the second annual meeting of the Society for Developmental Pediatrics, Williamsburg.

LUDLOW, CHRISTY L., AND JUDITH A. COOPER. 1983a. "Genetic Aspects of Speech and Language Disorders: Current Status and Future Directions," in *Genetic Aspects of Speech and Language Disorders,* eds. Christy L. Ludlow and Judith A. Cooper. New York: Academic Press.

———eds. 1983b. *Genetic Aspects of Speech and Language Disorders.* New York: Academic Press.

McKUSICK, VICTOR A. 1978. *Mendelian Inheritance in Man,* 5th ed. Baltimore: Johns Hopkins University Press.

MOESCHLER, JOHN B., et al. 1988. "Rett Syndrome: Natural History and Management," *Peds.,* 82, 1–10.

MOSES, KENNETH, L. AND M. V. VAN HECKE-WULATIN. 1981. "The Socio-Emotional Impact of Infant Deafness: A Counselling Model," in *Early Management of Hearing Loss,* ed. George T. Mencher and Sanford E. Gerber. New York: Grune & Stratton.

MYERS, EUGENE N., SYLVAN E. STOOL, AND PETER J. KOBLENZER. 1971. "Congenital Deafness, Spiny Hyperkeratosis, and Universal Alopecia," *Arch. Otolaryngol.,* 93, 68–74.

NELSON, SEVERINA E. 1939. "The Role of Heredity in Stuttering," *J. Peds.,* 14, 642–54.

———NAOMI HUNTER, AND MARJORIE WALTER. 1945. "Stuttering in Twin Types," *J. Speech Dis.,* 10, 335–43.

NOONAN, JACQUELINE A., AND DOROTHY A. EHMKE. 1963. "Associated Noncardiac Malformations in Children with Congenital Heart Disease," *J. Peds.,* 63, 468–70.

NORA, JAMES J., et al. 1974. "The Ullrich Noonan Syndrome (Turner phenotype)," *Amer. J. Dis. Child.,* 127, 48–55.

NORTHERN, JERRY L., AND MARION P. DOWNS. 1984. *Hearing in Children,* 4th ed. Baltimore: Williams & Wilkins.

OPITZ, JOHN M. 1969. "Genetic Malformation Syndromes Associated with Mental Retardation," in *Congenital Mental Retardation,* ed. William M. McIsaac, James Claghorn, and Gordon Farrell. Austin: University of Texas Press.

PAPARELLA, MICHAEL M. 1973. "Surgery of the Middle Ear, Eustachian Tube and Mastoid," in *Otolaryngology* vol. 2, ed. Michael M. Paparella and Donald A. Shumrick. Philadelphia: Saunders.

PERSAUD, T. V. N. 1985. "Brief History of Teratology," in *Basic Concepts in Teratology,* ed. T. V. N. Persaud, A. E. Chudley, and R. G. Skalko. New York: Alan R. Liss.

RECORDS, MARY ANN, KENNETH K. KIDD, AND JUDITH R. KIDD. 1977. "The Family Clustering of Stuttering." Paper presented at the annual meeting of the American Speech and Hearing Association.

REGEHR, SONYA M. 1987. "The Genetic Aspects of Developmental Dyslexia," *Can. J. Behav. Sci.,* 19, 240–53.

———AND BONNIE J. KAPLAN. 1988. "Reading Disability with Motor Problems May Be an Inherited Subtype," *Peds.,* 82, 204–10.

ROSS, MARK, AND THOMAS G. GIOLAS 1978. *Auditory Management of Hearing-Impaired Children.* Baltimore: University Park Press.

RUBEN, ROBERT J., AND THOMAS R. VAN DE WATER. 1983. "Recent Advances in the Developmental Biology of the Inner Ear," in *The Development of Auditory Behavior,* eds. Sanford E. Gerber and George T. Mencher. New York: Grune & Stratton.

SEIZINGER, BERND R., et al. 1987. "Common Pathogenetic Mechanism for Three Tumor Types in Bilateral Acoustic Neurofibromatosis," *Science,* 236, 317–19.

SMITH, ALEXANDER BROWNLIE. 1939. "Unilateral Hereditary Deafness," *Lancet,* 2, 1172–73.

SMITH, S. E., et al. 1983. "A Genetic Analysis of Specific Reading Disability," in *Genetic Aspects of Speech and Language Disorders,* ed. Christy L. Ludlow and Judith A. Cooper. New York: Academic Press.

SPARKS, SHIRLEY N. 1984. *Birth Defects and Speech-Language Disorders.* San Diego, CA: College-Hill Press.

STOOL, SYLVAN E., AND ROBERT HOULIHAN. 1977. "Otolaryngologic Management of Craniofacial Anomalies," *Otolaryngol. Clin. N. Amer.,* 10, 41–4.

SUMMITT, ROBERT L. 1969. "Familial Goldenhaar Syndrome," *Birth Defects Original Article Series,* 5, 106–109.

THOMPSON, MARGARET W. 1986. *Genetics in Medicine,* 4th ed. Philadelphia: Saunders.

USHER, C. H. 1914. "On the Inheritance of Retinitis Pigmentosa, with Notes of Cases," *Royal London Ophthal. Hosp. Report,* 9, 130–236.

VAN DER HOEVE, J. 1916. "Abnorme Länge der Tränenröhrchen mit Ankeloblepharon," *Klin. Mbl. Augenheilk.*, 56, 232.

VAN RIPER, CHARLES 1939. *Speech Correction*. Englewood Cliffs, NJ: Prentice-Hall.

VERNON, MCCAY. 1976. "Usher's Syndrome: Problems and Some Solutions," *Hearing and Speech Action*, 44, 6–13.

WAARDENBURG, P. J. 1948. "Dystopia Punctorum Lacrimalium, Blepharophimosis, en Partiele Irisatrophia bij een Doofstomme," *Ned. Tijdschr. Geneeskd.*, 92, 3463–66.

———1951. "A New Syndrome Combining Developmental Anomalies of the Eyelids, Eyebrows and Nose Root with Pigmentary Defects of the Iris and Head Hair and with Congenital Deafness," *Amer. J. Human Genetics*, 3, 195–253.

WEBSTER, DOUGLAS B., AND MOLLY WEBSTER. 1979. "Effects of Neonatal Conductive Hearing Loss on Brain Stem Auditory Nuclei," *Ann. Otol., Rhinol., Laryngol.*, 88, 684–88.

WENTHOLD, ROBERT J. 1980. "Neurochemistry of the Auditory System," *Ann. Otol., Rhinol., Laryngol.*, Suppl. 74, 121–31.

WEST, ROBERT. 1958. "An Agnostic's Speculations About Stuttering," in *Stuttering: A Symposium*. ed. Jon Eisenson New York: Harper & Row.

———MERLE ANSBERRY, AND ANNA CARR. 1957. *The Rehabilitation of Speech*, 3rd ed. New York: Harper & Row.

WEVER, ERNEST G., AND MERLE LAWRENCE. 1954. *Physiological Acoustics*. Princeton, NJ: Princeton University Press.

WHITE HOUSE CONFERENCE ON CHILD HEALTH AND PROTECTION. 1931. *Special Education, Report of the Committee on Special Classes*. New York: Appleton-Century-Crofts.

WILSON, MARGO, AND ALICE DYSON. 1982. "Noonan Syndrome: Speech and Language Characteristics," *J. Comm. Dis.*, 15, 347–52.

WITT-ENGERSTROM, INGEGERD, AND CHRISTOPHER GILLBERG. 1987. "Rett Syndrome in Sweden," *J. Autism Dev. Dis.*, 17, 149–50.

WIZNITZER, MAX, ISABELLE RAPIN, AND THOMAS R. VAN DE WATER. 1987. "Neurologic Findings in Children with Ear Malformations," *Intl. J. Ped. Otorhinolaryngol.*, 13, 41–55.

4

Teratogens, Mutagens, Infections, and Iatrogens

In brief, a *teratogen* is anything that causes a birth defect, a new phenotype. Schor (1984) defined teratogens as "agents in the environment of the developing embryo and fetus which cause structural or functional abnormalities." A *mutagen*, causes a new genotype; it increases the incidence of birth defects by producing changes in DNA. Hence, mutagens are a class of teratogens, and it is probable that mutations appear continuously in the course of exposure to environmental insults. *Iatrogens* include all drugs or other treatments provided by physicians (*iatros* is Greek for "physician") that may have adverse results prenatally or at any time of life.

Taken collectively teratogens account for 8 percent of all birth defects. Moreover, they have their most common effects early in prenatal life. An important distinction in the discussion of this chapter and the previous two is that here we discuss *exogenous* factors—that is, factors that come from outside the organism. In this chapter we consider infection, intoxication, and iatrogenic conditions.

INFECTION

Infections are teratogenic agents that occur naturally; they may be *bacterial*, *protozoal*, or *viral*. The difference is important with respect to teratogenicity.

Viruses are among the smallest living creatures; they are capable of passing through filters that retain bacteria. That doesn't mean, though, that we should be unconcerned about bacteria in prenatal life.

A pregnant woman can have a bacterial disease (e.g., tuberculosis) that is capable of affecting her unborn child. Viruses can and do cross the placental barrier, and the time (i.e., the fetus's gestational age) at which they do is closely related to their effects. Their frequencies are shown in Table 4–1 (Sever 1983). Moreover, a high frequency of infection may be associated with malnutrition and undernutrition; this is discussed later.

Congenital deafness, blindness, mental retardation, neuromotor abnormalities, seizure disorders, and many other adverse consequences for communication may result from prenatal disease. A special and peculiar problem is the one posed by syphilis. Syphilis is protozoal—that is, it is caused by a one-celled organism, a protozoon—and, among the bacteria, it is so small that it may act like a virus. For that reason, and many others, syphilis is often called "the great imitator."

Prenatal Viral Diseases

Any viral disease that occurs during the embryonic period may be damaging or lethal to the baby; however, the nature of communicative disorders caused by viral infection is not different in postnatal life from those acquired prenatally. It is the case, though, that there seem to be different incidence and prevalence rates between antenatal and postnatal viral disease sequelae. Among the viruses, two stand out as having communicative consequences for the survivors of prenatal disease. These are *rubella* and *cytomegalovirus*; thus, we concentrate the discussion more on these two than on others.

TABLE 4–1. Frequencies of Maternal and Fetal Infections Known to Damage the Central Nervous System

Infection	Mother/10,000	Child/10,000
Viral		
Cytomegalovirus	300–2,000	100–200
Rubella: Epidemic	200–400	20–40
Rubella: Nonepidemic	<10	<1
Herpes simplex	15–150	1–5
Varicella	2–8	<1
Bacterial/Protozoal		
Syphilis	2–60	1–3
Tuberculosis	<1–8	<1
Toxoplasmosis	<1–7	1–3

SOURCE: John L. Sever, "Maternal Infections," in Catherine Caldwell Brown, ed., *Childhood Learning Disabilities and Prenatal Risk* (Skillman, N.J.: Johnson and Johnson Baby Products, 1983), p. 32.

Rubella Rubella is popularly known as "German measles" or the "three-day measles." Rubella came to the attention of communicative disorders specialists as a result of an epidemic in Australia from 1939 to 1941. Gregg (1941) observed that many infants born during that period were visually impaired due to congenital cataracts. In 1944, Swann described the deafness of these same children. The consequences of the North American rubella epidemic of 1963–65 were described by numerous clinical scholars and summarized by Bordley et al. (1967), and a simultaneous epidemic was described by Baldursson et al. (1972). The importance of the rubella epidemic is evident from Table 4–1.

The rubella virus was first isolated by Weller and Neva in 1962. Until that time it was the most common viral cause of birth defects; as many as 1 in 200 live births presented with organ damage as a consequence of maternal rubella infection (Andersen et al. 1986). It usually produces a very mild disease marked by the enlargement of lymph nodes but with little fever or other bodily reactions. In fact, one of the reasons it is so dangerous is that a pregnant woman may be unaware that she has a rubella infection. Moreover, its effects in the patient are usually nil, but it can severely disrupt a developing embryo. Bordley et al. (1967) expressed their great concern that "prenatal rubella can damage a child while giving no clinical symptoms in the mother." Alford, Stagno, and Pass (1980) observed that gestational age is "influential" because of the prematurity of the fetal immune system in early pregnancy, and this seems to be especially true for rubella and toxoplasmosis. The effects, when they occur, may appear as deafness, cataracts, preterm birth, cardiac defects, mental retardation with or without microcephaly, or, in fact, any combination or all of these. The timing of the infection is associated with the form of the sequelae.

Bordley et al. examined 79 children with confirmed prenatal exposure to rubella virus, although 34 of the mothers had had a "subclinical" infection. At the time of their report, 47 of these children exhibited positive virus cultures. It is important to observe that, of these 47, it was possible to determine the time of infection for 45. Among these 45, 18 (40 percent) did *not* contract the disease in the first trimester, contrary to popular belief. Wolfson, Aghamohamadi, and Berman (1980) reported "hearing problems to be present in 68 percent of cases resulting from maternal infection in the first trimester, in 40 percent of those occurring in the second trimester, and in a smaller number in the third trimester."

Bordley et al. (1967) reported the results of hearing tests on 49 of the original 79 children, and 26 (53 percent) were found to be hearing impaired. In addition, 21 of the 79 (27 percent) were mentally retarded, of whom 15 exhibited microcephaly. Among the 26 hearing impaired children, 21 (81 percent) were also retarded and 15 (58 percent) had ocular defects. Eleven (42 percent) of the 26 hearing impaired children had both ocular defects and mental retardation. Twenty-three of the 79 children had normal hearing, but 10 (43 percent) were developmentally delayed and one also had ocular problems. This recitation of the numbers is to stress the fact that prenatal rubella, more often than not, results in communicative disorders and often in multiple handicaps.

Chess and Fernandez (1980) found a high incidence of neurologic damage among multiply handicapped rubella babies, but not among those with normal intelligence. In general, this additional handicap took the form of a behavior disorder. As a matter of fact, Chess (1971, 1977) found a high incidence of prenatal rubella among children diagnosed as autistic. She has argued repeatedly that "these data support the concept of organic causation of the syndrome of autism." Although they did not argue for a causal relationship between prenatal rubella and autism, Ornitz, Guthrie, and Farley (1977) found a history or probable history of prenatal rubella in 3 of 18 autistic children who were multiply handicapped. Wetherby (1985) observed, furthermore, that intrauterine viral infections and other congenital perinatal infections, among other factors, "contribute to a high risk for speech and language disorders in children . . . ." Unfortunately, she continued, "The predictive value of these high risk factors . . . remains to be determined."

The relationship between sequelae and time of infection was summarized by Dublin (1976):

> In the presence of infection during the first trimester of gestation there is a high probability of some degree of hearing loss. In cases of infection before the end of the sixth week of pregnancy, damage to the fetus is likely to be widespread and may involve eyes (microphthalmia, cataract, glaucoma, retinopathy), cardiovascular system (ventricular septal defect, patent ductus arteriosus) and brain (microcephaly, mental retardation). There may be stunting of growth. At the end of six weeks these organ systems may escape; even slightly later the cochlear duct and saccule may be affected while the utricle and semicircular ducts, structures that develop earlier, may be unaltered. The organ of Corti may fail to develop. . . .

Figure 4–1 displays the inner ear pathology mentioned by Dublin, Figure 4–2 is the type of audiogram frequently encountered in such a patient, and Figure 4–3 is a photograph of just such a multiply handicapped child.

Lindsay's (1973) description is entirely consistent with Dublin's; he found a normal middle ear and otic capsule with absence of the organ of Corti, including hair cells. However, Hemenway, Sando, and McChesney (1969) found, in addition, an anomalous stapes and cartilaginous fixation of the footplate. Cohn (1981) also noted the possibility of a middle ear anomaly.

FIGURE 4–1.   Basal turn of the cochlea in a case of congenital rubella deafness

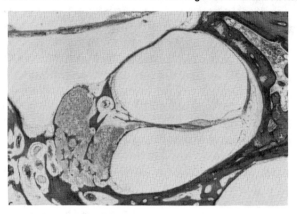

SOURCE: Michael M. Paparella and Mary Jayne Capps, "Sensorineural Deafness in Children–Nongenetic," in Michael M. Paparella and Donald A. Shumrick, eds., *Otolaryngology*, vol. 2: *Ear* (Philadelphia: W. B. Saunders, Co. 1973), p. 313. Reprinted by permission.

FIGURE 4–2.   Audiogram of a child with congenital rubella deafness

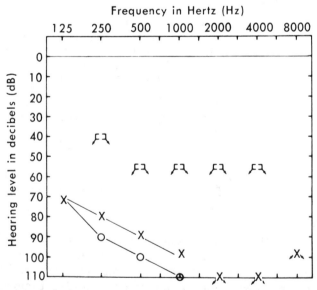

SOURCE: Fred H. Bess and Freeman E. McConnell, "Measurement of Auditory Function," *Audiology, Education, and the Hearing Impaired Child* (St. Louis, Mo.: Mosby, 1981), p. 51. Courtesy of Fred H. Bess.

FIGURE 4–3. A two-and-a-half-year-old deaf-blind child with congenital rubella

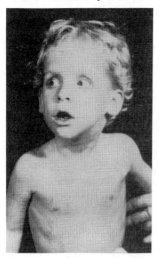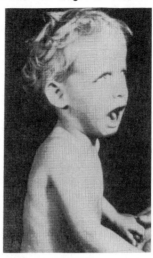

SOURCE: Jean M. Zadig and Allen C. Crocker, "A Center for the Study of the Young Child with Developmental Delay," in B. Z. Friedlander et al., eds., *Exceptional Infant: Assessment and Intervention* (New York: Brunner/Mazel, 1975), p. 9. Reproduced by permission.

What do we know, then, about the consequences of prenatal rubella? The answer to this question may be contained completely in Figure 4–3. The child is hearing impaired, visually handicapped, and developmentally delayed, and has a neuromotor disability, and probably a cardiac defect. The rubella-affected baby may be the epitome of the multiply handicapped child. It has been reported (Karchmer, Milone, and Wolk 1979) that 28 percent of all hearing impaired schoolchildren had an additional handicap and that 65 percent of these had severe-to-profound hearing losses. Mental retardation and visual impairment were the most common handicaps.

Rubella, however, has been one of the best examples of primary prevention of communicative (and other) disorders. Inoculation against rubella began in 1969; the beneficial consequences are apparent in Figure 4–4. In fact, the rubella vaccine is now combined with those to prevent rubeola (measles) and parotitis (mumps), and studies have been done to add a vaccine to prevent varicella (chicken pox) to that for these three viral diseases. Figure 4–5 is a dramatic illustration of the benefits of inoculation. This figure (Barr 1982) shows two important things: one, the incidence of congenital deafness varies with the incidence of prenatal rubella; and, two, the incidence of both dropped following the introduction of the vaccine. It also shows the effect of the epidemic of the mid-1960s.

FIGURE 4–4.   Rubella incidence in selected areas of the United States, 1929–1981

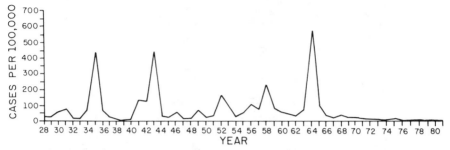

SOURCE: Walter A. Orenstein et al.,"Epidemiology of Rubella and Its Complications," in E. M. Gruenberg et al., *Vaccinating against Brain Syndromes: The Campaign against Measles and Rubella* (New York: Oxford University Press, 1986), p. 51.

FIGURE 4–5.   Incidence of congenital rubella and of deafness in different time periods

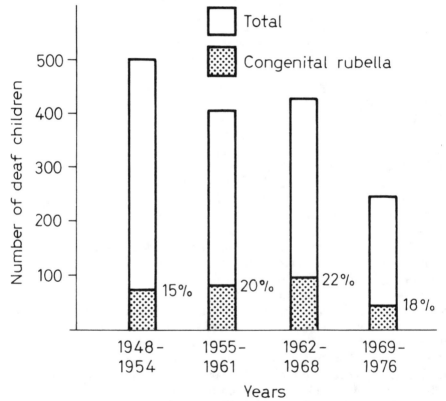

SOURCE: Bengt Barr, "Teratogenic Hearing Loss," *Audiology*, 21 (1982), p. 116. Courtesy of Bengt Barr.

It has been observed that genetic etiologies should increase in relative frequency as the incidence of these acquired etiologies diminishes (Nance and Sweeney 1975), but we may have become lax in our concern for prenatal rubella. Although Barr found 18 percent of the deaf babies who had been born by 1976 to be products of prenatal rubella, in 1984 Pappas and Schaibly found 20 percent of their deaf babies had confirmed diagnoses of viral etiologic agents. It does appear that the incidence of rubella may be increasing, and fewer and fewer children are being inoculated. On the other hand, Pappas and Schaibly's babies were products of "viral agents," not only of rubella. Still, "rubella vaccine should be included in all childhood immunization programs" (Andersen et al. 1986).

Cytomegalovirus Cytomegalovirus (CMV) is one of the most common diseases of humans. In 1975, Marx reported that 80 percent of the population of the United States by the age of 35 to 40 years were carrying CMV antibodies. Andersen et al. (1986) said that "nearly everyone" in the United States is infected before the age of 50. This does not mean that all of these people had had CMV, but it does mean that they had been exposed to it at some time. It is the most common viral disease among the newborn and the most common viral cause of mental retardation (see Table 4–1). Reynolds et al. (1974) estimated its prevalence in infants to approximate one in 400, and its incidence to be between 0.5 and 1.5 percent of all live births in the United States and in the United Kingdom. Andersen et al. claimed it to occur in almost 2 percent of all live births. Harris et al. (1984) found CMV in 0.5 percent of all births in one hospital in Sweden.

Sever (1983) summarized the situation this way:

> Congenital infection occurs in .5 to 1.5 percent of births. As many as 10 percent of these children exhibit permanent damage in the form of poor mental performance and high-tone hearing loss. Based on these figures for fetal damage and a birth rate of approximately 3.5 million in the United States, it has been estimated that some 3,000 children are damaged each year by this virus. Damage to the brain includes direct tissue destruction with mild to severe mental retardation, microcephaly, hydrocephaly, and deafness. . . .

There has even been a report of autism in a child with congenital CMV (Stubbs 1978). However, 90 to 95 percent of all infants born with this disease are asymptomatic.

The timing of the infection is pertinent not only to the severity of the sequelae but also to the actual occurrence of infection. Alford, Stagno, and Pass (1980) reported that 20 percent of the infants infected in utero are damaged. Infants infected at birth (e.g., due to the presence of the infection in the mother's genital tract) or later (e.g., by infected breast milk) usually suffer no sequelae. Johnson et al. (1986) reported that hearing impairment was not encountered in infants who were infected later than three weeks of age, a finding that confirms the expectation of Alford, Stagno, and Pass. In those infants who are infected prenatally, progressive deafness seems to result (Gerber, Mendel, and Goller 1979). Andersen et al. said that 10 to 15 percent of "infected-but-asymptomatic" infants develop sensory-neural hearing loss due to chronic CMV infection of the inner ear. The fact that hearing impairment is a common result of prenatal CMV infection has been known for some time (Medearis 1964). Alford, Stagno, and Pass found "significant auditory deficits" in 7 percent of the infants they studied. Their conclusion is very important:

> Present estimates from our longitudinal investigations of congenitally infected infants indicate that about 10% are afflicted with severe infection while another 10% or so develop late-appearing subtle defects, such as deafness. If these values hold in other populations then 0.2% of all live births are damaged annually as a result of intrauterine CMV infection. Consequently cytomegaloviruses are now a greater public health hazard than rubella virus was in the prevaccine era.

It must be stressed that virtually all infants born with a CMV infection have no symptoms. Their infections are described as "silent." There is a high mortality rate among those infants who do have symptoms of cytomegalic inclusion disease; typically, the survivors are severely and multiply handicapped with mental retardation, motor disabilities, seizures, blindness, and deafness. The etiology of the deafness that results from a congenital CMV infection is clearly a viral infection of the cochlea (Myers and Stool 1968). Cytomegaloviruses actually were isolated from the inner ear of an infant who died at one month of age (Davis et al. 1979).

At the present state of the virologist's art, there is no primary prevention: No vaccine exists to prevent or inhibit CMV. To be sure, efforts are underway to develop one, but none is available in a form useful for widespread inoculations. Secondary prevention is also difficult. Blackman (1984a) reported that 50 percent of women of childbearing age have no immunity. Moreover, women can be reinfected in successive pregnancies. Given that virtually all affected infants are asymptomatic, and given that the consequent handicaps are probably progressive, it may be impossible to detect the majority of those CMV-infected infants who will become handicapped. Andersen et al. recommended the practice of good hygiene among women of child-bearing age who may come into contact with children who could be shedding CMV.

Dahle et al. (1974) expressed a hope for secondary prevention via increased availability of methods to isolate the virus in newborns. There is a reluctance on the part of practitioners and public health agencies, however, to employ these methods even where they are available. The test known as TORCH (for toxoplasmosis, rubella, cytomegalovirus, and herpes) is available, but the reluctance to employ it arises from a risk of overinclusiveness. The fact remains that "at present there is no known effective treatment or preventative strategy" (Fischler 1985).

We also have a relatively newfound problem: the association of CMV with AIDS (acquired immune deficiency syndrome). Transplacental transmission has been reported to occur (Steis and Broder 1985); in fact, 77 percent of children with AIDS have mothers who have AIDS or are at risk for AIDS. Whether the AIDS infection is congenital or appears some time after birth, these children suffer the same consequences of immunosuppression as do adults. This puts them at high risk for CMV and/or other viral infections. In fact, Steis and Broder claimed that "cytomegalovirus infects nearly all AIDS patients . . . progression to blindness is not uncommon." To date there have been no reports of AIDS-related CMV with effects not expected among patients who have CMV but do not have AIDS. However, we should expect these effects to appear and we should be prepared for them. Ammann (1983) reported the onset of symptoms to be between the ages of three and six months among patients who have pediatric AIDS; and, again, CMV is common. This fact opens the possibility of secondary prevention insofar as communicative screening should be included among the services brought to such infants.

Other viruses Our historic and legitimate concern for rubella and CMV continues to be valid. However, we must be aware that other viruses can be contracted prenatally and that the effects of prenatal disease are essentially the same for all of them. Consequently, one can find reports of communicative sequelae of prenatal varicella (chicken pox), parotitis (mumps), herpes, rubeola (measles), and influenza.

Epstein et al. (1986) followed 36 children with a diagnosis of AIDS, AIDS-related complex, or asymptomatic infection with human immunodeficiency virus (HIV). Because these children were as young as two months post-partum, and 26 of them were products of risk factors in their mothers, one must conclude that these are congenital infections. The infection occurs in the intrauterine environment; one study found ten cesarean sections among 33 infants born with AIDS (Minkoff et al. 1987a). Some 30 to 50 percent of infants born to mothers with AIDS or HIV, or at risk to develop AIDS, will be infected. Many of these mothers are not evidently infected at the time of delivery (seven-eighths of them, in fact) even though maternal infection is implicit, but are at risk for later development of symptomatic illness (Minkoff et al. 1987b). There are few data on perinatal transmission—via the birth canal or breast milk, for example—but the risk is low compared to intrauterine transmission (AAP 1988).

If we broaden the definition of congenital to include onset early in life—expecting that the onset of symptoms was occasioned by a prenatal event or condition—then we must also broaden our concern to include these infants. The 34 infants followed by Minkoff et al. (1987b) had an average age for onset of symptoms of 5.7 months, but the youngest was two weeks of age. The American Academy of Pediatrics (1988) reported that the majority of infants who had perinatally acquired AIDS were normal at birth but displayed clinical symptoms within the first two years. These symptoms included "failure to thrive, generalized lymphadeno-pathy, hepatosplenomegaly, parotitis, persistent oral candidiasis and chronic or recurrent diarrhea. Developmental disabilities and neurologic dysfunc-tion are frequently seen." Kastner and Friedman (1988) predicted that AIDS will approximate the incidence of Down syndrome, and AIDS has been established as a cause of mental retardation. Moreover, there have been occasional reports of craniofacial dysmorphism. Twenty of the 36 children described by Epstein et al. had progressive encephalopathy that was "the result of primary and persistent infection of the brain with this retrovirus."

Some data exist on the communicative consequences of AIDS, but few on congenital and/or early onset AIDS. We have every reason to suppose that we will see more and more of these patients, and more and more of them will be children. The rate at which the number of AIDS cases doubles is now greater in children than in adults (Proujan 1988). Furthermore, children with AIDS are more subject to opportunistic and severe infections than adults because of the immaturity of their immune systems. Andersen et al. (1986) reported the symptoms of AIDS to be nonspecific and more variable in children than in adults. Still, they include hepatosplenomegaly (often associated with CMV), developmental delay, upper respiratory infections, pneumonia, and ear diseases. Infec-tious manifestations have been reported in the otorhinolaryngeal system. Kaposi's sarcoma has been seen in the external ear and in the oral cavity; herpes zoster oticus has appeared among the opportunistic infections which arise in AIDS patients; and as many as half of these patients have hearing losses (Flower and Sooy 1987).

Otolaryngologic data on pediatric AIDS have been published by Williams (1987). His summary is telling: "Ninety percent were micro-somic. Developmental delay occurred in 90%. Inflammatory ear disease occurred in 80%. Lymphocytic interstitial pneumonia and mucocutane-ous candidiasis each occurred in 80%, cortical atrophy in 60%, cervical adenopathy in 40%, and parotid enlargement in 40%." The children he studied ranged in age from 15 to 164 months.

About one-third of these pregnancies results in low birth weight infants (<2,500 g) with the risks usually attendant upon low birth weight.

Iosub et al. (1987) examined eight children, ranging in age from 4 to 33 months, who were diagnosed as having AIDS or AIDS-related complex. They hypothesized that there may be a distinct (dysmorphic?) facies in these children: *hypertelorism*, obliquity of eyes, long palpebral fissures, blue sclerae, depressed nasal bridge, and prominent upper vermilion border. In addition, sudden onset sensory-neural hearing loss has been known to occur (Real, Thomas, and Gerwin 1987).

Although we mentioned that rubella and CMV are by far the most frequent prenatal viral sources of congenital communicative disability, they are not the only ones. Lindsay (1973) observed the rare instance of varicella (chicken pox) virus as a source of congenital deafness, for example.

Herpes simplex has become quite common. Typically, the neonate is contaminated during its passage through the birth canal. The incidence of neonatal infection approximates 1 in 7,500 in the United States (Malvern 1980), and 1 in 10,000 will be seriously ill (Andersen et al. 1986). Malvern reported a high mortality rate (62 percent), but that has been reduced to 18 percent (Moon 1987). Half of all survivors had central nervous system lesions, but these too have been markedly reduced. These lesions appear most frequently in the frontal and temporal lobes, which often results in psychomotor seizures (Painter 1983). Dahle and McCollister (1988) also reported CNS involvement in 50 percent of their patients, but were the first to report the incidence of hearing impairment, 10 percent (2 of 20) in the group they studied. The two infants also had visual abnormalities, hydranancephaly, severe psychomotor retardation, and other handicaps.

Dublin (1976) commented that several infectious agents could lead to congenital encephalitis. But, as we observed at the beginning of the book, the topic of communicable disease—that is, infection—is the brightest spot from the viewpoint of primary prevention. The best, and best known, examples of vaccination for the prevention of disease are the smallpox and polio vaccines. Jenner's observations and his introduction of a smallpox vaccine date from 1798, but it was only in the middle of the twentieth century that smallpox finally disappeared. Poliomyelitis has yet to disappear, but the now routine inoculations have significantly diminished its incidence. Isolation of the rubella virus (Weller and Neva 1962) eventually led to the development of rubella vaccine; and, by 1980, there were fewer than 60 cases per year in the United States (Hanshaw 1980). Inoculations against measles and mumps are common. The varicella vaccine has had clinical trials and has been combined successfully with the measles, mumps, and rubella (MMR) vaccine (Arbeter et al. 1986). Vaccines against CMV and HIV are still to come, but substantial progress is being made toward a CMV vaccine.

Other Prenatal Diseases

Notable among the other diseases that can and do affect the developing infant are the protozoa (single-celled creatures) syphilis and toxoplasmosis. Additionally, there are bacterial disorders which, if they appear in a pregnant woman, can have adverse consequences for her baby. Malvern (1980) cautioned that bacteria, fungi, and viruses may all be found in the lower genital tract "and be potential sources of severe, occasionally lethal, perinatal infection." These would include, among others, the viruses discussed above and *Treponema pallidum* (the bacterium which causes syphilis), *Trichomonas* (which leads to vaginitis), and *Candida* (a yeast which can lead to meningitis, among other things). *Chlamydia* are now known to have the potential for blindness, even when they appear perinatally. The list is potentially a very long one; here we limit the discussion to syphilis and toxoplasmosis with mention of a few others.

Syphilis Today we recognize syphilis in women as a venereal disease, via a route that ascends through the cervix. Reports as far back as the sixteenth century suggested that it was a tropical disease related to *yaws*, and it is, but those observations may have been true due to sanitary conditions in the tropics at that time. It is produced by a bacterium, *Treponema pallidum*, which can pass the placental barrier. In general, it is claimed that bacteria don't cross the placental barrier because of their relatively (to viruses) large size. *Treponema pallidum*, however, is an extremely small bacterium, and has been identified in placental tissue. Its sequelae are manifold.

It is important to note that syphilis is a treatable disease, given that a correct and early diagnosis is made. *Treponema* does not pass to a fetus prior to the fourth month of gestation (Lederer 1973); therefore, the importance of early intervention is obvious. Blackman (1984a) made the point that untreated syphilis in the mother "whether contracted during pregnancy or years before" can be transmitted to her baby. He also noted that there is no risk in future pregnancies if she has been adequately treated.

It is also important to note that syphilis is called "the great imitator" and is often incorrectly diagnosed. Hence, Blackman apparently believed that all pregnant women should be tested for syphilis early on. In adults, it often presents with the symptoms of Ménière disease and a possibly incorrect diagnosis of endolymphatic hydrops is made. When treatment for Ménière disease fails, questions about the presence of syphilis arise. Proper and prompt diagnosis and treatment of a pregnant woman who has syphilis can prevent consequences for her child.

Perinatal syphilis has been reported to have a mortality rate of 3.2 per 1,000 deliveries; 72 percent of those were stillborn and the other 28 percent were early neonatal deaths (Ross et al. 1980). Blackman (1984a) reported that 25 percent die before birth. The surviving 75 percent may show no signs of infection after birth but have serious problems that appear later, even much later. These include sensory-neural deafness, mental retardation, blindness, psychosis, skeletal anomalies, and abnormalities of the teeth.

The issue of late appearing sensory-neural hearing loss is important. Zoller et al. (1978) concluded that syphilis must be considered in every case where the hearing impairment is of obscure origin. Indeed, the auditory symptoms resulting from congenital syphilis may appear in childhood, but half of all such cases have no symptoms until the age of 25, or even 35, years (Sando, Suehiro, and Wood 1983). The onset of the hearing loss is usually sudden, bilateral, and symmetrical and without vestibular difficulties. The degree and extent of nervous system damage determine the severity of neurologic sequelae, including mental retardation. The long-term consequences of congenital syphilis are usually in the form of multiple and progressive handicaps.

To repeat: Syphilis is a curable disease. Prevention insofar as curing syphilis in a pregnant woman may prevent consequences for the child. In such a case, it may be primary prevention for the baby and secondary prevention for the mother. The first problem, though, is to diagnose the disease. The most specific and sensitive means to detect the presence of *Treponema* is the flourescent treponemal antibody absorption (FTA-ABS) test. It has been suggested (e.g., Northern and Downs 1984) that FTA-ABS be added to the TORCH series discussed earlier. In some literature, therefore, one may see STORCH or TORCH + S.

The FTA-ABS test is a means to secondary prevention. What about primary prevention? One must be continually aware that syphilis is a venereal disease; it is transmitted by sexual contact. Hence, all of the advice we have been giving each other with respect to AIDS applies equally to syphilis. Primary prevention consists of safe sex practices, wise choice of sexual partners, use of adequate protection, and, above all, knowledge.

Toxoplasmosis Toxoplasmosis is the T (or TO) of TORCH. This disease is caused by the rather common protozoon *Toxoplasma gondii*, which is found in blood, in certain tissues, and even within certain kinds of cells. This is another of those infections with symptoms that are often inapparent but is extremely dangerous in prenatal life. It may result in death, and in survivors, it is common to find brain and eye disorders becoming apparent at several weeks of age. Sever et al. (1988) found bilateral deafness, microcephaly, and an IQ under 70 to be associated with the presence of high maternal antibody levels to toxoplasmosis.

The approximate incidence of toxoplasmosis is 1 to 2 per 1,000 live births. Among women who contract toxoplasmosis in the first trimester of pregnancy, about one-third of their babies dies in utero and half of the survivors are severely handicapped. As pregnancy proceeds, the risk of death diminishes along with the severity of complications. In the third trimester, most babies will suffer no consequences. Nevertheless, about 30 to 40 percent of infected women will have infected infants.

There are few reports of severe hearing loss in patients with congenital toxoplasmosis, and Wright's (1971) review found only a few "well documented cases of middle-ear disease" and those were in patients who had other severe sequelae. Nevertheless, it is wise to remember that "the congenital infection is so serious that there is no doubt that it may cause hearing loss" (Northern and Downs 1984). In fact, Theissing and Kittel (1962) claimed that toxoplasmosis is responsible for up to 20 percent of all profound childhood deafness. Whether or not hearing loss appears, the communicative consequences of toxoplasmosis are evident in that these children often have microcephaly or hydrocephaly. The mental retardation that results has its own speech and language properties, frequently compounded by the fact that such children are visually impaired.

Prevention of toxoplasmosis continues to elude us. The disease seems to arise most commonly from the presence of infected fecal matter of domestic cats, but it seems unreasonable to demand that pregnant women should be prohibited from keeping cats as pets. There has been some success in secondary prevention with the use of a drug called spiramycin, which is not available in the United States; the successes have been in France. The best summary of the situation, however distressing, was stated by Hanshaw (1980):

> Our strongest efforts should be directed towards control of cytomegalovirus, group B streptococcus, coliform bacteria, *Toxoplasma gondii*, and herpes simplex in the perinatal period. These relatively common infections are all characterized by a capacity for long-term sequelae and collectively represent significant morbidity and mortality for the newborn infant. The difficult problem of prevention of disease due to these perinatal agents is, quite appropriately, the subject of active and important investigation which could have an enormous impact on the quality of life for literally millions of people from many parts of the world.

In other words, we are not yet successful in preventing toxoplasmosis at the primary level, some progress is being made in secondary prevention, but tertiary prevention continues to be the most available choice.

Bacteria It is evident from Hanshaw's comments that other bacterial infections in the perinatal period are cause for concern. The so-called group B streptococcus (i.e., *Streptococcus agalactiae*) is acquired by an infant during the birth process, that is, during labor or delivery. An acute onset of disease appears usually within the first 24 hours of life, and is characterized by rapid deterioration, often leading to death. The disease has come to be called GBS infection, and now ranks ahead of *Staphyloccus pyogenes* and *Escherichia coli* as the dominant bacterial infection of the perinatal period (Reid and Lloyd 1980). In the United States, this disease appears in 12,000 to 15,000 babies each year; half die and half of the survivors develop neurologic sequelae (Hanshaw 1980).

GBS infection appears in 1.2 to 4 infants per 1,000 live births. Anthony and Okada (1977) reported a death rate of 55 percent, but Lloyd and Reid (1976) found only 28 percent; however, they agree that low birth weight infants are especially at risk. In fact, Reid and Lloyd (1980) alleged that 90 percent of the GBS deaths were infants with birth weights under 2,500 grams. Reid and Lloyd also defined a "late onset" variety that appears between 1 and 12 weeks of age. Survivors, in either case, commonly have pneumonia and meningitis, and we are well aware of the communicative consequences of meningitis. Moreover, Reid and Lloyd reported that *all* of the survivors of the late onset variety have meningitis. On the other hand, GBS, like other bacterial diseases, is treatable with antibiotics, specifically penicillin and gentamycin. Commercial pneumococcal vaccines are available, but their efficacy is unproven (Hanshaw 1980).

What is true of GBS is true of other bacterial disorders as well. For example, tuberculosis in a pregnant woman puts her child at risk. In general, bacterial infections in a mother may be "caught" by her baby usually during passage through the birth canal but sometimes by a transplacental route. Furthermore, the risk to the infant correlates with birth weight, which, in turn, correlates with nutritional and other environmental factors. And genetic predisposition or genetic resistance must always be considered. Not every baby born to an ill mother becomes ill.

Primary prevention of bacterial disorders is found generally in the area of public health, community hygiene, and sanitation. In other words, the goal is to eliminate these bacteria from the environment and thereby avoid prenatal infection. Because bacterial infections are usually treatable with antibiotics, it has been possible to reduce mortality due to perinatal disease; this is secondary prevention. On the other hand, some of the appropriate drugs for such treatment may be the source of iatrogenic disorders; for example, gentamycin is ototoxic. It is not possible in a given instance to determine if a sequela is of teratogenic or iatrogenic origin; we don't give drugs to well babies. In other words, most of the time we cannot know if certain sequelae are due to the disease or its treatment.

Maternal Disease

Ill women get pregnant; pregnant women get sick. Women who have chronic disorders—diabetes, hypothyroidism, epilepsy, kidney disease—can and do conceive. Many of these women take medications for their chronic conditions, as indeed they should, and these may or may not be teratogenic. Most important among these pre-existing disorders is diabetes both because of its frequency of occurrence and its potential consequences.

Diabetes Birth defects of all kinds appear far more frequently in children born to diabetic mothers than in the general population. For example, cardiovascular malformations appear in somewhat less than 8 per 1,000 births among mothers without diabetes; they appear in nearly 62 per 1,000 among mothers who have had diabetes for longer than five years (Heinonen 1976). More directly relevant to our clinical concerns is the fact that "overt maternal diabetes more than doubles the frequency of malformations including clefts" (Myrianthopoulos 1980). A syndrome of ear anomalies, deafness, and facial nerve palsy has been reported in offspring of diabetic mothers (O'Loughlin and Lillystone 1983). There has also been a report of congenital deafness and diabetes arising within a family apparently by a dominant mode of transmission (Hognestad 1967). Diabetes arising during pregnancy has been associated with Noonan syndrome and a variety of nonspecific anomalies appearing in multiple organ systems (Sparks 1984). Blackman (1984b) cautioned that diabetes may appear during pregnancy in women who have had no signs of the disease before.

It is not hard to understand why the infant of a diabetic mother is at such high risk. Yogman et al. (1982) pointed out that such a fetus is exposed to continuous changes in insulin output due to the mother oscillating between hypoglycemia and hyperglycemia. When such infants are born small, they are at increased risk of intellectual impairment. The more usual finding, though, is that diabetic mothers have large babies, and they are susceptible to respiratory distress. Ogata (1984) noted that insulin stimulates fetal growth, so the metabolic alterations that exist in the diabetic *gravida* have a direct effect on the growth of the fetus. The consequences for the infant were summarized in one phrase by Cornblath and Schwartz (1966): "congenital anomalies, respiratory distress syndrome, hypoglycemia, hypocalcemia, electrolyte abnormalities, hyperbilirubinemia, heart failure, renal vein thrombosis and hypoparathyroidism. . . ." Nearly 20 years later, Ogata repeated that list. Most important among these is respiratory distress syndrome, a topic discussed at length in Chapter 7, with its obvious risk of hypoxic encephalopathy and deafness. Especially significant is an increased risk of *hyalin membrane disease* because insulin limits the synthesis of surfactant.

Diabetes, although not curable, is controllable. And it has been shown that control of diabetes in pregnancy can and does reduce both mortality and morbidity in the perinatal period (Goldstein et al. 1978). It is interesting and important, however, that Goldstein et al. did not produce a decrease in the usually high rate of congenital malformations. They concluded that "the teratogenic factor has something to do with the abnormal biochemical environment the fetus is exposed to." They did minimize the rate of preterm delivery and the number of babies who were small for gestational age, and thereby reduced the morbidity associated with such infants. This is primary prevention. Secondary prevention would take the form of preparation for difficulties in the expectation that the diabetic mother does have such a high risk. This preparation could even take the form of arranging for cesarean section in case of intrapartum emergency and/or preparation for an infant in respiratory distress. The goal should and can be, however, "normalization of diabetes in a woman before conception" (Ogata 1984).

Thyroid disorders Notable among prenatal disorders or preexisting conditions are those of thyroid metabolism. Metabolic disorders are the subject of Chapter 8; here we are concerned with such disorders during prenatal life.

Congenital hypothyroidism occurs at least as often as 1 in 10,000 births, perhaps as frequently as 1 in 5,000 (Fisher and Burrow 1975). Man (1975) found that children born to mothers with thyroid disease that had been inadequately treated had significantly lower mean WISC IQs than those of adequately treated mothers (83 vs. 103). Although an I.Q. of 83 would probably not be considered an indication of mental retardation, it is certainly a sign of developmental delay. Moreover, Man's data show that adequate treatment can prevent (or at least inhibit) a potential for decreased intelligence. The earlier the hypothyroidism occurs in prenatal life, the more severe and lasting are its effects; and treatment must begin during the first month of life to prevent irreversible brain damage (Legrand 1984).

The association between prenatal hypothyroidism and mental retardation has been known for many, many years. In the extreme, it results in cretinism (Figure 4–6). Even the word "cretin" has been in the literature since the eighteenth century or possibly earlier. The disorder results in severe retardation of both physical and mental development and is frequently accompanied by hearing impairment.

FIGURE 4–6.   Characteristic face of a cretin

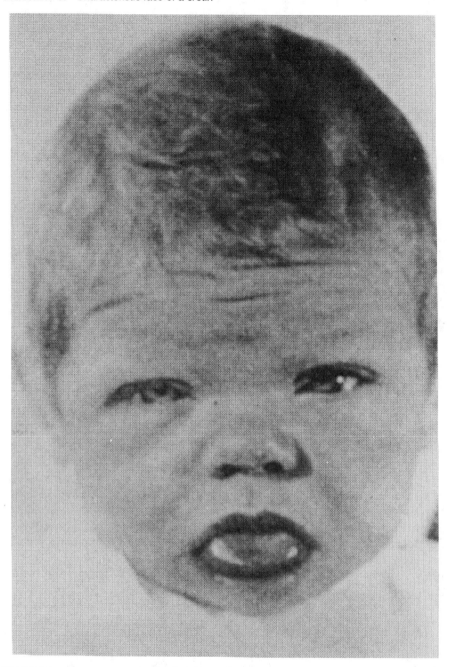

SOURCE: Richard E. Behrman and Victor C. Vaughn, eds., *Nelson Textbook of Pediatrics.*
Reprinted courtesy of W. B. Saunders Co.

In many parts of the world, cretinism is sufficiently common to be labeled as endemic cretinism, and the question has been raised if it is the same disorder as so-called sporadic cretinism (Hetzel 1972). In either case, patients sometimes have mixed hearing losses; Koenig and Neiger (1972) reported audiometric data on ten hearing impaired cretins, two of whom had conductive losses in addition to their "receptive-type hearing defects." Their review raises some confusion about the form of the otic pathology in that they claim that audiometric data reveal "receptive" impairment, whereas temporal bone studies always show middle ear pathology. The fact of hearing impairment in addition to the mental retardation means that a cretin is a multiply handicapped patient deserving of our attention. Happily, cretinism has become rare in most parts of the world. Generally, Western countries have addressed the issue of iodine shortage in water or food supplies, which, historically, have been the most common cause of cretinism.

Nevertheless, thyroid dysfunction remains a source of communicative disorders; significant among them is Pendred syndrome. In 1896, Vaughan Pendred first described the syndrome that now bears his name in an article only one paragraph long. Pendred did not know the genetic origin of this disease, although he described the combination of *goiter* and deafness that appeared in two of ten siblings. In fact, in his paper, he sought advice about its etiology. It was another 30 years until Brain (1927) postulated that the thyroid disease and the deafness resulted from the same abnormal gene. It is now well established that Pendred syndrome is due to autosomal recessive inheritance. The deafness is congenital—or at least of extremely early onset—but the goiter does not appear until some time later, usually in the preteen years (Fraser 1976). Sensory-neural hearing impairment is universal, and typically displays the falling audiogram expected.

Because the deafness appears in very early infancy, but the goiter does not appear until later, a thorough examination of the family history is essential. This is clearly illustrated in the pedigree of Brain's (1927) family, shown in Figure 4–7; the affected sisters (two of eight sibs) were the only family members in five generations shown to have this disorder and their daughters did not. It is for this reason that Pendred syndrome is a popular example of a recessively inherited disorder.

Fraser (1976) found that 7.8 percent of congenitally deaf persons in the British isles were products of Pendred syndrome; hence, it is one of the most common forms of congenital deafness. Moreover, Fraser observed that autosomal recessive deafness and thyroid disease could very well appear in the same person and not be Pendred syndrome. This observation is important for primary prevention; a genetic counselor must make this distinction. Vis-a-vis secondary prevention, the goiter is treatable, but the deafness is not curable. Secondary prevention of the

FIGURE 4–7.   Pedigree of a family with Pendred syndrome, as described by Brain (1927)

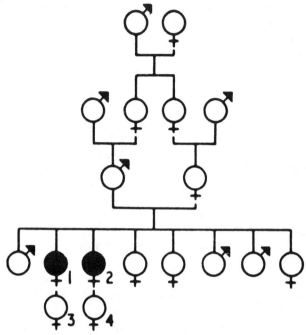

SOURCE: George R. Fraser, *The Causes of Profound Deafness in Childhood* (Baltimore, The Johns Hopkins University Press, 1976), p. 14.

consequences of Pendred syndrome is the same for other inherited hearing disorders: early identification and early intervention.

Prenatally acquired thyroid disease with communicative sequelae need not take the form of cretinism or of Pendred syndrome. Mathog (1973) noted that such thyroid dysfunction may result in deafness, ataxia, and sometimes mental retardation. In addition, anomalies of the thyroid area do occur in such a way that they could conceivably interfere with respiration or phonation. The primordium of the thyroid gland should reach the level of the larynx by the seventh gestational week, and the embryonic thyroglossal duct is obliterated. However, should this duct persist, then thyroglossal duct cysts and/or accessory thyroid tissue may appear (Atkins and Keane 1983). Such a cyst may also become infected and rupture, and must be surgically removed (Karmody 1983). This could become secondary prevention of a voice disorder in a child.

Hyperbilirubinemia   In its 1982 position statement (and in earlier ones as well), the Joint Committee on Infant Hearing cited neonatal *hyperbilirubinemia* as one of the seven relatively common conditions that would put a newborn at risk for the development of communicative disorder. The most common, but by no means the only, preexisting condition that would lead to hyperbilirubinemia of the newborn is Rh incompatibility. Rhesus (Rh) factor incompatibility between mother and fetus may lead to a disorder called *erythroblastosis fetalis*, which is characterized by a pathology known as *kernicterus* and a syndrome distinguished by hearing impairment and neuromotor disturbance. Simply stated, if the Rhesus factor appears in the fetal blood but the mother is Rh–, then an incompatibility arises such that the fetus may receive maternal antibodies to the Rhesus factor. If the antibodies exist in sufficient quantity, then the neonate is subject to this disorder. Deposits of kernicteric material have been found in the inner ear spaces, along the auditory nerve, and throughout the central nervous system.

Northern and Downs (1984) stated the consequences of this disorder most succinctly:

> This condition involves the destruction of Rh positive blood cells of the fetus by maternal antibodies. Complications of Rh incompatibility account for about 3% of profound hearing loss among school age deaf children. Clinical symptoms develop during the immediate neonatal period, and include elevated bilirubin, jaundice, and possible brain damage. Most infants having kernicterus die during the first week with 80% of those surviving having complete or partial deafness. Other common residuals reported include cerebral palsy, mental retardation, epilepsy, aphasia, and behavioral disorders.

Moreover, Gerber (1966) found that *all* of such children who have neuromotor disability also have hearing impairments.

Hyperbilirubinemia of the newborn, when it is due to Rhesus incompatibility, is subject to primary prevention. The drug Rhogam significantly inhibits the production of Rh antibodies in the mother in the immediate postpartum period, and thus she will not produce sufficiently more antibodies in a succeeding pregnancy to harm the baby. If Rhogam is administered following each delivery, the risk is reduced virtually to zero. Secondary prevention may take the form of an exchange transfusion of the baby's blood before or immediately after birth. In fact, "fetal transfusion has become standard therapy" (Harrison, Golbus, and Filly 1984). A more conservative, and probably more usual, method to achieve secondary prevention is with phototherapy. This is a procedure in which the infant is placed under a bank of lights that have the property of causing the excess bilirubin to exude through the skin. This is a very effective technique for those infants who are at somewhat lower risk than for those for whom transfusion would be needed. The incidence of sequelae of Rh incompatibility has dropped 80 percent since 1970 due to these means of primary and secondary prevention.

Acquired Diseases

Everything said so far about prenatal diseases is true of those same diseases when they are acquired postnatally. In addition, there are diseases that cannot be transmitted to an embryo or fetus (e.g., most bacterial infections) but can have serious effects later. The prevalence of postnatally acquired deafness due to infection has dropped from about 24 percent of deaf children in 1951, to about 21 percent in 1963, to some 18 percent by 1970. This figure of 18 percent seems to have remained fairly constant ever since, and the decrease since 1951 reflects the use of immunization. Years ago, the most common causes of acquired deafness in childhood were rubeola (measles) and mumps. Whether via direct viral

FIGURE 4–8. Reported measles incidence, United States, 1950–81

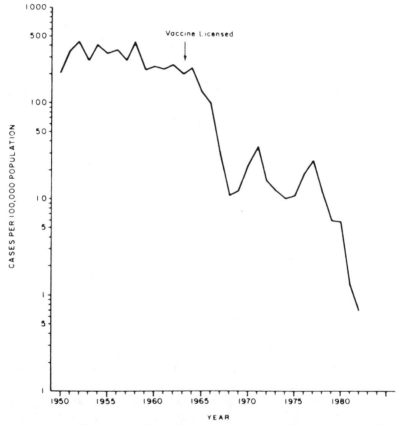

SOURCE: Alan B. Bloch et al., "Epidemiology of Measles and its Complications," in E. M. Gruenberg et al., *Vaccinating against Brain Syndromes: The Campaign against Measles and Rubella* (New York: Oxford University Press, 1986), p. 6.

invasion of the cochlea or by secondary bacterial infection of the ear, measles historically accounted for 3 to 10 percent of cases of deafness (Johnson and Griffin 1986). Today, we vaccinate children against measles and mumps with considerable success (Figure 4–8).

The U.S. Centers for Disease Control (CDC) define pediatric AIDS when the disease appears in children under the age of 13. Clearly, this includes the group discussed earlier of children born to women with AIDS or HIV. One may suppose that all cases of pediatric AIDS, as defined by the CDC, were contracted in utero, as the formal definition of AIDS is that it is a venereal disease and one hopes that venereal diseases are not often contracted by children under 13. The symptoms in such children are the same as those in adults: lymphadenopathy, parotitis, hepatosplenomegaly, interstitial pneumonitis, and Kaposi's sarcoma (Steis and Broder 1985)— and, of course, death. Premortem symptoms, one may note, should be those accompanying CMV, mumps, and respiratory disease; but they are resistant to treatment in the child with AIDS. However, work is being advanced in animal models of AIDS as part of the search for a vaccine (Check 1987).

We have learned some things recently about bacteria which cause meningitis and its sequelae. In a 1987 review, Gerber discovered that *Haemophilus influenzae* (H. flu) continues to be the most common source of bacterial meningitis, but permanent auditory sequelae are far more frequent from *Diplococcus pneumoniae* (Table 4–2). The implications for treatment during the acute phase of the disease could differ, therefore, and it behooves us to be alert to the consequences of neurotoxic and ototoxic drugs. Again, medicine is not given to babies who are well, but we must attend to the possibility that a patient may have a complete or partial recovery from the sequelae of the disease. This alone is secondary prevention.

TABLE 4–2. **Prevalence of Sensory-Neural Hearing Loss Secondary to Bacterial Meningitis**

	Number of Cases	Percent of Cases	Hearing Loss No.	Hearing Loss %
Haemophilus influenza	335	68	25	7
Neisseria meningitides	44	9	3	7
Diplococcus pneumoniae	63	13	15	24
Other or unknown	50	10	4	8

SOURCE: Sanford E. Gerber (1987), "The State of the Art in Pediatric Audiology, " in Sanford E. Gerber and George T. Mencher, eds., *International Perspectives on Communication Disorders.* (Washington, D.C.: Gallaudet University Press, 1987). Reprinted with permission.

INTOXICATION

A toxin is any poisonous or noxious substance; thus, we have already been discussing toxins of certain kinds. In this section, we consider toxins that arise naturally in the environment, are produced by the behavior of the individual, or appear in the practices of the community.

Natural and Environmental Toxins

Viruses and bacteria are naturally occurring toxins. Other natural toxins include those that affect our water or food supply (e.g., some metals), or they may appear from the flora and fauna of the area. Obvious examples of natural toxins from local flora are airborne allergenic substances, and from fauna, toxoplasmosis from cat feces.

Christian (1983) noted three populations at risk from reproductive hazard: males, females (pregnant or not), and conceptuses. She makes the strong point that "the conceptus is at risk from long before birth, and the risk persists long after birth." She listed these risks as follows:

1. "Production of defective cells, cells which have heritable changes (mutagenicity) or changes in normal development.
2. "The normal secretions of either the male or female genital tracts can be changed. Toxic agents may even enter these secretions and possibly affect the conceptus by direct exposure via these secretions.
3. "The pregnant woman is at risk and more vulnerable to toxic agents during gestation. . . . Changes in maternal susceptibility are interrelated to the potential hazard for the conceptus.
4. "Inability to define exact endpoints for anatomical, physiological, and 'behavioral' teratogenic effects reflects the fact that the organ systems of the conceptus continue to develop and grow not only after primary morphological development has occurred but also after birth.
5. "Toxins can alter maternal lactation and the response of the neonate. . . . The milk may be made unpalatable, or it may be toxic."

The volume edited by Christian et al. (1983) considers several classes of toxins: radiation, petroleum and petroleum products, foods and food additives, pharmaceuticals, and drugs. These are discussed in later sections.

Lead and other metals The President's Committee on Mental Retardation has found that 75 percent of the nation's retarded citizens come from poor, urban areas. Some of this retardation occurs because of environmental factors in such places, notably lead poisoning. Yet, too little is known about the prevalence of lead, the costs (both financial and human), and the means to locate sources. It is known that excessive exposure to lead can produce acute and chronic renal system damage, alteration of red blood cells, and damage to a developing brain and nervous system. Brackbill (1987) listed the persistent sequelae of elevated lead levels in children: "a bevy of unwelcome classroom behaviors: distractibility, lack of perseverance, dependence, disorganization, hyperactivity, impulsiveness, day dreaming, and inability to follow directions."

In California, it has been determined that as many as 4 percent of children have elevated blood lead levels; and California is probably one of the better states in that respect. Excessive levels of environmental lead are found where there is older housing (where lead-based paint had been used), where there are industries that emit lead, where there is exhaust of leaded gasoline from heavy automobile and truck traffic, where there are landfills with hazardous waste, and the like. It has been shown that the incidence of congenital malformations diminishes as distance from urban areas increases. Again, this is partly due to housing, but it is also due largely to automobile exhaust. In 1984, 120 million pounds of lead were discharged into the air in the United States. Therefore, the Environmental Protection Agency proposed to reduce the lead content of gasoline from 1.1 grams per gallon to 0.1 by the end of 1986—a goal that was met—and to eliminate lead from gasoline within a few more years.

Vorhees and Mollnow (1987) described the neurotoxic effects of lead, stressing that they are primarily postnatal. They noted that lead encephalopathy has been known since 1839, and that about 80 percent of such patients have permanent neurological damage. The symptom sequence is confusion, seizures, lethargy, vomiting, coma, and death. In survivors, the permanent sequelae are mental retardation and seizures.

Clearly, the consequences of lead neurotoxicity are totally preventable at the primary level. Lead-based paint is no longer in common use, and progress is being made to remove it from older buildings. Good progress has been seen in reducing lead concentrations in automobile exhaust, and attention is directed in many communities to hazardous waste disposal. There is, nevertheless, a continuing hazard: dishware. *Sunset* magazine reported that nearly half of the earthenware containers tested exceeded the lead content limit set by the Food and Drug Administration (Anonymous 1987). Some of these were made in the United States.

Lead is not the only metal that may be teratogenic, however. For example, Padmanabhan (1987) reported cadmium to have produced "fetal death, craniofacial, limb, and skeletal malformations" and "malformations of the external, middle, and inner ear" of experimental animals. He pointed out that cadmium is an environmental pollutant and that "humans are exposed through food, water, beverages, and cigarettes." Needleman (1983) observed that the effects of cadmium are essentially the same as those of lead.

Mercury has long been known to interfere with development of the human embryo; and the "Minimata disaster" resulted in large numbers of retarded children. According to Wilson (1977a), "Metals and related elements have frequently been found to cause malformations, intrauterine resorption and death, and intrauterine growth retardation in laboratory animals." Of course, many metals (e.g., iron) are essential for human survival; the problem is one of excess.

Radiation In Chapter 2, we observed that pregnant women are no longer exposed to X-radiation because of its teratogenicity. Hicks and D'Amato (1978) summarized the risks from ionizing radiation (including X-radiation):

> The public has become much aware, through the press, of the many sources of ionizing radiations and their multiple biological effects, especially in relation to atomic weapons, nuclear reactors, space exploration, and medical irradiation. Ionizing radiations can assure medical diagnosis, cure cancer, and advance science and technology, but in an overexposure or nuclear detonation, it can kill or produce lingering illness. Even small doses from any source may increase the risk of cancer in those exposed, and genetic diseases in their descendents . . . medical exposure of human fetuses to therapeutic doses of radiation caused them to develop small brains and mental deficiency.

The teratogenic nature of ionizing radiation results in mental retardation, the most common of all communicative disorders. Moreover, there is risk to the developing retina, and animal studies have revealed *anophthalmia* when radiation occurs early in somatic development. Also, peculiarities of gait have been known to occur, and rats exposed in the neonatal period seem to suffer deficits in fine motor control.

Finally, although data are, fortunately, scarce, Hicks and D'Amato observed similar results in humans. The example is the long-term consequences to persons exposed in utero to the 1945 bombings of Nagasaki and Hiroshima. The number of retarded adults, assessed 20 years after the intrauterine exposure, greatly exceeds the normal prevalence. In fact, Vorhees and Mollnow (1987), in their review 40 years later, reported it to be *five times* the expected rate. In addition to these extremes, teratogenic risks associated with X-radiation of a pregnant woman include a large increase in the rate of cardiovascular anomalies (Heinonen 1976) and increased incidence of leukemia in the first ten years of life (Laurence 1976). In general, though, the doses of X-radiation to which we are typically exposed (e.g., dental X-rays) are usually not sufficient to be teratogenic.

Petroleum and petroleum products   Today's plastic and mobile world is pervaded by the consequences (beneficial and not so beneficial) of petroleum and petroleum products. We have discussed the progress made toward removing lead from gasoline, but what about the petroleum products themselves? Here we include the menu given by Schreiner (1983):

> A petrochemical is an organic compound for which petroleum or natural gas is the ultimate material. This covers a multitude of compounds, including paraffins, olefins, aromatic hydrocarbons such as benzene, toluene, ethylene and plastics. Ethylene glycol can be considered a petrochemical because petroleum cracking produces ethylene. Synthetic fertilizers can also be petrochemicals.

Schreiner observed further that we are exposed to such substances in the workplace and generally in the environment. Domestic animals and wildlife (which may become food for humans) are similarly exposed.

Most chemical agents that enter the maternal circulation cross the placenta and enter the embryonic or fetal circulation as well. In such a case, it is possible for these substances to disrupt processes of cell differentiation, to interrupt growth, or to cause altered morphogenesis (Hutchings 1978).

Benzene is one of the most common solvents and has been tested frequently. The period of embryonic development when the contact occurs is relevant. In the mouse, it has been shown that early contact with benzene led to cleft palate, micrognathia, and even agnathia; still earlier contact produced embryonic absorption. Humans typically contact benzene by inhalation, but Schreiner observed that few developmental anomalies have been shown to occur in laboratory animals so affected. Those that have appeared have been limited in the main to skeletal malformations. Similarly, styrene (used in the manufacture of many plastic and rubber products) has not been shown to produce a significant number of malformations. On the other hand, acrylonitrile, also used in the production of plastics and certain fibers, has been shown to "interfere with embryonal and fetal development at doses which are not maternally toxic" (Schreiner 1983).

The American Petroleum Institute—which, one might argue, is not a neutral observer—has found no teratogenic effects by inhalations in rats for a rather large number of substances. However, the institute does report decreases in maternal and fetal weight from breathing benzene and that high levels of exposure to shale oil are embryotoxic. Moreover, given the legitimate and continuing concern about petroleum reserves, there is an ongoing search for substitute fuels. One that has great promise is methanol, but methanol is a potent neuropoison. It has been reported to be a behavioral teratogen unaccompanied by overt toxicity (Infurna and Weiss 1986).

What about postnatal risk? Fazen, Lovejoy, and Crone (1986) surveyed 90 patients with acute poisoning. Of those that were accidental, the most frequent (10 percent) were due to ingestion of petroleum distillates. The immediate consequence was aspiration pneumonia, although respiratory system effects were the most common consequences for the majority of poisonings. Furthermore, there have been numerous reports of "glue sniffing" or "gasoline sniffing" among young people. Their fumes contain methanol. Among the 90 cases of acute poisoning reported by Fazen, Lovejoy, and Crone, two were methanol poisoning resulting in retinal hemorrhage and abnormal liver function.

Again, the risk for a teratogenic effect is tied to some kind of genetic predisposition or threshold for the effect. The interaction is likely to be multifactorial, or polygenic. Motulsky (1975) observed: "There seems to be tacit assumption by many observers that many birth defects are caused by drugs or chemical agents. This concept is not proven at all. . . . " Birth defects are polygenic; nevertheless, there are more and more evident teratogens.

Pesticides and other chemicals In Chapter 5, we take up the topic of chemical trauma. Here, we limit our discussion to chemicals as teratogens. Significant among them are the pesticides. Although a federal law requires testing for teratogenicity of pesticides before they go on the market, 60 to 70 percent of those on the market today antedate that law. Thus, the teratogenicity of most commercially available pesticides is unknown. The Department of Food and Agriculture in California listed 200 ingredients used in 717 different pesticides that are likely to be hazardous; 95 percent of them had not been tested by their manufacturers.

Bodmer (1953) listed insecticides that contain selenium as etiologic for conjoined ("Siamese") twins in experimental animals. Guttmacher and Nichols (1967) stated that the agents cited by Bodmer "must be considered as theoretically significant in human embryology." It has been a fact, though, that "presently used pesticides at current use levels have not been shown to increase the risk of human embryotoxicity" (Wilson 1977b). Wilson's comment about herbicides was only slightly less optimistic; he described them as "relatively nonembryotoxic at ordinary use levels. " It is important to note his use of the terms "current use levels" and "ordinary use levels." There has been at least one instance where undiluted herbicide was sprayed onto a school ground, contrary to the manufacturer's instructions.

The medical toxicology branch of California's Department of Food and Agriculture lists 19 pesticide ingredients that have a high priority for assessment because of their teratogenicity and/or mutagenicity; 35 others have a lower priority. This is the result of a primary prevention program. State law (adopted in 1984) requires assessment for all pesticide ingredients registered in California.

Polychlorinated biphenyls (PCBs) and polybrominated biphenyls (PBBs) have been used in paint and other products for some time. Due to their established toxicity, PCBs are no longer in use. PBBs have been used in feed for chickens and cattle, with no evident teratogenicity resulting. PCBs, on the other hand, had gotten into waterways and had been consumed by food fish. Mothers who had been so exposed gave birth to children of somewhat less than normal birth weight and gestation, and there is evidence that these children may be learning disabled (Vorhees and Mollnow 1987).

Foods and food additives Three things are considered here: food, the things we put into food, and nutrition. Certain substances normally found in foods may be toxic to some people. Allergies are the obvious example, but there are others more immediately relevant to the study of communicative disorders. Probably the best known of these is *phenylketonuria*, or PKU.

Phenylalanine is an amino acid naturally found in high-protein foods, including meats and dairy products. PKU is an inherited metabolic error that results in an inability to convert phenylalanine to other amino acids with a natural, normal enzyme; people born with PKU lack this enzyme. If such infants are not treated, they will develop severe mental retardation and serious behavioral consequences. PKU appears in 1 in 10,000 to 20,000 live births, averaging about 1 in 14,000. If, soon after birth, such children are placed on a diet low in phenylalanine, they are healthy and near normal. But, as adults, women with PKU are at high risk for having children with microcephaly, heart disease, and mental retardation (Schultz 1984). Hence, diagnosis of PKU in the newborn nursery is secondary prevention; awareness of the risk of PKU in an affected family may be primary prevention. PKU is discussed further in Chapter 9.

Chemicals added to foods apparently have not had the attention they merit as potential mutagens. Table 4–3 is the list of Malling and Wassom (1977) of food and feed additives "which needed immediate evaluation." Notice that there are only seven of them. One, sodium cyclamate, is no longer employed, and has been replaced largely by aspertame. Many merchants and producers now avoid the use of nitrites in meat; many don't. Caffeine continues to be popular. EDTA, ethylene oxide, and nitrous acid have been shown to produce chromosomal aberrations. This is also true of caffeine, which, in addition, "potentiates activity of other mutagens by inhibiting repair enzymes. . . . " Schardein, in 1976, listed 91 food products, nutrients, and additives that have been shown to be teratogenic in a variety of mammals. These include some

TABLE 4–3. **Food and Feed Additives**

Compound	Use
Nitrous acid	Formed from the food preservative sodium nitrite
Caffeine	Food additive
EDTA	Food additive
Ethylene oxide	Food sterilant
Sodium cyclamate	Artificial sweetener
Sodium bisulfite	Food preservative
Hydroquinone	Food antioxidant

SOURCE: H. V. Malling and J. S. Wassom, "Action of Mutagenic Agents," in James G. Wilson and F. Clarke Fraser, eds., *Handbook of Teratology, Volume I: General Principles and Etiology* (New York: Plenum Press, 1977), p. 141.

quite common substances, such as gelatin, lactose, lysine, potato(!), sucrose, and many others. One must not interpret data from animal studies as being totally applicable to humans. For example, sucrose has produced skeletal defects in rabbits and guinea pigs but not in mice and rats. Again, the appearance of birth defects is multifactorial.

Primary prevention, is, naturally, to avoid using these products, and many people do. It means, more generally, for all of us to maintain basic good health, including consumption of proper diet. Unfortunately, some people have mistakenly believed that proper diet requires large doses of vitamins. Some vitamins are potentially teratogenic: A, B, and D.

Vitamin A hypervitaminosis has been described as a universal teratogen. Rosa, Wilk, and Kelsey, in their 1986 review, observed that *all* analogs of vitamin A are teratogenic in animals. They reported that, by 1986, 45 cases of craniofacial and nervous system anomalies in humans had been reported. Excessive vitamin A has resulted in head and face malformations, digital anomalies, tongue defects, eye abnormalities, and others in several mammalian species. Vitamin A taken during pregnancy seems to offer protection against defect if taken in proper amounts. This vitamin, in the form of retinol, is used as a commercial medicine (Accu-tane) for the treatment of severe acne. Perhaps it should be discussed later as iatrogenic, but the fact is that retinol has been known to cause birth defects in infants of women who use it (Figure 4–9). There is also a little evidence of teratogenicity from excessive use of vitamins B and D.

Clearly, lack of adequate vitamins (hypovitaminosis) is a nutritional issue for prenatal and postnatal development. Schardein (1976) claimed "virtually all vitamin deficiencies studied have teratogenic potential in pregnant animals." Vitamin A hypovitaminosis has resulted in

FIGURE 4–9. Birth defects caused by vitamin A when used in the form of retinol

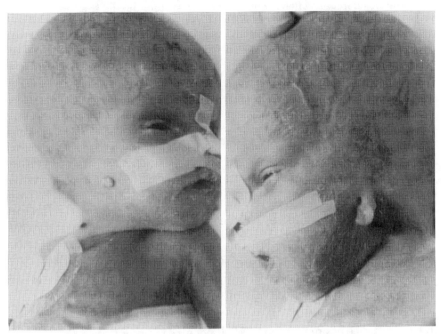

SOURCE: Elizabeth de la Cruz, Shyan Sun, Kamtorn Vangvanichyakorn, and Franklin Desposito, "Multiple Congenital Malformations Associated with Maternal Isoretinoin Therapy," *Pediatrics*, 74 (1984), p. 429. Reprinted by permission.

ocular defects; lack of vitamin B or E, in multiple defects; lack of vitamin C, in muscular defects; lack of vitamin D, in skeletal deformities; and lack of vitamin K, in brain hemorrhage.

In addition to vitamins, nutrients include carbohydrates, proteins, and minerals. Obviously, an essential requirement for normal fetal development is proper placental transfer of nutrients to the fetus (Zamenhof and van Marthens 1978). Iron, for example, is necessary for life; but iron in excess of that found in breast milk may facilitate bacterial infections in neonates. Zamenhof and van Marthens concluded that "environmental, rather than genetic, factors are of primary importance" during the prenatal period. These environmental factors include embryonal and fetal nutrition. "There is no doubt that undernutrition during the brain growth spurt can lead to permanent stunting of body and brain growth" (Leathwood 1978). What are the consequences? An immediate effect of prenatal undernutrition is a diminution of birth weight and the consequent risk of neurological damage. The course is clear.

It begins with nutritional deprivation of the mother, which interferes with the development of the central nervous system during the first trimester of pregnancy, leads to premature birth with low birth weight and ends either with perinatal death or with death from meningitis at later ages (perhaps complicating spina bifida or hydrocephalus) or with survival into adulthood, despite the presence of central nervous system anomalies . . . . chronic malnutrition has no clear effect on fertility, while it almost certainly does have an effect on adult stature, and it is possible that it may affect mental performance. (Stein and Susser 1976)

There is, then, an increased risk of mental retardation and other developmental disabilities in cases of undernutrition and malnutrition. Specifically, it appears that undernutrition of the brain will affect its chemistry as well as cell growth (Hurley 1977).

It is a fact, though, that the effects of undernutrition can often be overcome, at least in part. For one thing, gross undernutrition is customarily accompanied by severe social deprivation, and their effects are not easily separated. Studies of children who were adopted from such environments into those which are socially and nutritionally richer have demonstrated considerable, but not complete, recovery (Rutter 1987).

Undernutrition means, specifically, having too little to eat, so all nutrients are similarly diminished. Malnutrition, however, can exist even in the presence of enough food. We have already mentioned the effects of a lack of iodine (cretinism) and shortages of certain vitamins. In studies of protein-deficient rats, it has been found that certain organ systems were diminished in size or weight and others were enlarged. Of special importance is the decreased kidney weight at birth that may lead to "hormonal inadequacies" throughout life (Hurley 1977). Cerebral weight, number of cerebral cells, and cerebral protein content are decreased in animals bereft of even a single essential amino acid. Prenatal carbohydrate shortages have been shown to have effects on the visual system.

We can make some generalizations about nutrition and therefore about teratogenic effects of undernutrition and malnutrition. First, "the best time to start feeding the baby is prior to conception" (Lugo and Hershey 1979). The best insurance that one would have a healthy baby is the mother's nutritional status during and before the pregnancy. A gravida who has been living on a healthful diet and who continues to do so should have no concerns for her baby for that reason. This is primary prevention of the best kind: Take care of yourself. Statistics have shown that undernutrition occurs most often in women under the age of 20 independent of race or socioeconomic status. This is apparently due to a shortage of iron, especially during menstrual periods. The optimum age range for pregnancy is from 20 to 30 years to ensure healthy mothers and healthy babies.

Fetal Alcohol Syndrome

Alcohol has been omitted thus far from our discussion because it is the most common environmental teratogen and, therefore, stands out among teratogens. Alcohol is the most widely used, and abused, drug in the United States; in 1981, the equivalent of 2.77 gallons of absolute alcohol was sold per person over the age of 14. Fetal alcohol syndrome is a leading cause of birth defects and the third most common cause of mental retardation. It appears in 1.9 per 1,000 live births (Abel and Sokol 1986).

Obviously, children have suffered the consequences of their mothers' alcohol consumption since people began to drink alcohol; and, over many years, there were occasional reports of defective children born to alcoholic mothers. The Bible advises a pregnant woman to "drink no wine or strong drink." The now classic papers on the subject are those of Jones et al. (1973, 1974) that described the association between maternal alcohol ingestion and birth defects. Jones and his colleagues published several papers on the point, especially during the mid-1970s, as they expressed the wish to alert health professionals.

They described a pattern of altered morphogenesis that involved cardiovascular, craniofacial, and limb defects accompanied by prenatal growth deficiency and developmental delay. These morphogenetic features are now considered to be a distinct syndrome widely known as fetal alcohol syndrome (FAS). Remember that a syndrome is a collection of symptoms that appear simultaneously from a single cause. The characteristics of FAS are in three classes: (1) small size (<10th percentile), which persists throughout postnatal development; (2) permanent developmental delay (i.e., microcephaly <3rd percentile) and (usually) other central nervous system involvement; and (3) facial abnormalities (microphthalmia, underdeveloped philtrum, thin upper lip, maxillary hypoplasia).

If all three characteristics appear and if there is evidence of alcohol consumption during the pregnancy, a diagnosis of fetal alcohol syndrome may be made (Figure 4–10). If one or two, but not all three, of the characteristics appear and are associated with maternal alcohol consumption, then the term "Fetal Alcohol Effects" (FAE) is used. The U.S. Centers for Disease Control estimate that FAS appears in 1 in 750 live births and FAE appears in 1 in 125. This means that FAS is among the most common birth defects, and that FAE could well be the most common—hence, their great importance. FAS is among the three leading causes of mental retardation; the others are Down syndrome and neural tube defects.

FAS and FAE are now known to be a common cause of cleft palate; Majewski and Goecke (1982) found clefts of the palate in 7 percent of their

FIGURE 4–10.   Fetal alcohol syndrome at birth

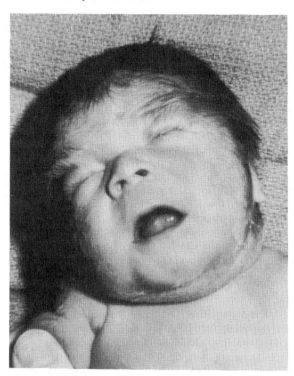

SOURCE: Kenneth L. Jones and David W. Smith, "Recognition of the Fetal Alcohol Syndrome in Early Infancy," *Lancet*, 2 (1973), p. 999. Reprinted by permission.

babies with FAS, and Young (1987) reported palatal clefts in one of eight children with FAS.   Apparently, it rarely leads to cleft lip, however (Melnick, Bixler, and Shields 1980). Clarren and Smith (1978) reported malformations of the ear also; Hanson, Jones, and Smith (1976) considered ear anomalies to be a common feature of FAS.   One investigation (Flint 1983) found that 1.5 percent of deaf babies studied had evidence of FAS, and Young claimed that one-third of babies with FAS had a hearing loss. Church and Gerkin (1988) reported an even greater incidence. They examined 14 children with FAS and found that 13 of them (93 percent) had had recurrent bilateral otitis media and four (29 percent) also had bilateral sensory-neural losses.

Clearly there are at least two major areas of concern for communicative disorders specialists.   One is the language delay (and perhaps dysfunction) accompanying the more general developmental delay of FAS; the other is the incidence of cleft palate and other altered facial features. The incidence of FAS or FAE among infants born with clefts may be as high as 20 or 25 percent. Grundfast (1983) reported a case of a submucous cleft in a child with FAS, and this child had recurrent otitis media both acute and effusive. In our clinic, we have seen an obvious case of FAS with all the features of the Pierre Robin sequence (see Chapter 6). Sparks (1984) claimed that the speech of children with FAS is characterized by problems with articulation and fluency.

Young (1987) listed several possible consequences of drinking when pregnant, which include mental retardation. In fact, fetal alcohol is a major source of retardation. As many as 40 percent of FAS babies suffer heart disease. Young further observed that the incidence of miscarriage or stillbirth increases when a pregnant woman drinks. As many as 50 percent of children born to mothers who drink heavily suffer from FAS; hence, one out of 650 babies born in the United States and Europe suffers from FAS. Furthermore, women who both smoke and drink are four times as likely as women who do neither to have a low-birth-weight infant. The consequences and characteristics of FAS and FAE are summarized in Table 4–4.

It is critical to stress that FAS is *not* limited to children born to mothers with frank alcoholism. Earlier literature on this point (e.g., Wilson 1977a) indicated that "severe chronic alcoholism" is often associated with this pattern of malformations. Although this is true, it is not the whole truth. In fact, a safe minimum level of alcohol consumption by a pregnant woman has never been determined. Thus, most authorities and practitioners advise complete abstinence from all alcoholic beverages during pregnancy. Occasionally one encounters a mother of a child with FAS or FAE who reports drinking "only" beer or wine, as if beer and wine contain no alcohol. Again, there is no known safe amount of alcohol (in any form) that may be consumed during pregnancy (Persaud 1985).

There has been legitimate concern that FAS appears because of its association with smoking and/or malnutrition. Animal studies have failed to establish this connection. When animals have had ethanol (the underlying constituent of alcohol) added to their otherwise adequate diets, they have produced malformed offspring. Women who smoke during pregnancy but who do not drink do have small babies, but these babies catch up; women who drink, whether or not they smoke, have small babies who never catch up. Some infants seem to be drunk at birth; they are irritable, have tremors and sometimes seizures, and apparently undergo withdrawal from ethanol intoxication.

In any case, FAS and FAE do appear in children whose mothers are not alcoholic, who are occasional and social drinkers. No difference has been found in frequency of congenital malformations in children whose mothers consumed more than 40 centiliters (about 1.5 ounces) of wine per day and those whose mothers drank wine in smaller quantities (Kaminski, Rumeau, and Schwartz 1978); the risk is 10 percent for a gravida who consumes no more than 2 ounces of alcohol daily. But there does seem to be a threshold effect: Thirty to 45 percent of infants born to

Table 4-4.   Fetal Alcohol Effects

Principal Fetal Alcohol Effects
  (Seen in More Than 50% of Patients)
Facial Features:
  Short, palpebral fissures
  Short, upturned nose with flat nasal bridge
  Maxillary hypoplasia
  Hypoplastic philtrum with thin upper lip
  Micrognathia or relative prognathia
    due to midface deficiency

Prenatal and Postnatal Growth Deficiency:
  Less than 2 standard deviations below
    mean for both length and weight
  Absence of signficant catch-up growth
  Disproportionately diminished adipose
    tissue

Central Nervous System Dysfunction:
  Microcephaly
  Altered muscle tone, especially hypotonia
    in infancy
  Poor fine and gross motor coordination

Frequent Fetal Alcohol Effects
  (Seen in 26–50% of Patients)
Facial Features:
  Ptosis, strabismus, epicanthal folds
  Posteriorly rotated ears
  Prominent lateral palatine ridges

Malformations:
  Cardiac murmurs, especially septal defects
  Pectus excavatum
  Labial hypoplasia
  Aberrant palmar creases
  Hemangiomas

Occasional Fetal Alcohol Effects
  (Seen in 25% of Patients or Less)
Facial Features:
  Myopia, microphthalmia,
    blepharophimosis
  Altered helical form
  Cleft lip and/or palate
  Small teeth with faulty enamel

Malformations:
  Great-vessel anomalies, tetralogy of Fallot
  Hypospadius, renal anomalies
  Limited joint movements, especially fingers
    and elbows
  Radioulnar synostosis
  Nail hypoplasia, polydactyly
  Pectus carinatum, bifid xiphoid
  Hernias of diaphragm, umbilicus, or groin
  Diastasis recti

SOURCE: Sterling K. Clarren and David W. Smith, "The Fetal Alcohol Syndrome," *New England Journal of Medicine*, 298 (1978), p. 1065. Reprinted by permission.

mothers who consume more than three ounces per day will have overt FAS (Persaud 1985).

FAS and FAE are totally preventable. Alcoholism itself is a treatable disease (secondary prevention), and social drinking can be avoided (primary prevention) (See Figure 4–11).

FIGURE 4–11. Education: primary prevention of FAS and FAE

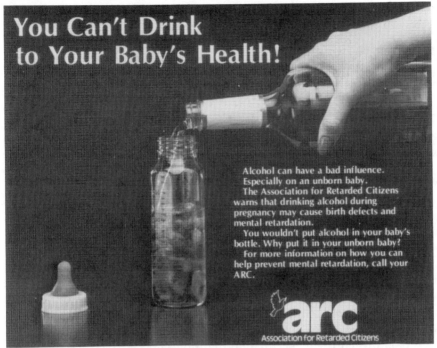

SOURCE: Courtesy of the Association for Retarded Citizens–United States.

How, then, would one prevent FAS and FAE? The answer lies in education, and specifically education of those who have yet to come to childbearing age. This is a most serious matter due to the ever increasing rate of teenage pregnancy. A prevention curriculum for schools beginning in the fourth grade (or even sooner) is expected to reduce the incidence of FAS and all other high-risk conditions. The California Department of Developmental Services reported a steady increase of problem drinkers from the seventh to the twelfth grade (Hickman and California Prevention Task Force 1984). Therefore, education for prevention must begin earlier.

Drugs

Teratogenic drugs fall into two general classes: social (or street) drugs and medicines. Teratogenic medicines are implicitly iatrogenic and, therefore, discussed in the next section.

One of the most commonly used of all social drugs is alcohol. Hence, what was said about prevention of alcohol-related birth defects and appropriate educational programs applies in this section as well. What needs to be covered here are the effects of the more common "recreational" drugs. Schardein (1976) estimated that "1 to 5% of congenital defects in the human are drug-related." But he was including both social and medicinal drugs, and drug use has increased since his writing. Even at that time, he reported that in one New York City hospital in 1972, 1 in every 27 births was heroin addicted!

In general, it seems that social drugs are behavioral teratogens rather than structural pathogens. That is to say, there have been no clearly defined, common morphologic changes associated with prenatal ingestion of any given drug (except alcohol). On the other hand, it is obvious that people who take psychotropic drugs do so because of their effects on the nervous system, and it is reasonable to assume that some of these drugs must have some effect on the baby's developing nervous system. Mothers who are addicted to heroin or methadone give birth to babies who are addicted to heroin or methadone. These infants show signs of narcotic withdrawal at birth, they display hyperirritability for several months after birth, and may be hyperactive until at least the age of three (Hoar 1983). Persaud (1985) reviewed the effects of cannabis (i.e., marijuana). These included embryonic death; among survivors, there were behavioral disturbances like those indicated for heroin. Infants prenatally addicted to marijuana display the symptoms of narcotic withdrawal (Fried et al. 1987)

It is difficult—in fact, it may be impossible—to assess the direct effect of any one drug on the children of a woman who uses it. Most such mothers "smoke cigarettes, drink alcohol, use more than one illicit drug, eat poor diets, live near or below the poverty level, and receive poor medical care before and after giving birth" (Young 1987). Hence, we need to rely on animal studies in the main, and one cannot always and/or easily interpret animal research data onto a human population. For example, marijuana has been shown to be teratogenic to the nervous system, the liver, and limbs in an assortment of mammals; the evidence with respect to humans is not complete. Young said that there is no "absolute evidence."

The better evidence in regard to marijuana use is that these babies are born too soon and too small with all the risks attendant upon preterm birth. Studies on human populations (summarized by Brown and Fishman 1984) have indicated that marijuana is a behavioral teratogen, at least early in life. Babies born to women who consider themselves heavy users of marijuana had diminished light responsiveness and a relatively high incidence of tremors with failed habituation of startle responses, and are said to have a cry reminiscent of the cri-du-chat syndrome. Even after infancy, these infants' visual behavior was noticeably different from controls.

The data on cocaine use are not complete. Young (1987) reported that cocaine use in a gravida increases the risk of perinatal mortality. Madden, Payne, and Miller (1986) described eight babies born to mothers who abused cocaine; no significant defects were found. However, they did stress that these data were early and on only eight babies. A study of 18 babies born to women who had abused cocaine revealed abnormalities of the auditory brainstem response suggestive of neurologic impairment (Shih, Cone-Wesson, and Reddix 1988). It has been reported that cocaine accounts for more than 60 percent of drug-addicted babies exclusive of the nearly 40 percent who abort spontaneously. These babies show signs of prenatal brain oxygen deprivation. There is also a report of an infant born to a mother who abused both cocaine and alcohol during pregnancy. The baby was evidently born normal, but was admitted to a hospital emergency room at two weeks of age suffering cocaine intoxication from breast milk (Chasnoff, Lewis, and Squires 1987).

There are more data on humans with other drugs. For example, PCP (phenylcyclidine or angel dust) has been demonstrated to cross the placenta to reach the fetus. Although the cause and effect relationship between PCP and birth defects is not clearly established, it is certain that users of PCP give birth to sick babies with poor attention skills and decreased reflexes. LSD (lysergic acid diethylamide) has been known to produce limb and eye malformations.

There are medications that would be iatrogenic if they were given by physicians, but people take them without prescription and in excessive doses as psychoactive drugs. These include, especially, the *uppers* (amphetamines) and the *downers* (barbiturates). Amphetamines increase the risk of low birth weight, and these infants seem prone to emotional disturbances. There may also be increased risk of lip and palate clefts. Long-term behavioral problems have been associated with barbiturates taken during pregnancy and it may be that this is due to prenatal death of brain cells.

As is the case with alcohol, primary prevention may be characterized by one word: don't. This is not as simple as it sounds, of course, for some users. Those who pretend that the drug taking is a form of recreation may be able to stop. Those who are genuinely addicted—whether the addiction is psychological or physiological—are another problem; in fact, they constitute a major social predicament. Not only do they endanger their own health and well-being but also that of the next generation. Moreover, addicted parents are high-risk parents; they are no more able to cope with a baby's problems than with their own.

In our clinic, we have seen the heroin-addicted infant born to a heroin-addicted daughter of a heroin addict. Public authorities have been reluctant to intervene in such a family, although we would agree that they should do so and do so vigorously. Moreover, such a family is likely to be resistant to secondary prevention. Secondary prevention is found in the fact that drug-addicted newborns, if treated, do seem to become more nearly normal past the time of early infancy. But this family would, and probably did, treat the baby's normal crying and fussiness with heroin. There is no secondary prevention except that, in some communities, these infants are removed from parental care and placed in foster homes with trained care givers.

What about smoking? According to Young (1987), the potential consequences of smoking during pregnancy can include Sudden Infant Death Syndrome (SIDS), increased risk of *abruptio placentae* (premature separation of the placenta from the uterus wall), and/or increased chances of *placenta previa* (attachment of the placenta too low in the uterus). There is also increased risk of intrauterine growth retardation, and consequently a premature or low-birth-weight baby, and also slowed growth in infancy and childhood. Physical and mental defects, learning disabilities, and behavior problems have been reported.

It is distressing that as many as 30 percent of women smoke during pregancy. Intrauterine growth retardation, with its consequence of small and early babies, may be universal (see, e.g., Table 4–5). Again, small babies are at risk for learning disabilities, including mental retardation. No, filters and so-called low nicotine cigarettes do not reduce the risk because they do not reduce carbon monoxide intake, and it is carbon monoxide that interferes with oxygen transfer to the baby. Prenatal cigarette exposure has been shown to be associated with "hypertonicity and increased nervous system excitation"at 30 days postpartum (Fried et al. 1987).

TABLE 4–5. Correlation Matrix: Birth Weight, Prepregnant Weight, Weight at Final Clinic Visit, Length of Gestation, and Number of Cigarettes per Day Smoked at Registration (n = 221)

	Prepregnant Weight	Final Weight	Gestation	No. Cigarettes per Day
Birth weight	0.16	0.38	0.39	− 0.21
Prepregnant weight		0.73	0.12	0.11
Final weight			0.19	0.08
Length of gestation				− 0.09
$p < 0.05$ if $r > 0.13$				
$p < 0.01$ if $r > 0.17$				

SOURCE: David Rush, "Cigarette Smoking during Pregnancy: The Relationship with Depressed Weight Gain and Birth weight," in Kelly et al., eds., *Birth Defects, Risks and Consequences* (New York: Academic Press, 1976), p. 162.

The conclusion is simple: Smoking during pregnancy is the most common cause of low birth weight (such babies average >200 g less than babies of nonsmoking mothers). Low birth weight is the most common cause of learning disabilities, including mental retardation, and mental retardation is the most common communicative disorder. Smoking accounts for at least 20 percent of low birth weight infants born in the United States. The effects of smoking during pregnancy have been documented to include long-term sequelae such as impaired neurological and intellectual development, including minimal brain dysfunction and abnormal ECGs; growth retardation at least up to age 11; measurable emotional, behavioral, and intellectual deficits; abnormal infant behavior patterns; and hyperkinesis (Klingberg et al. 1984).

So: don't smoke. That is primary prevention. Secondary prevention is don't teach your children to smoke (Figure 4–12).

FIGURE 4–12. Primary prevention: Don't teach your children to smoke

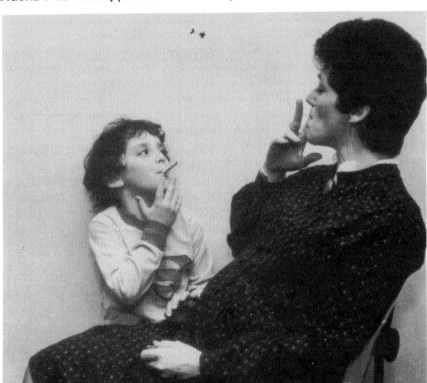

SOURCE: Jim Anderson/Stock, Boston.

IATROGENS

Iatrogens are medicines, prescription drugs, or other medical treatments that have unwanted effects. The word *iatrogenic* means "physician caused." Those of us in the communication sciences are too familiar with ototoxic drugs, medications that cause deafness. That is not quite the point here. This chapter deals with teratogens, substances that cause birth defects. Therefore, we now turn our attention to things that physicians may have to do but that have a high risk of affecting the unborn. It must be understood that there are very few teratogenic iatrogens, for the obvious reason that they don't get used. Sometimes, though, the teratogenic risk is unknown or exclusion of the drug is not feasible. As Young (1987) observed:

> Some medications are clearly necessary during pregnancy. They may be needed to protect or save the life of the mother, or to prevent damage or death to the fetus . . . the physician must weigh . . . the potential benefits of the drug treatment for the mother versus the possible risks to her unborn child.

Some medications are proven to be teratogenic; the classic example, as we all know, was *thalidomide*. This drug was popular during the '50s and early '60s as a treatment for the morning sickness which often accompanies early pregnancy, but it was never in widespread use in the United States. This is also the prime example of our occasional inability to predict human effects from animal studies: Thalidomide was not shown to be teratogenic in animals.[1] In humans, however, it was later found that the teratogen was a metabolite of the mother that breaks down this drug. Thalidomide babies typically have no arms, often have no legs, and are frequently deaf (Figure 4–13).

As specialists in communicative disorders, we must be concerned with iatrogens that may produce them. Although we are familiar with ototoxic drugs, it happens that the majority of them are not teratogenic. That is, those medications that could produce deafness in you or me usually do not deafen the unborn. There are two important exceptions, however: quinine and streptomycin. According to Schardein (1976), quinine had been reported to be teratogenic for many years, and half of these births were deaf due to hypoplasia of the auditory nerve. They also had other birth defects, including limb malformations, visual defects, and hypoplasia of other nerves. He also reported that 11 percent of births to mothers who took streptomycin or dihydrostreptomycin in pregnancy were hearing impaired. In fact, he concluded "The known ototoxicity associated with these drugs when they are administered after birth should serve to demonstrate that they have potential prenatal effects as well." We should take that as a warning.

---

[1]The opposite has occurred too: Cortisone is very teratogenic in rodents, but not in humans.

FIGURE 4–13. Thalidomide babies

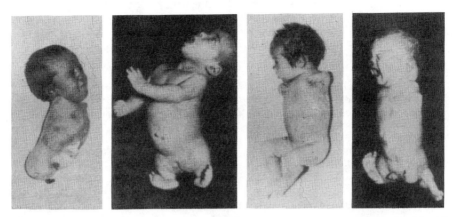

SOURCE: H. B. Taussig, "A Study of the German Outbreak of Phocomelia: The Thalidomide Syndrome," *American Medical Association Journal,* 180 (1962), p. 1110.

Of more frequent concern are those drugs that produce facial malformations. We have already discussed alcohol. Prime among the drugs that can lead to facial dysmorphogenesis are the anticonvulsants. It appears, in fact, that there may be a distinct syndrome consisting of facial clefts and cardiac defects among such infants. It is essential, of course, to ascertain if it is the drug and not the disease that produces the defects.   Lowe (1973) found that 6.7 percent of the infants born to mothers who took anticonvulsants during the first trimester were malformed, whereas only 2.7 percent of the infants born to epileptic mothers who did not take medication were so affected. Also, Wilson (1974) gave anticonvulsant drugs to pregnant monkeys that did not have a seizure disorder, and reported that "several" of them were defective.

Most common among the anticonvulsants are the hydantoins, particularly dilantin. In fact, Smith (1982) used the term "fetal dilantin syndrome" to describe a complex of growth deficiency, borderline to mild mental deficiency, craniofacial alterations, including cleft lip and palate, hypoplasia of digits and nails, and occasional other skeletal anomalies. These effects are summarized in Table 4–6 (Hill et al. 1974). It is clear, therefore, that such children will present with a risk of both language disorder and the possibility of phonologic dysfunction.   There is no evident reason why their treatment should be different from that done for other children with clefts and/or delayed development, but primary prevention may take the form of changing the mother's medication.

Hydantoins are not the only anticonvulsants used. Among the more common ones is phenobarbitol (see the previous discussion of the teratogenic effects of barbiturate abuse). However, phenobarbitol in clinical doses does not seem to produce structural defects. It may be a behavioral

TABLE 4–6   Congenital Malformations Occurring in 1,653 Infants Born to Women Who Received Anticonvulsants During Pregnancy

Malformation	Incidence (%)
Cleft lip, cleft palate, or both	3.8
Skeletal anomalies	1.9
Congenital heart disease	1.7
CNS malformations	1.3
Facial or ear anomalies	1.3
Gastrointestinal malformations	0.9
Mental retardation	0.8
Genitourinary malformations	0.8
Intrauterine growth retardation	0.2

SOURCE: R. M. Hill et al., "Infants Exposed *in Utero* to Antileptic Drugs: A Prospective Study," *American Journal of Diseases of Children*, 127 (1974), p. 651.

teratogen, however. Schardein (1976) claimed that it has an "addiction liability." In postnatal life, phenobarbitol has been shown to have unfavorable behavioral consequences that do not appear in children taking valproic acid, another common anticonvulsant and one that is equally effective in preventing seizures (Vining et al. 1987). However, valproic acid has been implicated as a teratogen in the production of *spina bifida* (Bjerkedal et al. 1982; Robert and Gulbaud 1982).

Anticoagulants, also, have been known to lead to facial deformities. Among these, warfarin has produced nasal hypoplasia and optic atrophy. Mental deficiency has also appeared.

Another area to be considered in certain circumstances is anesthesia. Pregnant women do have dental work, sometimes come to surgery for reasons unrelated to the pregnancy, and sometimes (as physicians, nurses, or other health workers) are exposed to anesthetic gases. A wisely cautious conclusion was stated by Harrison, Golbus, and Filly (1984) to the effect that there are too few data "to support a categorical statement that anesthetic agents are not teratogenic."

In summary, we find that many medications are neurotoxic, even if behavioral teratogens and not necessarily structural teratogens. Learning disabilities, language dysfunctions, attention deficit disorders, and the like have been found in babies born to mothers who had had certain essential iatrogens. As communication clinicians, it behooves us to be aware of such phenomena and to plan treatment strategies accordingly. These disorders are not solely behavioral. Moreover, primary prevention may not be possible; the drug may be life-sustaining for the mother (e.g., those with cardiovascular disease). Secondary prevention, then, arises from our awareness of the potential iatrogen.

CONCLUSION

This chapter has discussed many, but by no means most, of the teratogens in our environment and their effects. In summary:

> Drugs . . . at any stage of gestation may induce teratogenic effects that are detected at birth or later. To produce a defect, the drug must be given to a genetically susceptible individual during a particular developmental stage of gestation and must cross the placenta to achieve embryonic or fetal concentrations of appropriate dosage. Each organ and each system undergoes a critical stage of differentiation during which vulnerability to teratogens is greatest and specific malformations can be produced. In humans, the first trimester appears to be the most vulnerable period. (Harrison, Golbus, and Filly 1984).

There are several essential points in that summary: (1) The individual must be genetically susceptible; as before, birth defects are polygenic. (2) The drug must cross the placenta in sufficient dose to have an effect. (3) Critical and vulnerable periods interact with the appearance of particular defects.

What, then, about prevention? Primary prevention of many, probably most, teratogens is available. Natural teratogens, the viruses and bacteria, are becoming vulnerable to inoculation in ever increasing number. Smallpox has disappeared; polio is going; rubella has been greatly reduced, as have measles and mumps. Sexually transmitted diseases can be prevented by intelligent sexual behavior. Social drugs can be avoided if one chooses to do so, and this choice arises (one hopes) from education. Even iatrogens can be manipulated; a prescription can be changed. We can usually avoid radiation hazards and environmental metals, and we can assist our communities in ridding themselves of such teratogens.

Many teratogens are also mutagenic. This means that persons who are born with a given malformation have a risk of passing on that disorder to their offspring. Their knowledge of that fact can be primary or secondary prevention. They may choose not to reproduce, and thereby eliminate that particular mutagenic effect from their family line; or they may alert primary care providers to the need for secondary prevention, early identification.

Secondary prevention efforts arise from knowing that a risk of teratogenicity exists. We should be prepared to test the hearing of neonates if we know of prenatal viral disease or other maternal conditions (e.g., diabetes) that may put a newborn at risk. We should be alert to minor alterations of facial structure, and look for submucous clefts, for example. We want to know if the Apgar score is low enough for concern and fails to rise with sufficient haste.

In short, primary and secondary prevention are possible to minimize teratogenic effects. Programs to do so are the substance of Chapter 9.

GLOSSARY

abruptio placentae: premature detachment of a normally situated placenta.

anophthalmia: congenital absence of one or both eyes.

bacteria, bacterium: microscopic, unicellular organisms at the lower limit of an optical microscope and responsible for a number of serious diseases, including tuberculosis and syphilis.

candida albicans: a yeast like organism often producing infection of the oropharynx, vagina, or gastrointestinal tract and sometimes leading to pneumonia or meningitis.

chlamydia: a bacterium commonly implicated in trachoma or conjunctivitis and often leading to blindness if untreated; it is a common venereal disease.

cytomegalovirus: a group of herpes viruses commonly infecting humans and other animals; it has been identified as the most common viral cause of mental retardation and as a common cause of congenital progressive hearing impairment.

diplococcus pneumoniae: the *Streptococcus pneumoniae* or pneumococcus bacterium of which there are 32 types, one of which accounts for 40 to 60 percent of cases of pneumonia; often implicated in meningitis deafness.

erythrobastosis fetalis: a grave hemolytic disease of the newborn that usually results from development of antibodies to the Rh (rhesus) factor in a mother carrying an Rh+ fetus.

escherichia coli (E. coli): a bacterium that appears normally in the intestines of humans and other vertebrates; it is a frequent cause of infection in newborns.

exogenous: originating or produced from outside an organism.

goiter: a chronic enlargement of the thyroid gland that occurs endemically in some communities but may appear as a sporadic genetic trait.

gravida: a pregnant woman.

haemophilus influenzae: the influenza bacillus, also called Pfeiffer's bacillus or Kotch-Weeks bacillus; it causes acute respiratory infections leading to purulent meningitis in children and, hence, a major cause of neurosensory and/or neuromotor impairments.

hyaline membrane disease: a condition that appears in preterm neonates with respiratory distress associated with reduced amounts of lung surfactant.

hyperbilirubinemia: the presence of a large amount of bilirubin in the blood that results in clinically apparent jaundice at sufficiently high concentrations.

iatrogen(ic): an abnomal state or condition produced by a physician by inadvertent or erroneous treatment; sometimes an unavoidable negative by-product of medical procedures.

in utero: not yet born; i.e., within the womb.

kernicterus: a grave form of jaundice (i.e., icterus) of the newborn that may lead to neurosensory and/or neuromotor disability.

mutagen(ic): any agent that causes a mutation, an alteration of a genotype.

phenylketonuria: also known as Folling disease, a deficiency of phenylalanine metabolism such that it results in brain damage characterized by mental retardation, often with seizures and other neurologic abnormalities; it is transmitted as an autosomal recessive trait.

placenta previa: a condition in which the placenta implants in the lower segment of the uterus extending sometimes as far down as the cervix.

protozoa: an animal phylum including all unicellular forms (e.g., the syphilis spirochete).

rubella: the German or three-day measles caused by an RNA virus and marked by enlargement of lymph nodes but usually without fever or other reaction; it is distinguished by the high incidence of abnormalities that results.

spina bifida: a defect in which the spinal cord forms in a way such that it bulges out in a sac; children with this disorder lack muscle control and sensation below the level of the defect and may also show hydrocephalus and mental retardation.

staphylococcus aureus: a common bacterium found on skin and nasal mucosa; it is often found in suppurative wounds.

staphylococcus pyogenes albus: a name formerly applied to organisms now known to be mutants of *Staphylococcus aureus.*

streptococcus agalactiae: a bacterium found in milk and associated with a variety of infections in humans, especially those of the urogenital tract.

teratogen(ic): any drug or other agent that causes abnormal development.

thalidomide: a tranquilizing drug that, if taken early in pregnancy, may cause infants to be born with defective or incomplete development of limbs; sometimes associated with deafness.

toxoplasma gondii: small protozoan parasites that may multiply in host tissue resulting in bursting of the host cells.

treponema pallidum: the organism that causes syphilis.

trichomonas: a genus of protozoa found as parasites in the mouth, the intestinal tract, or the urogenital tract of humans; may appear as infection in a gravida.

virus: a group of microscopic organisms that, with few exceptions, can pass through filters that retain bacteria; they are incapable of growth or reproduction outside living cells.

yaws: an infectious tropical disease caused by *Treponema pertenue*; similar to syphilis but does not have its effects on the central nervous system and the cardiovascular system; it is characterized by ulcers on the extremities and it may involve bone.

REFERENCES

ABEL, E. L., AND R. J. SOKOL. 1986. "Fetal Alcohol Syndrome is Now Leading Cause of Mental Retardation," *Lancet*, 2, 1222.

ALFORD, CHARLES A., SERGIO STAGNO, AND ROBERT F. PASS. 1980. "Natural History of Perinatal Cytomegaloviral Infection," in *Perinatal Infections*, ed. Katherine Elliot, Maeve O'Connor, and Julie Whelan. Amsterdam: Excerpta Medica.

AMERICAN ACADEMY OF PEDIATRICS, TASK FORCE ON PEDIATRIC AIDS. 1988. "Policy Statement: Perinatal HIV Infection (AIDS)," *AAP News*, 4 (9), 6–7.

AMMANN, ARTHUR J. 1983. "Is There an Acquired Immune Deficiency Syndrome in Infants and Children?" *Peds.*, 72, 430–32.

ANDERSEN, RICHARD D., et al. 1986. *Infections in Children*. Rockville, MD: Aspen.

ANONYMOUS. 1987. "Still Some Serious Questions About Lead in Pottery," *Sunset*, July, 168.

ANTHONY, B. F., AND D. M. OKADA. 1977. "The Emergence of Group B Streptococci in Infections of the Newborn Infant," *Ann. Rev. Med.*, 28, 355–69.

ARBETER, ALLAN M., et al. 1986. "Combination Measles, Mumps, Rubella, and Varicella Vaccine," *Peds.*, 78, Suppl. 742–47.

ASSALI, N. S. 1972. *Pathophysiology of Gestation*, vol. II. New York: Academic Press.

ATKINS, JOSEPH P., AND WILLIAM M. KEANE. 1983. "Embryology and Anatomy," in *Pediatric Otolaryngology*, vol. II, ed. Charles D. Bluestone and Sylvan E. Stool. Philadelphia: Saunders.

BALDURSSON, GYLFI, et al. 1972. "Maternal Rubella in Iceland 1963–1964," *Scand. Audiol.*, 1, 3–10.

BARR, BENGT. 1982. "Teratogenic Hearing Loss," *Audiol.*, 21, 111–27.

BJERKEDAL, T., et al. 1982. "Maternal Valproic Acid and Spina Bifida," *Lancet*, 2, 1096.

BLACK, FRANKLIN O., LAVONNE BERGSTROM, MARION DOWNS, AND WILLIAM HEMENWAY. 1971. *Congenital Deafness*. Boulder, CO: Colorado Associated University Press.

BLACKMAN, JAMES A. 1984a. "Congenital Infections," in *Medical Aspects of Developmental Disabilities in Children Birth to Three*, ed. James A. Blackman. Rockville, MD: Aspen.

———1984b. "Perinatal Injury," in *Medical Aspects of Developmental Disabilities in Children Birth to Three*, ed. James A. Blackman. Rockville, MD: Aspen.

BLOCH, ALAN B., et al. 1986. "Epidemiology of Measles and Its Complications," in *Vaccinating Against Brain Syndromes*, ed. Ernest M. Gruenberg, Carol Lewis, and Stephen E. Goldston. New York: Oxford University Press.

BODMER, H. C. 1953. "Delivery of Thoracopagus Twins," *J. Mich. Med. Soc.*, 152, 200.

BORDLEY, JOHN E., et al. 1967. "Observations on the Effect of Prenatal Rubella in Hearing," in *Deafness in Childhood*, ed. Freeman McConnell and Paul H. Ward. Nashville, TN: Vanderbilt University Press.

BRACKBILL, YVONNE. 1987. "Behavioral Teratology Comes to the Classroom," *Topics in Early Childhood Special Education*, 6, 33–48.

BRAIN, W. R. 1927. "Heredity in Simple Goitre," *Quart. J. Med.*, 20, 303.

BROWN, ROGER M., AND RACHELLE H. B. FISHMAN. 1984. "An Overview and Summary of the Behavioral and Neural Consequences of Perinatal Exposure to Psychotropic Drugs," in *Neurobehavioral Teratology*, ed. Joseph Yania. Amsterdam: Elsevier Science.

CHASNOFF, IRA J, DOUGLES E. LEWIS, AND LIZA SQUIRES. 1987. "Cocaine Intoxication in a Breast-Fed Infant," *Peds.*, 80, 836–838.

CHECK, WILLIAM. 1987. "Nonhuman Primates Serve as Subjects in AIDS Research," *Research Resources Reporter*, 11, No. 7 (July), 13–18.

CHESS, STELLA. 1971. "Autism in Children with Congenital Rubella," *J. Autism Child. Schiz.*, 1, 33–47.

———1977. "Follow-up Report on Autism in Congenital Rubella," *J. Autism Child. Schiz.*, 7, 69–81.

———AND PAULINE FERNANDEZ. 1980. "Neurologic Damage and Behavior Disorder in Rubella Children," *Amer. Ann. Deaf*, 125, 998–1001.

CHRISTIAN, MILDRED S. 1983. "Statement of Problem," in *Advances in Modern Environmental Toxicology*, vol. III: *Assessment of Reproductive and Teratogenic Hazards*, ed. Mildred S. Christian et al. Princeton, NJ: Princeton Scientific Publishers.

———et al. 1983. *Advances in Modern Environmental Toxicology*, vol. III, *Assessment of Reproductive and Teratogenic Hazards*. ed. Mildred S. Christian et al. Princeton, NJ: Princeton Scientific Publishers.

CHURCH, M. W., AND K. P. GERKIN. 1988. "Hearing Disorders in Children with Fetal Alcohol Syndrome: Findings from Case Reports," *Peds.*, 82, 147–154.

CLARREN, STERLING K., AND DAVID W. SMITH. 1978. "The Fetal Alcohol Syndrome," *N. Engl. J. Med.*, 298, 1063–67.

COHN, ARNOLD. 1981. "Etiology and Pathology of Disorders Affecting Hearing," in *Medical Audiology*, ed. Frederick N.Martin. Englewood Cliffs, NJ: Prentice-Hall.

CORNBLATH, MARVIN AND ROBERT SCHWARTZ. 1966. "Infant of the Diabetic Mother," in *Disorders of Carbohydrate Metabolism in Infancy*, Vol. III, ed. Marvin Cornblath and Robert Schwartz. Philadephia: Saunders.

DAHLE, ARTHUR J., et al. 1974. "Subclinical Congenital Cytomegalovirus Infection and Hearing Impairment," *J. Speech Hear. Dis.*, 39, 320–29.

———AND FAYE P. MCCOLLISTER. 1988. "Audiological Findings in Children with Neonatal Herpes," *Ear and Hearing*, 9, 256–58.

DAVIS, LARRY E., et al. 1979. "Cytomegalovirus Isolation from a Human Inner Ear," *Ann. Otol., Rhinol., Laryngol.*, 88 424–26.

DE LA CRUZ, ELIZABETH, SHYAN SUN, KAMTORN VANGVANICHYAKORN, AND FRANKIN DESPOSITO. 1984. "Multiple Congenital Malformations Associated with Maternal Isotretinoin Therapy," *Peds.*, 74, 428–430.

DUBLIN, WILLIAM B. 1976. *Fundamentals of Sensorineural Auditory Pathology*. Springfield, IL: Chas. C Thomas.

EPSTEIN LEON G., et al. 1986. "Manifestations of Human Immunodeficiency Virus Infection in Children," *Peds.*, 78, 678–87.

FAZEN, LOUIS E., III, FREDERICK H. LOVEJOY, JR., AND ROBERT K. CRONE. 1986. "Acute Poisoning in a Children's Hospital: A 2-Year Experience," *Peds.*, 77, 144–51.

FISCHLER, RONALD S. 1985. "The Pediatrician's Role in Early Identification," in *Hearing-Impaired Children and Youth with Developmental Disabilities*, ed. Evelyn Cherow. Washington, DC: Gallaudet College Press.

FISHER, DELBERT A., AND GERARD N. BURROW, eds. 1975. *Perinatal Thyroid Physiology and Disease*. New York: Raven Press.

FLINT, EWEN F. 1983. "Severe Childhood Deafness in Glasgow," *J. Laryngol. Otol.*, 97, 421–25.

FLOWER, WILDA M., AND C. DANIEL SOOY. 1987. "AIDS: An Introduction for Speech-Language Pathologists and Audiologists," *Asha*, 29 (11), 25–30.

FRASER, GEROGE R. 1976. *The Causes of Profound Deafness in Childhood*. Baltimore: Johns Hopkins University Press.

FRIED, PETER A. et al. 1987. "Neonatal Neurological Status in a Low-Risk Population after Prenatal Exposure to Cigarettes, Marijuana, and Alcohol," *J. Dev. Beh. Peds.*, 8, 318–26.

GERBER, SANFORD E., 1966. "Cerebral Palsy and Hearing Loss," *Cerebral Palsy J.*, 6, 6–7.

———1987. "The State of the Art in Pediatric Audiology," in *International Perspectives on Human Communication Disorders,* ed. Sanford E. Gerber and George T. Mencher. Washington, DC: Gallaudet University Press.

———MAURICE I. MENDEL, AND MONICA GOLLER. 1979. "Progressive Hearing Loss Subsequent to Congenital Cytomegalovirus Infection," *Human Comm.*, 4, 231–34.

GOLDSTEIN, ARTHUR I., et al. 1978. "Perinatal Outcome in the Diabetic Pregnancy," *J. Reproductive Med.*, 20, 61–6.

GREGG, N. M. 1941. "Congenital Cataract Following German Measles in the Mother," *Trans. Ophth. Soc.* (Austral.), 3, 35–46.

GRUNDFAST, KENNETH M. 1983. "The Role of the Audiologist and Otologist in the Identification of the Dysmorphic Child," *Ear and Hearing,* 4, 24–30.

GUTTMACHER, A. F., AND B. L. NICHOLS. 1967. "Teratology of Conjoined Twins," *Birth Defects Original Article Series,* 3, 3–9.

HANSHAW, JAMES B. 1980. "Perinatal Infections: Prevention of Long-Term Sequelae," in *Perinatal Infections,* ed. Katherine Elliot, Maeve O'Connor, and Julie Whelan. Amsterdam: Excerpta Medica.

HANSON, JAMES W., KENNETH L. JONES, AND DAVID W. SMITH. 1976. "Fetal Alcohol Syndrome: Experience with 41 Patients," *J. Amer. Med. Assn.*, 235, 1458–60.

HARRIS, STEN, et al. 1984. "Congenital Cytomegalovirus Infection and Sensorineural Hearing Loss," *Ear and Hearing,* 5, 352–55.

HARRISON, MICHAEL R., MITCHELL S. GOLBUS, AND ROY A. FILLY. 1984. *The Unborn Patient.* Orlando, FL: Grune & Stratton.

HEINONEN, OLLI P. 1976. "Risk Factors for Congenital Heart Disease," in *Birth Defects: Risks and Consequences,* ed. Sally Kelly et al. New York: Academic Press.

HEMENWAY, W. GARTH, ISAMU SANDO, AND D. McCHESNEY. 1969. "Temporal Bone Pathology Following Maternal Rubella," *Arch. Klin. Exp. Ohren-, Nasen-, Kehlk. Heilk.*, 193, 287–300.

HETZEL, BASIL S. 1972. "Similarities and Differences between Sporadic and Endemic Cretinism," in *Human Development and the Thyroid Gland (Relation to Endemic Cretinism),* ed. John Stanbury and Robert L. Kroc. New York: Plenum Press.

HICKMAN, MARY LU, AND CALIFORNIA PREVENTION TASK FORCE. 1984. *Prevention 1990: California's Future.* Sacramento: California Health and Welfare Agency, Department of Developmental Services.

HICKS, SAMUEL P., AND CONSTANCE J. D'AMATO. 1978. "Effects of Ionizing Radiation on Developing Brain and Behavior," in *Studies on the Development of Behavior and the Nervous System,* vol. 4: *Early Influences,* ed. Gilbert Gottlieb. New York: Academic Press.

HILL, R. M., et al. 1974. "Infants Exposed *in Utero* to Antiepileptic Drugs: A Prospective Study," *Am. J. Dis. Child.,* 127, 645–53.

HOAR, RICHARD M. 1983. "Pharmaceuticals, Drugs and Birth Defects," in *Advances in Modern Environmental Toxicology,* vol. III: *Assessment of Reproductive and Teratogenic Hazards,* ed. Mildred S. Christian et al. Princeton, NJ: Princeton Scientific Publishers.

HOGNESTAD, S. 1967. "Hereditary Nerve Deafness Associated with Diabetes," *Acta Oto-Laryngol.*, 64, 219–25.

HURLEY, LUCILLE S. 1977. "Nutritional Deficiencies and Excesses," in *Handbook of Teratology,* vol. 1, *General Principles and Etiology,* ed. James G. Wilson and F. Clarke Fraser. New York: Plenum Press.

HUTCHINGS, DONALD E. 1978. "Behavioral Teratology: Embryopathic and Behavioral Effects of Drugs during Preganancy," in *Studies on the Development of Behavior and the Nervous System,* vol. 4: *Early Influences,* ed. Gilbert Gottlieb. New York: Academic Press.

INFURNA, ROBERT, AND BERNARD WEISS. 1986. "Neonatal Behavioral Toxicity in Rats Following Prenatal Exposure to Methanol," *Teratol.*, 33, 259–65.

IOSUB, SILVIA , et al. 1987. "More on Human Immunodeficiency Virus Embryopathy," *Peds.*, 80, 512–16.

JOHNSON, RICHARD T., AND DIANE E. GRIFFIN. 1986. "The Neurospsychiatric Sequelae of Measles," in *Vaccinating Against Brain Syndromes*, ed. Ernest M. Gruenberg, Carol Lewis, and Stephen E. Goldston. New York: Oxford University Press.

JOHNSON, SALLY J., et al. 1986. "Prevalence of Sensorineural Hearing Loss in Premature and Sick Term Infants with Perinatally Acquired Cytomegalovirus Infection," *Ear and Hearing*, 7, 325–27.

JOINT COMMITTEE ON INFANT HEARING. 1982. "Position Statement. 1982," *Peds.*, 70, 496–97.

JONES, KENNETH L., AND DAVID W. SMITH. 1973. "Recognition of the Fetal Alcohol Syndrome in Early Infancy," *Lancet*, 2, 999–1001.

JONES, KENNETH L., et al. 1973. "Pattern of Malformation in Offspring of Chronic Alcoholic Mothers," *Lancet*, 1, 1267–71.

————1974. "Outcome in Offspring of Chronic Alcoholic Women," *Lancet*, 1, 1076–78.

KAMINSKI, M., C. RUMEAU, AND D. SCHWARTZ. 1978. "Alcohol Consumption in Pregnant Women and the Outcome of Pregnancy," *Alcoholism: Clin. Exp. Res.*, 2, 155–63.

KARCHMER, M. A., M. N. MILONE, AND S. WOLK. 1979. "Educational Significance of Hearing Loss at Three Levels of Severity," *Amer. Ann. Deaf*, 124, 97–109.

KARMODY, COLLIN S. 1983. "Developmental Anomalies of the Neck," in *Pediatric Otolaryngology*, vol. II, ed. Charles D. Bluestone and Sylvan E. Stool. Philadelphia: Saunders.

KASTNER, TED, AND DEBORAH FRIEDMAN. 1988. "Pediatric Acquired Immune Deficiency Syndrome and the Prevention of Mental Retardation," *J. Dev. Beh. Peds.*, 9.(1988), 47–48.

KLINGBERG, MARCUS A., et al. 1984. "The Etiology of Central Nervous System Defects," in *Neurobehavioral Teratology*, ed. Joseph Yanai. Amsterdam: Elsevier Science.

KOENIG, M. P. AND M. NEIGER. 1972. "The Pathology of the Ear in Endemic Cretinism," in *Human Development and the Thyroid Gland (Relation to Endemic Cretinism)*, ed. John B. Stanbury and Robert L. Kroc. New York: Plenum Press.

LAURENCE, K. MICHAEL. 1976. "Prenatal Diagnosis of Anencephaly and Spina Bifida," in *Birth Defects: Risks and Consequences*, ed. Sally Kelly et al. New York: Academic Press.

LEATHWOOD, PETER. 1978. "Influence of Early Undernutrition on Behavioral Development and Learning in Rodents," in *Studies on the Development of Behavior and the Nervous System*, Vol. 4: *Early Influences*, ed. Gilbert Gottlieb. New York: Academic Press.

LEDERER, FRANCIS L. 1973. "Granulomas and Other Specific Diseases of the Ear and Temporal Bone," in *Otolaryngology*, Vol. 2: *Ear*, ed. Michael M. Paparella and Donald A.Shumrick, Philadelphia: Saunders.

LEGRAND, JACQUES. 1984. "Effects of Thyroid Hormones on Central Nervous System Development," in *Neurobehavioral Teratology*, ed. Joseph Yanai. Amsterdam: Elsevier Science.

LINDSAY, JOHN R. 1973. "Profound Childhood Deafness: Inner Ear Pathology," *Ann. Otol., Rhinol., Laryngol.*, Supplement. No. 5. (1973).

LLOYD, DAVID J., AND THOMAS M. S. REID. 1976. "Group B Streptococcal Infection in the Newborn. Criteria for Early Detection and Treatment," *Acta Ped. Scand.*, 65, 585–91.

LOWE, C. R. 1973. "Congenital Malformations Among Infants Born to Epileptic Women," *Lancet*, 1, 1979. 9–10.

LUGO, JAMES O., AND GERALD L. HERSHEY. 1979. *Human Development*, 2nd ed. New York: Macmillan.

MADDEN, JOHN D., TERRENCE F. PAYNE, AND SUE MILLER. 1986. "Maternal Cocaine Abuse and Effect on the Newborn," *Peds.*, 77, 209–11.

MAJEWSKI, F., AND T. GOECKE. 1982. "Alcohol Embryopathy," in *Fetal Alcohol Syndrome*, vol. II: *Human Studies*, ed. E. L. Abel. Cleveland, OH: CRC Press.

MALLING, H. V., AND J. S. WASSOM. 1977. "Action of Mutagenic Agents," in *Handbook of Teratology*, vol. 1: *General Principles and Etiology*, ed. James G.Wilson and F. Clarke Fraser. New York: Plenum Press.

MALVERN, JOHN. 1980. "Perinatal Infections: The Obstetrician's Viewpoint," in *Perinatal Infections*, ed. Katherine Elliot, Maeve O'Connor, and Julie Whelan. Amsterdam: Excerpta Medica.

MAN, EVELYN B. 1975. "Maternal Hypothyroxinemia: Development of 4-and-7-Year-Old Offspring," in *Perinatal Thyroid Physiology and Disease*, ed. Delbert A. Fisher and Gerard N. Burrow. New York: Raven Press.

MARX, JEAN L. 1975. "Cytomegalovirus: A Major Cause of Birth Defects," *Science*, 190, 1184–86.

MATHOG, ROBERT H. 1973. "Otologic Manifestations of Retrocochlear Disease," in *Otolaryngology*, vol. 2: *Ear*, ed. Michael M. Paparella and Donald A. Shumrick. Philadelphia: Saunders.

MEDEARIS, D. N., JR. 1964. "Observations Concerning Human Cytomegalovirus Infection and Disease," *Bull. Johns Hopkins Hosp.*, 114, 181–211.

MELNICK, MICHAEL, DAVID BIXLER, AND EDWARD D. SHIELDS, eds. 1980. *Progress in Clinical and Biological Research*, Vol. 46, *Etiology of Cleft Lip and Cleft Palate*. New York: Alan R. Liss.

MINKOFF, HOWARD et al. 1987a. "Pregnancies Resulting in Infants with Acquired Immunodeficiency Syndrome or AIDS-Related Complex," *Obst. Gynecol.*, 69, 285–87.

———1987b. "Pregnancies Resulting in Infants with Acquired Immunodeficiency Syndrome or AIDS-Related Complex: Follow-up of Mothers, Children, and Subsequently Born Siblings," *Obst. Gynecol.*, 69, 288–91.

MOON, MARY ANN. 1987. "Research Highlights," *Research Resources Reporter*, 11, 10–12.

MOTULSKY, ARNO G. 1975. "Pharmacogenetics, Enzyme Polymorphisms, and Teratogenesis," in *Methods for Detection of Environmental Agents that Produce Congenital Defects*, ed. Thomas H. Shepard, James R. Miller, and Maurice Marois. Amsterdam: North-Holland.

MYERS, EUGENE N., AND SYLVAN E. STOOL, 1968. "Cytomegalic Inclusion Disease of the Inner Ear," *Laryngoscope*, 78, 1904–14.

MYRIANTHOPOLOUS, NTINOS C. 1980. "The Human Population Data: Critique II," in *Progress in Clinical and Biological Research*. vol. 46, *Etiology of Cleft Lip and Cleft Palate*, ed. Michael Melnick, David Bixler, and Edward D. Shields. New York: Alan R. Liss.

NANCE, WALTER E., AND ANNE SWEENEY. 1975. "Genetic Factors in Deafness of Early Life," *Otolaryngol. Clin. N. Amer.*, 8, 19–48.

NEEDLEMAN, HERBERT L. 1983. "Environmental Pollutants," in *Childhood Learning Disabilities and Prenatal Risk*, ed. Catherine Caldwell Brown. Skillman, NJ: Johnson & Johnson Baby Products Co.

NORTHERN, JERRY L., AND MARION P. DOWNS. 1984. *Hearing in Children*, 3rd ed. Baltimore: Williams & Wilkins.

OGATA, EDWARD S. 1984. "Diabetes-Related Problems of the Newborn," *Perinatol. Neonatol.*, 8, 48–53.

O'LOUGHLIN, E. V., AND D. LILLYSTONE. 1983. "Ear Anomalies, Deafness and Facial Nerve Palsy in Infants of Diabetic Mothers," *Austral. Ped. J.*, 19, 109–11.

ORENSTEIN, WALTER A., et al. 1986. "Epidemiology of Rubella and Its Complications," in *Vaccinating Against Brain Syndromes*, ed. Ernest M. Gruenberg, Carol Lewis, and Stephen E. Goldston. New York: Oxford University Press.

ORNITZ, EDWARD M., DONALD GUTHRIE, and ARTHUR J. FARLEY. 1977. "The Early Development of Autistic Children," *J. Autism Child. Schiz.*, 7, 207–29.

PADMANABHAN, R. 1987. "Abnormalities of the Ear Associated with Exencephaly in Mouse Fetuses Induced by Maternal Exposure to Cadmium," *Teratol.*, 35, 9–18.

PAINTER, MICHAEL J. 1983. "Neurologic Disorders of the Mouth, Pharynx, and Esophagus," in *Pediatric Otolaryngology*, vol. II, eds. Charles D. Bluestone and Sylvan E. Stool. Philadelphia: Saunders.

PAPPAS, DENNIS G., AND MARY SCHAIBLY. 1984. "A Two-Year Diagnostic Report of Bilateral Sensorineural Hearing Loss in Infants and Children," *Amer. J. Otol.*, 5, 339–43.

PENDRED, VAUGHAN. 1896. "Deaf-mutism and Goitre," *Lancet*, 2, 532.

PERSAUD, T. V. N. 1985. "Causes of Developmental Defects," in *Basic Concepts in Teratology*, ed. T. V. N. Persaud, A. E. Chudley, and R. G. Skalko. New York: Alan R. Liss.

PROUJAN, BARBARA J. 1988. "AIDS in Children," *Research Resources Reporter*, 12, 1–5.

REAL, RANDY, MICHELLE THOMAS, and JOHN M. GERWIN. 1987. "Sudden Hearing Loss and Acquired Immunodeficiency Syndrome," *Otolaryngology—Head and Neck Surgery*, 97, 409–12.

REID, THOMAS M. S., AND DAVID J. LLOYD. 1980. "Neonatal Group B Streptococcal Infection," in *Perinatal Infections*, ed. Katherine Elliot, Maeve O'Connor, and Julie Whelan. Amsterdam: Excerpta Medica.

REYNOLDS, DAVID W., et al. 1974. "Inapparent Congenital Cytomegalovirus Infection with Elevated Cord IgM Levels," *New Engl. J. Med.*, 290, 291–96.

ROBERT, K. E., AND P. GULBAUD. 1982. "Maternal Valproic Acid and Congenital Neural Tube Defects," *Lancet*, 2, 937.

Rosa, Franz W., Ann L. Wilk, and Frances O. Kelsey. 1986. "Teratogen Update: Vitamin A Congeners," *Teratol.*, 33, 355–64.

Ross, S. M., et al. 1980. "The Genesis of Amniotic Fluid Infections," in *Perinatal Infections*, ed. Katherine Elliot, Maeve O'Connor, and Julie Whelan. Amsterdam: Excerpta Medica.

Rush, David. 1976. "Cigarette Smoking During Pregnancy: The Relationship with Depressed Weight Gain and Birthweight," in *Birth Defects, Risks and Consequences*, ed. Sally Kelly et al. New York: Academic Press.

Rutter, Michael. 1987. "Continuities and Discontinuities from Infancy," in *Handbook of Infant Development* 2nd ed., ed. Joy Doniger Osofsky. New York: John Wiley.

Sando, Isamu, Susumo Suehiro, and Raymond P. Wood, II. 1983. "Congenital Anomalies of the External and Middle Ear," in *Pediatric Otolaryngology*, vol. I, ed. Charles D. Bluestone and Sylvan E. Stool. Philadelphia: Saunders.

Schardein James L. 1976. *Drugs as Teratogens*. Cleveland, OH: CRC Press.

Schor, David P. 1984. "Teratogens," in *Medical Aspects of Developmental Disabilities in Children Birth to Three*, ed. James A. Blackman. Rockville, MD: Aspen.

Schreiner, C. A. 1983. "Petroleum and Petroleum Products: A Brief Review of Studies to Evaluate Reproductive Effects," in *Advances in Modern Experimental Toxicology*, vol. III: *Assessment of Reproductive and Teratogenic Hazards*, ed. Mildred S. Christian, et al. Princeton, NJ: Princeton Scientific Publishers.

Schultz, Frederick R. 1984. "Phenylketonuria and Other Metabolic Diseases," in *Medical Aspects of Developmental Disabilities in Children Birth to Three*, ed. James A. Blackman. Rockville, MD: Aspen.

Sever, John L. 1983. "Maternal Infections," in *Childhood Learning Disabilities and Prenatal Risk*, ed. Catherine Caldwell Brown. Skillman, NJ: Johnson and Johnson Baby Products.

———et al. 1988. "Toxoplasmosis: Maternal and Pediatric Findings in 23,000 Pregnancies," *Peds.*, 82, 181–192.

Shih, Lucy, Barbara Cone-Wesson, and Bruce Reddix. 1988. "Effects of Maternal Cocaine Abuse on the Neonatal Auditory System," *Intl. J. Ped. Otorhinolaryngol.*, 15, 245–51.

Smith, David W. 1982. *Recognizable Patterns of Human Malformation*, 3rd ed. Philadelphia: Saunders.

Sparks, Shirley, N. 1984. *Birth Defects and Speech-Language Disorders*. San Diego, CA: College-Hill Press.

Stein, Zena, and Mervyn Susser. 1976. "Maternal Starvation and Birth Defects," in *Birth Defects: Risks and Consequences*, ed. Sally Kelly et al. New York: Academic Press.

Steis, Ronald, and Samuel Broder. 1985. "AIDS: A General Overview," in *AIDS: Etiology, Diagnosis, Treatment, and Prevention*, ed. Vincent T. DeVita, Jr., Samuel Hellman, and Steven A. Rosenberg. Philadelphia: Lippincott.

Stubbs, E. G. 1978. "Autistic Symptom in a Child with Congenital Cytomegalovirus Infection," *J. Autism Child. Schiz.*, 8, 37–43.

Swann, C. 1944. "Congenital Malformations in Infants Following Maternal Rubella During Pregnancy: Review of Investigations Carried Out in South Australia," *Trans. Ophthal. Soc. (Austral.)*, 4, 132–41.

Taussig, H. B. 1962. "A Study of the German Outbreak of Phocomelia. The Thalidomide Syndrome," *J. Am. Med. Assoc.*, 180, 1106–14.

Theissing, G., and G. Kittel. 1962. "Die Bedeutung der Toxoplasmose in der Atiologie der Connatalen und Fruh Erworbenen Horstorungen," *Arch. Ohren-, Nasen-, Kehlk-. Heilk.*, 180, 219.

Vining, Eileen P. G., et al. 1987. "Psychologic and Behavioral Effects of Antiepileptic Drugs in Children: A Double Blind Comparison Between Phenobarbitol and Valproic Acid," *Peds.*, 80, 16574.

Vorhees, Chas. V., and Elizabeth Mollnow. 1987. "Behavioral Teratogenesis: Longterm Influences on Behavior from Early Exposure to Environmental Agents," in *Handbook of Infant Development*, 2nd ed. ed. Joy Doniger Osofsky. New York: John Wiley.

Weller, T. H., and F. A. Neva. 1962. "Propagation in Tissue Culture of Cytopathic Agents from Patients with Rubella-Like Illness," *Proc. Soc. Exp. Biol. Med.*, 111, 215–25.

Wetherby, Amy Miller. 1985. "Speech and Language Disorders in Children—An Overview," in *Speech and Language Evaluation in Neurology: Childhood Disorders*, ed. John K. Darby. Orlando, FL: Grune & Stratton.

WILLIAMS, MICHAEL A. 1987. "Head and Neck Findings in Pediatric Acquired Immune Deficiency Syndrome," *Laryngoscope*, 97, 713–16.

WILSON, JAMES G. 1974. "Teratologic Causation in Man and its Evaluation in Non-Human Primates," in *Birth Defects*, ed. A. G. Motulsky and W. Lenz. Amsterdam: Excerpta Medica.

———1977a. "Environmental Chemicals," in *Handbook of Teratology*, vol. 1: *General Principles and Etiology*, ed. James G.Wilson and R. Clarke Fraser. New York: Plenum Press.

———1977b. "Embryotoxicity of Drugs in Man," in *Handbook of Teratology*, vol. 1: *General Principles and Etiology*, ed. James G. Wilson and R. Clarke Fraser. New York: Plenum Press.

WOLFSON, ROBERT J., ALI M. AGHAMOHAMADI, AND STEVEN E. BERMAN. 1980. "Disorders of Hearing," in *Child Development and Developmental Disabilities*, ed. Stewart Gabel and Marilyn T. Erickson. Boston: Little, Brown.

WRIGHT, MARY INGLE. 1971. *The Pathology of Deafness*. Manchester: Manchester University Press.

YOGMAN, M. W. et al. 1982. "Behavior of Newborns of Diabetic Mothers," *Infant Beh. Dev.*, 5, 331–40.

YOUNG, PATRICK. 1987. *Drugs and Pregnancy*. New York: Chelsea House.

ZADIG, JEAN M., AND ALLEN C. CROCKER. 1975. "A Center for Study of the Young Child with Developmental Delay," in *Exceptional Infant*. vol. 3: *Assessment and Intervention*, ed. Bernard Z. Friedlander, Graham M. Sterritt, and Girvin E. Kirk. New York: Brunner/Mazel.

ZAMENHOF, S. E., AND E. VAN MARTHENS. 1978. "Nutritional Influences on Prenatal Brain Development," in *Studies on the Development of Behavior and the Nervous System*, vol. 4: *Early Influences,* ed. Gilbert Gottlieb. New York: Academic Press.

ZOLLER, MICHAEL et al. 1978. "Detection of Syphilitic Hearing Loss," *Arch. Otolaryngol.*, 104, 631–165.

5

Trauma

The word *trauma* comes from the Greek meaning "to wound." Thus, trauma applies to any injury caused outside the organism. In this chapter, we consider the kinds of traumas (or traumata) that befall children and the means to prevent them. Three categories of trauma are covered: mechanical trauma, chemical trauma, and burns. It is important to observe that traumata appear in children at rates different from those in adults (Table 5–1).

MECHANICAL TRAUMA

One-third of all permanent disabilities among children is caused by accidents, and accidents are the leading cause of death among persons under the age of 15 years (Table 5–1). Motor vehicle accidents are the major contributor, being the leading cause of death and disability to persons between the ages of 1 and 45 (Table 5–2). In 1983, 43,000 children under the age of 5 were injured or killed in automobile accidents; 80,000 from 5 to 15 years of age were injured or killed (Wagenaar and Webster 1986). In 1985, more than a half-million people in the United States were injured in bicycle accidents, 70 percent of them under the age of 15 years; however, of course, the vast majority of cyclists are children. If the bicycle accident involves an automobile, then (obviously) the risk increases: fifteen percent of these children died or were discharged from hospital with severe and permanent damage.

Traumata to the head, face, and/or neck are very much the concern of communicative disorders specialists. Some traumata may even be

TABLE 5–1.　Major Causes of Death (1979), Illness (1980), and Accident (1980):
Total U.S. Population and U.S. Children.

Deaths

Total U.S. Population	*Percent*	*U.S. Children*	*Percent*
(N = 1,913,841)		(N = 19,254)	
1. Heart disease	38.3	1. Accidents	46.9
2. Cancer	21.1	2. Cancer	11.1
3. Stroke	8.8	3. Congenital anomalies	8.3
4. Accidents	5.5	4. Homicide	3.7
5. Pulmonary disease	2.6	5. Heart disease	2.8
6. Pneumonia and influenza	2.4	6. Pneumonia and influenza	2.4
7. Diabetes	1.7	7. Meningitis	2.2
8. Cirrhosis of the liver	1.6	8. Anemias	.8
9. Ateriosclerosis	1.5	9. Suicide	.8
10. Suicide	1.4	10. Stroke	.7
11. All other	15.1	11. All others	20.3

Incidents of Acute Illness

(N = 484,159,000)		(N = 189,629,000)	
1. Respiratory conditions	52.3	1. Respiratory conditions	52.7
2. Injuries	15.0	2. Infectious and parasitic	14.1
3. Infectious and parasitic	11.1	disease	
disease		3. Injuries	11.8
4. Digestive system	5.1	4. Digestive system	4.6
5. All other	16.5	5. All other	16.5

Accidents

(N = 68,089,000)		(N = 21,693,000)	
1. Home-related	39.2	1 Home-related	46.1
2. Work-related	15.9	2. Moving vehicle	4.2
3. Moving vehicle	6.4	3. Work-related	0.0
4. All other	41.4	4. All other	49.7

SOURCE:　Dorothy Noyes Kane, *Environmental Hazards to Young Children* (Phoenix, Ariz.:
Oryx Press, 1985), p. 2. Copyright © 1985 by the Oryx Press. Used by permission

Ages 1–14 for deaths based on National Center for Health Statistics data (1982), ages 0–16 for
illness and accidents based on National Center for Health Statistics data (1981).
Note that totals in data source are inconsistent: thus, some percentage columns exceed 100
percent.

described as acquired craniofacial disorders. You may recall your parents
telling you don't run with a stick in your mouth; they knew that some
palatal clefts are traumatic. They also told you to stay out of the street,

TABLE 5–2. Motor Vehicle Deaths and Injuries by Type, Location, and Age, 1983

	Age Group		
Deaths	*0–1*	*5–14*	*Under 15*
Total	1,200	1,500	3,700
Pedestrian	540	1,070	1,610
Pedalcycle[a]	20	440	460
Other types	640	990	1,630
Total: Urban	500	1,100	1,600
Pedestrian	430	840	1,270
Pedalcycle	[b]	170	170
Other types	70	90	160
Total: Rural	700	1,400	2,100
Pedestrian	110	230	340
Pedalcycle	20	270	290
Other types	570	900	1,470
Injuries			
Total	50,000	130,000	180,000
Pedestrian	7,000	30,000	37,000
Pedalcycle	1,000	21,000	22,000
Other types	42,000	79,000	121,000

SOURCE: Dorothy Noyes Kane, *Environmental Hazards to Young Children* (Phoenix, Ariz: Oryx Press, 1985), p. 14. Copyright © 1985 by the Oryx Press. Used by permission. National Safety Council estimates based on reports from the National Center for Health Statistics and state traffic authorities.

[a] Pedalcycle excludes mopeds.
[b] Less than five deaths in this group.

out of the way of cars. And, in our clinic, we have seen at least one child whose cerebral palsy (with its accompanying *dysphasia* and *dysarthria*) was the result of an automobile accident in which he hit his head on the dash. In fact, it is sure that any one could mention a familiar case like these.

Head Injuries

Head injuries have been reported as a cause of death in more than 41 percent of cases of pediatric mortality, five times the mortality incidence of leukemia, which ranks second (Ewing-Cobbs et al. 1985). Half of all head injuries in adults are due to motor vehicle accidents at high speed; but half of pediatric head injuries are due to falls, including low-speed automobile-pedestrian accidents (Billmire and Myers 1985). Among preschool-aged children, accidents in the home constitute a significant proportion, but falls are more frequent among school-age children. However, head-injured children are not a random sample of the population; they tend to have been premorbidly "impulsive, aggressive, attention-seeking, and behaviorally disturbed" (Rutter, Chadwick, and Shaffer 1983).

Automobile crashes are obvious sources of mortality and morbidity in children. But one must be aware of non-crash injuries resulting in pediatric morbidity in instances of sudden stopping, rapid acceleration, or abrupt turns. Agran and Dunkle (1982) found that 15 percent of the children they saw who were injured in automobiles were not in crashes, and that these children tended to be younger than those injured in crashes. These incidents include being ejected from the car, falling in the car and striking a dashboard, windshield, or steering wheel, or colliding with another passenger. Of these children, 64 percent had minor injuries (e.g., abrasions or lacerations), but the remainder had moderate or serious injuries, as serious as skull fracture.

The chronic results of head (i.e., brain) injuries in children were listed by Birch (1964): disordered behavior, short attention span, emotional lability, social incompetence, defective work habits, impulsiveness and meddlesomeness, and specific learning disorders. Some years later, Gabel and Erickson (1980) published essentially the same list: distractibility, hyperkinesis, lability of mood, and learning disorders. However, they also pointed out that the relationship is inconsistent. The characteristics of closed head injury (therefore, diffuse rather than focal) in children were summarized by DePompei and Blosser (1987), as shown in Table 5–3.

TABLE 5–3. Characteristics of Closed Head Injury in Children

Physical:	Impairments can exist in mobility, strength, coordination, vision, and/or hearing.
Communication:	Problems can occur in language, articulation, word-finding (anomia), reading, writing, computation, abstraction.
Cognitive:	Difficulties can be found with long- and short-term memory, thought processes, conceptual skills, problem solving.
Perceptual motor:	Involvement can include visual neglect, visual field cuts, motor apraxia, motor speed, motor sequencing.
Behavior:	Problems can account for impulsivity, poor judgment, disinhibition, dependency, anger outbursts, denial, depression, emotional lability, apathy, lethargy, poor motivation.
Social:	Impairments can result in the CHI student not learning from peers, not generalizing from social situations, behaving like a much younger child, withdrawing, distracting in noisy surroundings, and becoming lost even in familiar surroundings.

SOURCE: Roberta DePompei and Jean Blosser, "Strategies for Helping Head-Injured Children Successfully Return to School, " *Language, Speech, and Hearing Service in Schools,* 18 (1987), p. 293. © American Speech-Language-Hearing Association.

Prime among the sequelae of brain injury is language dysfunction, what has sometimes been called acquired aphasia. Swisher (1985) reported that most children whose aphasia is a result of a cerebral insult are nonfluent at first and then become agrammatic and telegraphic; in 1981, the same observation was made by Satz and Bullard-Bates. Swisher predicted prognosis as anywhere from poor to "possibly complete"; Alajouanine and Lhermitte (1965) claimed that two-thirds of patients recover and that this fact is "one very particular to children." In 1977, van Dongen and Loonen summarized the factors that contribute to the prognosis. It is directly related to the age of onset, traumatic etiologies have better prognoses than vascular disease, but prognosis is not good if there was an experience of coma longer than seven days.

Swisher also summarized the differences between such aphasias in children and traumatic aphasias in adults as follows: The younger the child at the time of onset, the more likely that right hemisphere or bilateral insult (rather than a left hemisphere insult) has occurred; fluent aphasias do not appear to occur in children; recovery tends to be more rapid and to a higher level (than in adults); and academic deficiencies that remain have been attributed to general brain damage and to residual language problems.

Rutter (1987) also discussed the effect of age. He concluded that there is increased probability of a generalized deficit if the injury occurs in infancy, whereas specific deficits (such as dysphasia) appear later in childhood. This, he apparently believed, is due to the greater susceptibility of the relatively immature brain coupled with its increased ability to recover due to neural plasticity, including interhemispheric transfer of language functions. On the other hand, the damaged immature brain may be less capable of acquiring new skills and knowledge, leading to a persistent learning disability.

Kinsbourne and Caplan (1979) had come to essentially the same conclusion:

> The immature brain has considerable compensatory potential. Only if brain damage is very widespread will there be no available brain areas to compensate for those that are damaged, and only then will general mental retardation supervene. If restricted brain damage, however severe, occurs early, it will always prompt some compensation by the residual intact brain, so that the individual will not be totally and permanently deprived of the affected cognitive skill.

In fact, mild cognitive impairments without aphasia were found among children whose left hemisphere injury occurred in the perinatal period, whereas there was aphasia among children whose injuries appeared later (Woods and Carey 1979).

The permanence of effects is related to the severity of the injury. Rutter, Chadwick, and Shaffer (1983) observed that those who had severe injuries had a phase of "marked cognitive recovery" that was not apparent in children with mild injuries. They concluded, though, that severe injuries lead to permanent intellectual impairment and mild injuries do not. There is, in fact, a "significant decline" of intellect in cases of pediatric head trauma (Fletcher et al. 1985).

As specialists who deal with communicative disorders, we are confronted with any or all of four kinds of problems. First, and perhaps foremost, is the generalized developmental delay or disability—even mental retardation—with its usual communication problems. Second is the language dysfunction, the dysphasia, which may be a consequence of the developmental dysfunction, which may extend beyond the consequence of the developmental dysfunction, or may exist instead of a developmental disability. Third is the dysarthria and/or *dyspraxia*, which would result in phonologic dysfunction; severe dysarthria is known to follow head injuries with increased intracranial pressure (Brown 1985). And fourth is the possibility of sensory-neural hearing loss due to temporal bone fracture.

In discussing head injury in children, it is important to remember that the issue here is one of accident. Indeed, children do have strokes (happily, very rarely) and do have brain disease. But we are concerned with traumata, with closed head injuries. However, very little is known about how (or if) closed head injuries affect children in ways different from their effects on adults except insofar as prognosis seems to be better. In her 1987 review, Mentis summarized the properties of closed head injuries' effects in adults and discovered that the "predominant problem" displayed by these patients is their "inappropriate pragmatic and discourse abilities. . . ." Mentis and Prutting (1987) described the conversation of head-injured adults as fragmented, tangential, and irrelevant. Perhaps it is this inappropriate behavior that was described by earlier observers (e.g., Birch 1964) with such terms as lability, social incompetence, impulsiveness, or meddlesomeness. In other words, the lasting effects of brain injuries in children are pragmatic ones, and the persistent learning disabilities may appear in the form of odd conversation.

Temporal bone fracture, however, is quite a different case. Fractures of the temporal bone are of two kinds, longitudinal or transverse. Longitudinal fractures account for 80 percent of the incidence (Parisier 1983). Table 5–4 is Parisier's summary of temporal bone fractures. In brief, longitudinal fractures usually result from a circumscribed blow to the temperoparietal area, whereas transverse fractures occur from forceful blows over the frontal or the occipital areas. From the table, one may see that transverse fractures are more important for our purposes, as they result in profound sensory-neural hearing losses and frequent severe vertigo. To be sure, these consequences may appear with longitudinal fractures, but they are less common. Electronystagmographic distur-

TABLE 5–4. Classification of Temporal Bone Fractures

	Longitudinal Fractures	Transverse Fractures
Percent of temporal bone fractures	80%	20%
Point of impact	Temperoparietal area	Frontal or occipital area
Force of impact	Moderate to severe	Severe
Loss of conciousness	Not always present	Present
	Associated Otologic Findings	
Ear canal bleeding	Frequent	Infrequent
Tympanic membrane perforation	Frequent	Infrequent
Hemotympanum	Common	Less common
Hearing loss	Variable: conductive, mixed, and neurosensory	Profound neurosensory loss
Vertigo	Variable frequency and severity	Frequent; severe
Facial nerve:		
Injury	Variable severity	Severe
Incidence	25%	50%
Paralysis	May be incomplete;	Immediate onset

SOURCE: Simon C. Parisier, "Injuries of the Ear and Temporal Bone," in Charles D. Bluestone and Sylvan E. Stool, eds., *Pediatric Otolaryngology,* Vol. I (Philadelphia: W. B. Saunders Co., 1983), p. 624.

bances have been reported to persist as long as eight years after blunt head injury in children (Vartiainen, Karjalainen, and Karja 1985). In addition, injuries to the facial nerve are both more common and more severe following transverse fractures, and such injuries may result in phonologic handicaps.

We must be conscious, however, that head trauma resulting in brain injury is more serious than injuries limited to the temporal bone. It was a wise and thoughtful caution made by Bordley, Brookhouser, and Tucker (1986) that "serious head injury, of course, can pose a threat to life, and neurosurgical concerns regarding possible intracranial injury must take precedence over otologic considerations." Safety helmets, after all, must be worn, and they are primary prevention.

At this point in our discussion of head injury, we must, unfortunately, consider child abuse. In 1985, there were nearly 1.9 million reported instances of child abuse, and two-thirds of these were cases of neglect. However, it has also been reported that more than half of all such cases remain unsubstantiated; in fact, one study found that 87.6 percent were unfounded (Silverman 1987).

In one pediatric hospital, it was reported that 64 percent of all head injuries and 95 percent of serious intracranial injuries in children under one year of age had resulted from child abuse (Billmire and Myers 1985). The mean age of those who were abused was four months, and five months for accident victims. Relevant to the comments about temporal bone injuries, Billmire and Myers found that 87 percent of the infants with skull fractures had linear parietal fractures. The tragic point is that 19 of their infants had serious intracranial injuries; 18 of them were abused. They concluded, therefore, that "child abuse is the most common cause of serious head injury in children less than 1 year of age."

What if the child is older and/or the head trauma less severe? Casey, Ludwig, and McCormick (1986) defined "minor" head traumas as those without the symptoms of concussion, namely, altered conciousness, loss of memory, or neurologic impairment. In their study of children from 6 months to 14 years of age who met these criteria in their hospital ($n = 1,072$), they found "substantial functional morbidity" in the absence of physical morbidity. What does that mean? Among other things, it means that 27 percent of these children had behavioral problems, and 29 to 40 percent had a high rate of school absenteeism and high deviance scores on standardized tests. It was their conclusion, however, that this so-called functional morbidity "probably reflects parental overreaction and possibly family dysfunction." Nevertheless, these children did exhibit symptoms, at least for a while, and the accident may be a result of a stressful family environment which itself merits treatment.

Psychosocial and socioeconomic factors also are relevant in the occurrence of accidents and therefore in the prevention of injury to children. A survey by Rivara and Barber (1985) identified a number of variables related to pedestrian injuries. Highest on their list of relevant demographic variables was crowded housing per acre leading to increased environmental exposure. In other words, the children played in the street. This conclusion is supported by their other findings: Most of the children were struck between street intersections, most of them were from nonwhite and single-parent families, and most lived below the poverty level. Prevention, then, is a social issue, just as it is in cases of child abuse.

Primary prevention can be of two kinds: manipulating the environment and educating the community. The environment may be altered by providing playgrounds, for example, so that children need not play in the street. The community can be educated, to some extent, about avoiding accidents, and child abusers require treatment themselves. Automobile restraints do work. There was a 25 percent reduction in the number of young children injured in automobile accidents within five years after the introduction of Michigan's restraint law (Wagenaar and Webster 1986). Figure 5–1 summarizes the status of such restraint laws in the United States.

The American Academy of Pediatrics has a stated goal of having every newborn strapped into an appropriate car seat upon leaving the hospital of birth. In fact, the American Hospital Association has considered a policy of prohibiting discharge of an infant unless proper restraint,

FIGURE 5–1.   Child passenger protection laws, by state, 1984

State	Original Year Enacted	Original Effective Date	Restraint Requirement Age	Safety Seat Required	May Substitute Safety Belt	Safety Belt Required
Alabama	1982	7/82	Under 3	Under 3	No	
Alaska	1984	6/85	Under 6	Under 4	Between 4 & 6	
Arizona [1] [*]	1983	8/83	Thru 4 [2]	Thru 4 [2]	No	
Arkansas	1983	8/83	Under 5	Under 3	Between 3 & 5	**
California [1]	1982	1/83	Under 4 [2]	Under 4 [2]	If not in parent's vehicle	**
Colorado	1983	1/84	Under 4 [2]	Under 4 [2]	No	**
Connecticut	1982	5/82	Under 4	Under 4	Between 1 & 4 in rear seat	
Delaware [1]	1982	6/82	Under 4	Under 4	No	**
Florida [*]	1982	7/83	Under 6	Under 4	Between 4 & 6	
Georgia	1983	7/84	Under 4	Under 3	Between 3 & 4	**
Hawaii	1983	7/83	Under 4	Under 3	Between 3 & 4	**
Idaho [1]	1984	1/85	Under 4 [2]	Under 4 [2]	No	**
Illinois [1] [*]	1982	7/83	Under 6	Under 4	Between 4 & 6	**
Indiana	1983	1/34	Under 5	Under 3	Between 3 & 5	**
Iowa [*]	1984	1/85	Under 6	Under 3	Between 3 & 6	**
Kansas [1] [*]	1981	1/82	Under 4 [4]	Under 4 [4]	No	
Kentucky [1]	1982	7/82	Under 40″	Under 40″	No	**
Louisiana	1984	9/84	Under 5	Under 5	Between 3 & 5 in rear seat	
Maine [1] [*]	1983	9/83	Under 12	Under 4	Between 1 & 4 if not in parent's vehicle	4 thru 11
Maryland	1983	1/84	Under 5	Under 3	Between 3 & 5	**
Massachusetts [*]	1981	1/82	Under 12	Under 5	Under 5	5 thru 11
Michigan	1981	4/82	Thru 4	Thru 4	1 thru 4 in rear seat	**
Minnesota [*]	1982	8/83	Under 4	Under 4	No	
Mississippi	1983	7/83	Under 2	Under 2	No	
Missouri	1983	1/84	Under 4	Under 4	Under 4 in rear seat	**
Montana [1] [*]	1983	1/84	Under 4 [2]	Under 2	Between 2 & 4	**
Nebraska	1983	8/83	Under 4	Under 1	Between 1 & 4	
Nevada	1983	7/83	Under 5	Under 5	Under 5 in rear seat	**
New Hampshire [*]	1983	7/83	Under 5	Under 5	Under 5	
New Jersey	1983	4/83	Under 5	Under 5	Between 1½ & 5 in rear seat	
New Mexico [*]	1983	6/83	Under 11	Under 5	Between 1 & 5 in rear seat	5 thru 10 **
New York [*]	1981	4/82	Under 10	Under 4	Between 4 & 10 in rear seat	4 thru 9 **
North Carolina [*]	1981	7/82	Under 6	Under 3	Between 3 & 6	**
North Dakota [*]	1983	1/84	Thru 5	Under 3	3 thru 5	
Ohio	1982	3/83	Under 4 [2]	Under 4 [2]	Between 1 & 4 if not in parent's vehicle	**
Oklahoma [*]	1983	11/83	Under 5	Under 4	Under 4 in rear; 4-5 in front or rear	**
Oregon [*]	1983	1/84	Under 16	Under 1	Between 1 & 5	5 thru 15**
Pennsylvania [*]	1983	1/84	Under 4	Under 4	Between 1 & 4 in rear seat	
Rhode Island [*]	1980	7/80	Thru 12	Thru 3	No	4 thru 12
South Carolina	1983	7/83	Under 4	Under 4	Between 1 & 4 in rear seat	
South Dakota [*]	1984	7/84	Under 5	Under 2	Between 2 & 5	**
Tennessee [*]	1977	1/78	Under 4	Under 4	No	**
Texas	1984	10/84	Under 4	Under 2	Between 2 & 4	**
Utah [1]	1984	7/84	Under 5	Under 2	Between 2 & 5	
Vermont [*]	1984	7/84	Under 5	Under 5	Between 1 & 5 in rear seat	
Virginia [*]	1982	1/83	Under 4	Under 3	Between 3 & 4 or over 40 pounds	**
Washington [1]	1983	1/84	Under 5	Under 1	Between 1 & 5	5 thru 8
West Virginia [*]	1981	7/81	Under 9	Under 3	Between 3 & 5	
Wisconsin [*]	1982	11/82	Under 4	Under 2	Between 2 & 4	
Wyoming	1985	4/85	Under 3 [2]	Under 3 [2]	No	**
Dist. of Col.	1982	7/83	Under 6	Under 3	Between 3 & 6	

NOTES: [1] Law applies only to parents and legal guardians
  [2] Or less than 40 pounds
  [3] Most states waive fines upon proof of safety seat acquisition
  [4] Kansas law applies only to children riding in front seat.
  [*] States which have upgraded laws since original enactment.
  ** Covered by State Safety Belt Laws

SOURCE: Courtesy of the National Safety Council.

properly applied, is employed. Of course, parents need to be educated to the need for restraint and how to use car seats, and this applies equally to the parents' use of seat belts.

Secondary prevention is problematic because many cases of abuse or accident go undiscovered or at least unreported. Secondary prevention would be in the form of prompt emergency treatment and correct diagnosis. The children who never appear in the hospital's emergency room don't get the treatment they need when they need it.

Facial Injuries

Don't run with a stick in your mouth! Head and neck traumata amount to some two-thirds of all injuries sustained by children in accidents, but facial fractures are far less frequent in children than in adults (Bailey 1979). Injuries to the hard palate are uncommon because it is a firm, bony structure and is difficult to penetrate. However, a maxillary fracture can occur in a case of a severe injury, and trauma to the midface is a relatively common childhood injury.

Although trauma is common, fracture is not. Fracture of the maxillofacial area accounts for only some 10 percent of facial fractures in children (Yarington 1977). Marlowe (1983) believed that this is due to the relative elasticity of the facial bones of a young child. On the other hand, Marlowe continued, when such a fracture does occur, it must be taken seriously, especially in light of concomitant central nervous system damage.

Soft tissue injuries may result in hematomas, lacerations, crush wounds, and the like, and may lead to cellulitis (Gatot, Tovi, and Moshiashvili 1986). The greater risk is penetration of the soft palate, as it is composed of muscle and mucosa, not bone. There is danger of acute bleeding; but, otherwise, spontaneous healing should be expected without consequent hypernasality. If a persistent fistula were to remain, it could be repaired surgically (Maisel and Mathog 1983). The fact is, though, that there are frequent injuries to the oral and pharyngeal mucosae in the form of lacerations and punctures from sticks, pencils, toys, and so on. Hypernasality from inadequate healing or hyponasality from improper repair are always possible. One needs to be alert to a possible asymmetry of facial movement following injury, as this could be indicative of facial nerve injury. Also, teeth may be lost. Loss of teeth and/or permanent injury to the facial nerve have clear consequences for articulation.

Finally, facial injury opens a possibility of obstruction of the airway. For example, Marlowe (1983) observed that fracture of the mandible may cause posterior displacement of the tongue with a consequent occlusion of the airway. Although respiratory problems are the subject of Chapter 7, here we are reminded that sometimes such problems may be of traumatic origin. Furthermore, fractures of the mandible rank second only to those of the nose as the most common facial fractures.

Laryngeal Injuries

If injury to the face opens the possibility of respiratory difficulty, then injury to the larynx must be still more significant. For example, it is possible for the epiglottis to occlude the airway, or the hyoid bone may be fractured. There can be lacerations of the larynx, which may lead to paralysis or scarring of the vocal folds. Scarring, according to Maisel and Mathog (1983), may cause a contracture of the glottis and fixation of the vocal folds. Vocal dysfunction results, which usually may be alleviated surgically. Moreover, there are iatrogenic instances where injury is caused by an instrument employed, for example, to remove a foreign body from the airway. Some 8 percent of injuries due to animal bites are to the face and/or neck, and one must be concerned also with the risk of tetanus or rabies.

Aronson (1985) described three kinds of larynx injury: (1) blunt or penetrating injuries such as those that result from automobile accidents in which the patient is thrown forward striking the neck region; (2) penetrating wounds as from gunshot or knives; and (3) collision with wires or cables as might occur in boating or motorcycle accidents. He considered all of the following as simultaneous injuries: edema, hematoma, fractures, dislocations, lacerations, and paralysis.

Fortunately, external trauma to the larynx is rare in the youngest children. However, as children get older and begin to ride bicycles or other wheeled contrivances, the incidence of laryngeal injury increases. Gross injury to the larynx may lead to emphysema and respiratory distress. Bordley, Brookhouser, and Tucker (1986) said that this "is obviously a major catastrophe and may require tracheotomy" due to discontinuity of the airway, especially if the injury extends also to the trachea.

How, then, may we prevent injuries to the neck region? Thoughtful education of the very young is bound to be the most fruitful form of primary prevention: Don't hurt yourself. It is too often the case that secondary prevention is the only kind available, and it may have to be in the form of emergency surgical intervention such as intubation or tracheotomy. Airway injuries can be lethal.

CHEMICAL TRAUMA

In this section we consider chemical substances in addition to those discussed in Chapter 4. These may be neurotoxic, and, furthermore, we discuss substances that do direct damage to the face and neck.

Lead Poisoning

Lead poisoning has already been discussed as a teratogen. It is also a common and potent toxin leading to *encephalopathy*. Approximately 85 percent of cases are children between one and three years of age, and nearly 40 percent of those children have permanent neurologic sequelae (Grant 1981). Dreifuss (1975) concluded that lead intoxication is "uniformly followed by significant interference with learning ability, and is associated with findings suggestive of widespread neurologic dysfunction."

In 1987, the American Academy of Pediatrics, in recognition of this environmental hazard, issued a statement on the subject. The academy stressed that lead is a significant hazard to children's health. Lead has no biological value; hence, the ideal blood lead level is zero, none at all. Nevertheless, it had been found that blood lead levels approximated 16 μg/dL in preschool-aged children. At this blood lead level, children do not display overt signs of lead poisoning, but do eventually display behavioral changes and diminutions of intellectual function. There are also physical signs: short stature, decreased weight, and diminished circumference of the chest in children under the age of seven. By 1980, 4 percent of American children between the ages of six months and five years had blood lead levels in excess of 30 μg/dL. The academy estimated that more than three-fourths of a million people had excess levels of lead in their blood, in spite of the fact that blood lead levels had decreased to this amount since 1974.

Table 5–5, modified from the American Academy of Pediatrics' publication, shows the sources of lead commonly and less commonly found. The academy observed that lead is ubiquitous; it is found in the earth's crust, in drinking water, in soil, and in vegetation. It is also a useful substance employed in ways that are not inherently dangerous, such as radiation shields. It becomes dangerous when it is used improperly and

TABLE 5–5. Sources of Lead

Common	*Uncommon*
Low dose	Metallic objects
Food	Lead glazed ceramics
Ambient air	Old toys and furniture
Drinking water	Storage battery casings
Intermediate dose	Gasoline sniffing
Household dust	Lead plumbing
Interior paint removal	Exposed lead solder in cans
Soil contaminated by automobile accident	Imported canned foods and toys
Industrial sources	Folk medicines (e.g., azarcon, Greta)
Improper removal of exterior paint	Leaded glass artwork
High dose	Cosmetics
Interior and	Antique pewter
exterior paint	Farm equipment

SOURCE: American Academy of Pediatrics, "Statement on Childhood Lead Poisoning," *Pediatrics*, 79 (1987), pp. 458-59. Copyright 1987. Reprinted by permission.

discarded without proper attention. Also, biological reasons for increased lead susceptibility appear when other metals are lacking in one's diet. Deficiencies of iron, calcium, and zinc have all been shown to increase lead absorption. Iron is especially important because as many as 15 percent of infants are deficient in iron, and this deficiency increases the gastrointestinal absorption of lead.

The American Academy of Pediatrics made five recommendations to public agencies to combat the widespread and dangerous problem of lead toxicity: (1) mandate reporting of all cases of lead poisoning; (2) systematic screening of lead hazards in housing; (3) "prompt, vigorous, and safe abatement of all environmental lead hazards"; (4) funding for screening, for identification of hazard, and for abatement of lead hazard; and (5) insistence on proper standards for laboratory blood testing. In general, the academy recommended that all children who are at risk of exposure should be screened at approximately 12 months of age.

One must add, however, that efforts toward identification and abatement of hazard have been conducted, and sometimes vigorously, in many places. For example, some communities have reduced the lead content of drinking water by reducing water acidity and/or eliminating lead-based solder in plumbing. The proportion of lead in gasoline—and therefore in vehicle exhausts—has been greatly reduced. Removal of lead-based paint has been carried out in many places, but too often the means for such removal create another hazard, that of airborne lead particles or lead dust. Proper and intensive care must be taken to ensure that we do not substitute one lead hazard for another. Finally, lead waste products must be properly discarded in an appropriate hazardous waste site.

The Centers for Disease Control revised its definition of lead poisoning downward from 30 µg/dL to 25 µg/dL. Recall that the "major tragedy of subclinical lead poisoning is that its neurologic consequences are permanent and irreversible" (Landrigan and Graef 1987). Pursuit of ever downward blood lead levels is the goal of primary prevention.

Other Metals

Iron is essential for life. Consequently, many people take iron in tablet or liquid form because they are indeed iron deficient or because they imagine they are. Attractive packaging may lead small children to these products, and evidence is that this is the case. Although there is no indication of large numbers of children ingesting overdoses of iron, it has been reported that 13 percent of such incidents have resulted in hospitalization (Kane 1985).

One of the most dangerous metals is mercury, a fact known for centuries. Among toxic metals, mercury ranks first in the ratio of emissions into the atmosphere produced by humans to those that occur naturally. Mercury reaches the environment by release into the air from certain manufacturing processes such as those involving shale, copper, iron, gas, and coal. From the air, then, it can find its way into soil and water and, therefore, into food. It is indeed teratogenic, and may also be absorbed via the respiratory system, the gastrointestinal system, and even the skin. Hearing, speech, and language disorders have been reported in cases of mercury poisoning, and the evidence is that it, like lead, produces irreversible encephalopathy. Fortunately, we have all benefited from the general awareness of mercury's toxicity. As a consequence of this primary prevention, there is rather little hazard from mercury in ambient air except in particular instances.

Cadmium—discussed earlier as a teratogen—also is commonly used in industry and is found in the environment. Cadmium levels in soil in areas where smelting operations are conducted have been reported to be unacceptably high (Fleischer et al. 1974). There have been cases of adverse alterations of brain metabolism in addition to symptoms less directly involved in communication. Kane (1985) claimed that excess cadmium reduces verbal IQ scores, but lead seems to have a greater effect on nonverbal scores. However, cadmium excesses seem to appear in the same children as excess levels of lead, so cadmium adds to the negative effect of blood lead.

Poison

More than 60,000 American children under the age of five years ingested prescription drugs in 1985; 75 percent of these children were between the ages of one and a half and three and a half. Almost always (80 percent of the incidents) such unintentional ingestions take place in the child's home. In fact, medicines account for the highest prevalence among toxic substances ingested by children (Table 5–6), some 40 percent of all cases. In 1978, in the United States, nearly 94,000 children under the age of five ingested toxins; and, in 1980, nearly 34,000 children under the age of five years were seen in hospital emergency rooms after having ingested medications.

Although medications are the most common source of toxic ingestion, exposure to petroleum products accounts for the largest number of hospital admissions. Poisoning is the most common medical emergency, but it has been claimed that only 2 percent of cases are reported (Mofenson and Greensher 1979). Nevertheless, morbidity following treatment is less common in children than in adults, and 50 percent of pediatric patients treated in hospitals are discharged the next day (Fazen, Lovejoy, and Crone 1986).

TABLE 5–6. Toxicity of Nine General Categories of Substances Ingested in 1978 by U.S. Children under the Age of Five

Category	Total	Number Hospitalized	Percent Hospitalized	Number Fatal
Medicines	37,664	1,042	2.76	2
Cleaning and polishing agents	14,009	141	1.00	0
Plants and plant substances	11,804	57	0.05	0
Cosmetics	10,372	48	0.05	0
Miscellaneous or unknown	7, 573	91	1.20	0
Pesticides	5,385	140	2.59	2
Turpentine and paints	4,124	86	2.08	0
Petroleum products	2,727	154	5.64	0
Gases and vapors	106	8	7.50	0
All other	93,764	1,870	1.99	4

SOURCE: Adapted from Dorothy Noyes Kane, *Environmental Hazards to Young Children* (Phoenix, Ariz.: The Oryx Press, 1985), p. 132.

What are the consequences? One study reported that, of 14 patients under the age of 17 treated in a pediatric intensive care unit, three were discharged to a psychiatric hospital, one to a foster home, one to another hospital, and one died (Fazen, Lovejoy, and Crone 1986). In other words, 6 of the 14 children (43 percent) had an unfavorable outcome. This group was described as having "significant CNS depression," but long-term sequelae were not cited by those authors.

Poisoning can be prevented at both the primary and secondary levels. Prompt emergency response to the ingestion of poisons is secondary prevention, and we have seen that the majority of cases are treated successfully in the emergency room of a local hospital. Moreover, there are evidently no long-term sequelae in these cases. The emergency room also provides a venue for primary prevention. Woolf et al. (1987) used the opportunity that necessarily arises in the emergency room to provide education to parents, advising them of two things: to keep syrup of ipecac (an emetic) in the home for emergency treatment and to keep the phone number of a poison center at their telephones. They found that a larger number of families who received this brief advice did so than did the number of control (i.e., unadvised) families. The best primary prevention, of course, is to store potentially dangerous substances where children cannot reach or find them.

BURNS

Burns account for more fatalities and crippling injuries each year than did polio at its peak. Burns will damage those structures required for the production of speech. In fact, both acid and alkali are common causes of chemical burns to the oral cavity. Burns from fire, flame, and great heat may destroy structures of the face. In addition, there is some risk from radiation hazard.

Chemical Injuries

In the 1970s, there were as many as 5,000 accidental lye ingestions per year in the United States by children under the age of five (Riding and Bluestone 1983). In fact, children at that age are the most common victims of lye ingestion (Zwiren, Andrews, and Hester 1985). This was in spite of warning labels mandated by federal regulations since 1970. The largest number of such burns was caused by alkalis, followed by phenols, bleaches, and acids. In one year, 1969, there were 76,155 accidental ingestions of caustic substances by children under the age of five.

According to Zwiren, Andrews, and Hester (1985), immediate treatment of lye burns is ineffective. Still, there is a risk of communicative sequelae. This risk arises from upper airway obstruction due to burns of the larynx. Of course, a marked obstruction of the upper airway demands immediate surgical attention. Nevertheless, burns of the vocal folds and/or other tissue in the glottal area must be expected to threaten phonatory function. There can be destruction of laryngeal tissue, and surgery may be necessary, especially if strictures develop. Burns in the area of the larynx can cause permanent respiratory—and, hence, phonatory—problems. It is important to know that these can occur even in the absence of burns to the mouth because swallowing is a normal reflex. Hence, the child will be likely to swallow the substance before it does harm to oral mucosa. Burns of the oral mucosa should be expected to heal. The greatest concern is for permanent damage to the esophagus, and many patients require lifelong treatment. Zwiren, Andrews, and Hester recommend banning the sale of liquid lye: primary prevention.

Thermal Injuries

Ingestion of very hot fluids is the most probable risk for thermal injuries. In addition to fluids, there is a risk from electrical hazards, from fire itself, and, occasionally, from radiation. Kane (1985) claimed that excessive heat is a greater threat to children than to adults because their skin is "thin, soft, and tender. . . ." Moreover, due to the relative immaturity of their immune systems, children are at increased risk of infection following burn trauma.

Most burns occur at home, and 80 percent of those are in the kitchen. Toddlers are at highest risk, as they are the ones most likely to pull a pot off a stove or bite an electrical cord. Furthermore, in children, burn injuries occur most often in the facial area, but sometimes extensive surgical repair succeeds (Figure 5–2). Electrical burns of the mouth are more common before the age of four—again, toddlers. There is usually

FIGURE 5–2.   Facial burn constrictions (A and B) and some years after repair (C and D)

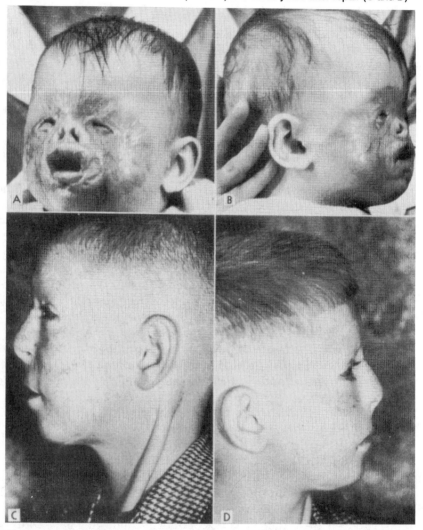

SOURCE: Blair O. Rogers, *Facial Disfigurement* (Washington, D.C.: U.S. Department of Health, Education, and Welfare, 1963), p. 55.

considerable tissue destruction (Bordley, Brookhouser, and Tucker 1986). The consequences for speech production are obvious. Similarly, ingestion of hot liquids or inhalation of hot gases can damage the vocal folds (Aronson 1985). Finally, a child's nervous system may be vulnerable to both ionizing and nonionizing radiation.

Primary prevention of thermal injuries is certainly not difficult; it is a matter of proper child care and sensible home behavior patterns. Just as we wish to store caustics where children cannot reach them, we would store matches in the same place. We would be alert to toddlers in the kitchen, and we would protect electrical outlets. We would employ flame-retardant materials for our children's clothes, and we might lower the temperature on our water heaters. Secondary prevention is found in emergency treatment both prompt and efficacious.

For older children, education about hazards may lead to primary prevention. Public education has been shown to be effective: McLoughlin et al. (1982) found a reduction in burn rates in their community, although a direct cause-effect relationship is difficult to measure.

CONCLUSION

In general, trauma to children is less of a problem than it has been in the past. At the beginning of the twentieth century, only 77 percent of births were expected to reach maturity; it is now 98 percent. This, of course, is due largely to the great progress in the fight against infectious disease, but there have been positive advances in prevention of trauma. In the first third of the century 75 children of every 100,000 died by accident; in the last third, only some 26 children under the age of five per 100,000 died accidentally and just 15 between the ages of 5 and 14. Removal of environmental toxins such as lead will lead to a reduction of morbidity. Similarly, public education and intelligent behavior will lead to a reduction of the number of accidental injuries. We are getting better at using automobile restraints for our children, and also for ourselves. An area in which we are not improving is that of near drowning, and we have a new hazard, hot tubs. Tron, Baldwin, and Pirie (1985) reported two children who drowned in hot tubs. What about survivors? Of 31 nearly drowned children described by Nussbaum and Maggi (1988), 7 later died and 12 (of the 24) survivors had serious neurologic consequences "characterized by severe mental deterioration, generalized spasticity, major motor seizures, or unresponsiveness to family members." Clearly, these children merit our attention as clinicians, but it is obviously much more important that we do everything possible in our communities to prevent these accidents. Perhaps the major problem that is not yet addressed adequately is that of abuse and neglect.

GLOSSARY

cellulitis: inflammation of cells or connective tissue.
dysarthria: any of several motor speech disorders that originate in the central or peripheral nervous system; hence, any disturbance of articulation due to paralysis, noncoordination,and the like.
dysphasia: a disorder caused by damage to the brain and characterized by an impairment of language production and/or comprehension.
dyspraxia: a disorder caused by damage to the brain and characterized by an inability to execute a motor response, especially a speech act.
encephalopathy: a general term meaning any brain disease.
hematoma: a localized mass of blood completely or partly confined within an organ or tissue.

REFERENCES

AGRAN, PHYLLIS A., AND DEBORA E. DUNKLE. 1982. "Motor Vehicle Occupant Injuries to Children in Crash and Noncrash Events," *Peds.,* 70, 993–96.
ALAJOUANINE, TH., AND F. LHERMITTE. 1965. "Acquired Aphasia in Children," *Brain,* 88, 653–62.
AMERICAN ACADEMY OF PEDIATRICS. 1987. "Statement on Childhood Lead Poisoning," *Peds.,* 79, 457–65.
ARONSON, ARNOLD E. 1985. *Clinical Voice Disorders,* 2nd ed. New York: Thieme.
BAILEY, BYRON J. 1979. "Facial Skeletal Injuries in Children," in *Pediatric Otorhinolaryngology,* ed. Basharat Jazbi. Amsterdam: Excerpta Medica.
BILLMIRE, M. ELAINE, AND PATRICIA A. MYERS. 1985. "Serious Head Injury in Infants: Accident or Abuse?" *Peds.,* 75, 340–42.
BIRCH, HERBERT G. 1964. *Brain Damage in Children. The Biological and Social Aspects.* Baltimore: Williams & Wilkins.
BORDLEY, JOHN E., PATRICK E. BROOKHOUSER, AND GABRIEL FREDERICK TUCKER, JR. 1986. *Ear, Nose, and Throat Disorders in Children.* New York: Raven Press.
BROWN, J. KEITH. 1985. "Dysarthria in Children: Neurologic Perspective," in *Speech and Language Evaluation in Neurology: Childhood Disorders,* ed. John K. Darby. Orlando, FL: Grune & Stratton.
CASEY, ROSEMARY, STEPHEN LUDWIG, AND MARIE C. McCORMICK. 1986. "Morbidity Following Minor Head Trauma in Children, " *Peds.,* 78, 497–502.
DePOMPEI, ROBERTA, AND JEAN BLOSSER. 1987. "Strategies for Helping Head-Injured Children Successfully Return to School," *Lang. Speech Hear. Serv. Schools,* 18, 292–300.
DREIFUSS, F. E. 1975. "The Pathology of Central Communicative Disorders in Children," in *The Nervous System,* vol. 3, *Human Communication and Its Disorders,* ed. Eldon L. Eagles. New York: Raven Press.
EWING-COBBS, LINDA, et al. 1985. "Language Disorders after Pediatric Head Injury," in *Speech and Language Evaluation in Neurology: Childhood Disorders,* ed. John K. Darby. Orlando, FL: Grune & Stratton.
FAZEN, LOUIS E., III, FREDERICK H. LOVEJOY, JR., AND ROBERT K. CRONE. 1986. "Acute Poisoning in a Children's Hospital: A 2-Year Experience," *Peds.,* 77, 144–51.
FLEISCHER, M. et al. 1974. "Environmental Impact of Cadmium: A Review by the Panel on Hazardous Trace Substances," *Environmental Health Perspectives,* 29, 253–323.
FLETCHER, JACK M. et al. 1985. "Cognitive and Psychosocial Sequelae of Head Injury in Children: Implications for Assessment and Management," in *The Injured Child,* ed. Benjy Frances Brooks. Austin: University of Texas Press.
GABEL, STEWART, AND MARILYN T. ERICKSON. 1980. *Child Development and Developmental Disabilities.* Boston: Little, Brown.
GATOT, ALBERT, FERIT TOVI, AND ABRAHAM MOSHIASHVILI. 1986. "Periorbital Cellulitis: Presenting Feature of Undiagnosed Old Maxillary Fracture," *Intl. J. Ped. Otorhinolaryngol.,* 11, 129–34.

GRANT, MURRAY. 1981. *Handbook of Community Health,* 3rd ed. Philadelphia: Lea & Febiger.
KANE, DOROTHY NOYES. 1985. *Environmental Hazards to Young Children.* Phoenix, AZ: Oryx Press.
KINSBOURNE, MARCEL, AND PAULA J. CAPLAN. 1979. *Children's Learning and Attention Problems.* Boston: Little, Brown.
LANDRIGAN, PHILIP J., AND JOHN W. GRAEF. 1987. "Pediatric Lead Poisoning in 1987: The Silent Epidemic Continues," *Peds.,* 79, 582–83.
MAISEL, ROBERT H., AND ROBERT H. MATHOG. 1983. "Injuries of the Mouth, Pharynx, and Esophagus," in *Pediatric Otolaryngology,* vol. II., ed. Charles D. Bluestone and Sylvan E. Stool. Philadelphia: Saunders.
MARLOWE, FRANK I. 1983. "Injuries of the Nose, Facial Bones, and Paranasal Sinuses," in *Pediatric Otolaryngology,* vol. I, ed. Charles D. Bluestone and Sylvan E. Stool. Philadelphia: Saunders.
MCLOUGHLIN, E., et al. 1982. "Project Burn Prevention: Outcome and Implications," *Amer. J. Pub. Health,* 72, 241–47.
MENTIS, MICHELLE. 1987. "The Study of Aphasia and Closed Head Injury from a Philosophy of Science Perspective," unpublished monograph, University of California, Santa Barbara.
———AND CAROL A. PRUTTING. 1987. "Cohesion in the Discourse of Normal and Head-Injured Adults," *J. Speech Hear. Res.,* 30, 88–98.
MOFENSON, H. C., AND J. GREENSHER. 1979. "Poisonings—An Update," *Clin. Peds.,* 18, 144–46.
NUSSBAUM, ELIEZER, AND J. CARLOS MAGGI. 1988. "Pentobarbital Therapy Does Not Improve Neurologic Outcome in Nearly Drowned, Flaccid-Comatose Children," *Peds.,* 81, 630–34.
PARISIER, SIMON C. 1983. "Injuries of the Ear and Temporal Bone," in *Pediatric Otolaryngology,* vol. I. ed. Charles D. Bluestone and Sylvan E. Stool. Philadelphia: Saunders.
RIDING, KEITH H., AND CHARLES D. BLUESTONE. 1982. "Burns and Acquired Strictures of the Esophagus," in *Pediatric Otolaryngology,* vol. I. ed. Charles D. Bluestone and Sylvan E. Stool. Philadelphia: Saunders.
RIVARA, FREDERICK P., AND MELVIN BARBER. 1985. "Demographic Analysis of Childhood Pedestrian Injuries," *Peds.,* 76, 375–81.
ROGERS, BLAIR O. 1963. "Some Congenital and Acquired Deformities Causing Facial Disfigurement," in *Facial Disfigurement,* ed. Blair O. Rogers. Washington, DC: U.S. Department of Health, Education, and Welfare.
RUTTER, MICHAEL. 1987. "Continuities and Discontinuities from Infancy," in *Handbook of Infant Development* 2nd ed., ed. Joy Doniger Osofsky. New York: John Wiley.
———OLIVER CHADWICK, AND DAVID SHAFFER. 1983. "Head Injury," in *Developmental Neuropsychiatry,* ed. Michael Rutter. New York: Guilford Press.
SATZ, PAUL, AND CAROL BULLARD-BATES. 1981. "Acquired Aphasia in Children," in *Acquired Aphasia,* ed. Martha Taylor Sarno. New York: Academic Press.
SILVERMAN, FREDERICK N. 1987. "Child Abuse: The Conflict of Underdetection and Over-reporting," *Peds.,* 80, 440–43.
SWISHER, LINDA. 1985. "Language Disorders in Children," in *Speech and Language Evaluation in Neurology: Childhood Disorders,* ed. John K. Darby. Orlando, FL: Grune & Stratton.
TRON, V. A., V. J. BALDWIN, AND G. E. PIRIE. 1985. "Hot Tub Drownings," *Peds.,* 75, 789–90.
VAN DONGEN, H. R., AND M. C. B. LOONEN. 1977. "Factors Related to Prognosis of Acquired Aphasia in Children," *Cortex,* 13, 131–36.
VARTIAINEN, EERO, SEPPO KARJALAINEN, AND JUHANI KARJA. 1985. "Vestibular Disorders Following Head Injury in Children," *Intl. J. Ped. Otolaryngol.,* 9, 135–41.
WAGENAAR, ALEXANDER C., AND DANIEL W. WEBSTER. 1986. "Preventing Injuries to Children through Compulsory Automobile Safety Seat Use," *Peds.,* 78, 662–72.
WOODS, BRYAN T., AND SUSAN CAREY. 1979. "Language Deficits after Apparent Clinical Recovery from Childhood Aphasia," *Ann. in Neurol.,* 6, 405–49.
WOOLF, ALAN, et al. 1987. "Prevention of Childhood Poisoning: Efficacy of an Educational Program Carried Out in an Emergency Clinic," *Peds.,* 80, 359–63.
YARINGTON, C. THOMAS, JR. 1977. "Maxillofacial Trauma in Children," *Otolaryngol. Clin. N. Amer.,* 10, 25–32.

ZWIREN, GERALD T., H. GIBBS ANDREWS, AND THOMAS RODERICK HESTER, JR. 1985. "Progress in Treating Lye Burn Injuries of the Esophagus in Children," in *The Injured Child,* ed. Benjy Frances Brooks. Austin: University of Texas Press.

6

Complex Craniofacial Disorders

"Prevention" is a brush with a broad stroke. At its most obvious and effective level, prevention can refer to the eradication of an infectious disease with the use of a vaccine, as in the dramatic reduction in rubella embryopathy that has occurred because of the widespread use of rubella vaccine in children (see Chapter 4). At another level, the recognition of teratogenic agents—such as alcohol, hydantoin, thalidomide, trimethadione, and warfarin—can lead to making certain drugs (such as thalidomide) unavailable, or warning pregnant women to avoid exposure to potential teratogens such as alcohol. At yet another level, prevention can be applied by providing good prenatal care. Endemic cretinism, caused by a severe iodine deficiency, is rarely seen any more, thus eliminating a potent contributor to the population of hearing impaired and cognitively disordered children. At a more controversial level, chromosomal disorders can now be easily and safely detected prenatally, and mothers who have balanced translocations that could predispose them to having children with aneuploidies (abnormal chromosome complements) can be identified by karyotypes.

In the types of cases cited above (rubella embryopathy, fetal alcohol effects, cretinism, trisomy 21) pregnancies result in children with multiple malformations (including major craniofacial anomalies) that are totally preventable. However, there are many conditions involving major craniofacial anomalies that are difficult or impossible to detect with today's state of the art and that contribute largely to the pool of children

This chapter was written by Robert J. Shprintzen, Ph.D., director, Center for Craniofacial Disorders, Montefiore Medical Center, and professor of plastic surgery and professor of otolaryngology, Albert Einstein College of Medicine, Yeshiva University, Bronx, New York.

with disorders of resonance, articulation, voice, and hearing. Most of these conditions are rare, so that even the most experienced clinicians may have seen only a few cases. Others are more common among the communicatively impaired population, yet often go unrecognized as specific diagnostic entities because the sciences of *dysmorphology* and syndromology are not a part of the speech-language-hearing curricula. The combination of inexperience and an inability to recognize many disorders has led to a relatively sparse contribution to the process of syndrome delineation from clinicians in the communicative sciences.

The purposes of this chapter are to provide the reader with a conceptual framework regarding the relationship of communicative impairment to congenital anomalies of the craniofacial complex and to discuss prevention in a somewhat different way than elsewhere in this volume.

Individuals who study children with congenital anomalies are referred to as dysmorphologists or syndromologists. Dysmorphologists tend to characterize anomalies in several different ways—for example, according to severity. Minor anomalies are those that are abnormal, yet do not of necessity require treatment or affect the quality and/or quantity of life. Accessory ear tags, missing fingernails, supernumerary teeth, and patches of depigmented or hyperpigmented skin are examples of minor anomalies. Major anomalies, then, are those that do affect the quantity or quality of life and usually require treatment. Cleft palate, hydrocephalus, microtia, missing limbs, and *aglossia* are examples of major anomalies. Even disorders of function are regarded as anomalies; thus, disorders of speech, hearing, language, and cognition are also considered to be birth defects by dysmorphologists. Clearly, the assumption made by the dysmorphologist or syndromologist is that such functional deficits have their roots in structural (or organic, if you prefer) abnormalities.

Dysmorphologists also categorize anomalies according to other parameters, such as etiology, the body part or system affected, and age of onset. All of these ways of looking at complex multiple anomaly syndromes are important because they give the clinician the power of insight and the power of prediction.

INSIGHT AND PREDICTION

In attempting to reach a firm diagnosis of a syndrome (i.e., trying somehow to relate the multiple problems observed in one child), clinicians try to determine the exact extent of the problem with which they are presented, what to do about the problem, and what the expected outcome might be. Therefore, an insight toward the full clinical picture must somehow be developed. Syndromologists call the full clinical picture the phenotypic spectrum. The future course of the disorder and how it will respond to treatment is known as the natural history of the syndrome. The eventual outcome is referred to as the prognosis. By knowing the phenotypic spectrum, natural history, and prognosis, the clinician has actually achieved insight and prediction.

Phenotypic Spectrum

Phenotypic spectrum refers to all of the problems—observed, probable, or possible—associated with a particular syndrome. For example, velocardiofacial (Shprintzen) syndrome (Figure 6–1) is a relatively common genetic multiple anomaly syndrome with over 30 known traits (Shprintzen 1988b; Shprintzen et al. 1979, 1981; Williams, Shprintzen, and Goldberg 1985). Among the traits are severe hypernasality, learning disabilities, language impairment, congenital heart disease, cleft palate (most frequently submucous or occult submucous cleft palate), eye anomalies, mild growth deficiency, immunologic and metabolic abnormalities,

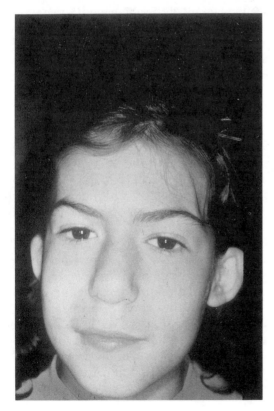

FIGURE 6–1.
Eight-year-old girl with velocardiofacial (Shprintzen) syndrome
SOURCE: All illustrations for this chapter were provided by Dr. Robert J. Shprintzen.

and a characteristic face. Many of the anomalies associated with this syndrome are minor and difficult to detect. Among the major anomalies, some require laboratory investigation, radiographic studies, and other specialized tests. Therefore, if not looked for specifically, many of these hard-to-detect anomalies would go unnoticed.

If a clinician were to be presented with a child who had a history of hypernasal speech in the absence of overt cleft palate, a ventriculoseptal defect (a congenital heart lesion), and language impairment, that clinician might suspect velocardiofacial syndrome. Therefore, referrals would be made to the appropriate professionals to look for suspected abnormalities reported to be found in this syndrome. Nasapharyngoscopy could be done to determine if a submucous or occult submucous cleft were present (Croft et al. 1978; Lewin, Croft, and Shprintzen 1980) and to determine if the internal carotid arteries were in a position making pharyngeal flap surgery excessively risky (MacKenzie-Stepner et al. 1987). Thymic hormone studies could be performed to see if the patient has an immunologic deficiency predisposing to chronic infections such as serous otitis and pneumonia. Complete cognitive testing could be ordered—and so on. In other words, a search would be made for all of the abnormalities reported to be associated with the syndrome. By thoroughly investigating the phenotypic spectrum, the clinician has helped to confirm the diagnosis and has identified all possible problems. A problem discovered can be treated, whereas one left uncovered could turn out to be an unpleasant surprise at a later date.

Natural History

Once a disorder has been identified, its course over time should be known so that necessary diagnostic efforts and treatments can be applied at the appropriate times. In the velocardiofacial syndrome example, learning disabilities have been reported in all known cases to date (Golding-Kushner, Weller, and Shprintzen 1985; Shprintzen 1988b; Shprintzen et al. 1978, 1981; Williams, Shprintzen, and Goldberg 1985). However, in early cognitive testing, the majority of patients with velo-cardiofacial syndrome have normal scores. The cognitive dysfunctions do not become obvious until school age and are specific to the abstraction abilities necessary for reading comprehension and mathematical reasoning (Golding-Kushner, Weller, and Shprintzen 1985; Shprintzen 1988b). If the clinician knows that the natural history of velocardiofacial syndrome predicts the development of these learning problems, appropriate educational supervision can be provided, and the child will not be delayed in the immediate application of proper class placement or resource room help.

Prognosis

If one can predict the eventual outcome of a disorder, realistic long-range goals can be made and appropriate counseling applied. In velocardiofacial syndrome, the reading and mathematical skills of these children can be improved with intensive educational efforts. However, regardless of the time and energy spent on remediating these learning disabilities, they will remain lifelong problems. Abstraction in general will always be a weakness, so the adult life of a patient with the syndrome needs to be planned in order to keep daily events concrete and simple. The prognosis for the complete habilitation of these problems is very poor. Therefore, rather than perpetually attempting to remediate these specific learning problems, educational and vocational efforts should be restructured to exclude unsuccessful confrontations with abstract concepts.

A NEW PERSPECTIVE ON PREVENTION

By arriving at a primary diagnosis for the child with multiple anomalies and delineating the disorder's phenotypic spectrum, natural history, and prognosis, a new perspective on prevention becomes evident. This new perspective takes several different forms: (1) the prevention of frustration, (2) the prevention of unnecessary or dangerous treatments, (3) the prevention of missed opportunities, (4) the prevention of progression, and (5) the prevention of uncertainty.

The Prevention of Frustration

When a child is born with multiple anomalies, it is usual for each abnormality to be studied separately by the specialist who would customarily evaluate or treat that problem. For example, a child with *Stickler syndrome* (Stickler et al. 1965) often presents with micrognathia, a cleft palate, and upper airway obstruction (Figure 6–2). This combination often prompts the diagnosis of *Pierre Robin syndrome,* an essentially nonexistent disorder (Shprintzen 1988a). More appropriately named the Robin sequence (Sadewitz and Shprintzen 1986), it is a nonspecific association of clinical findings with multiple etiologies. True syndromes have only a single etiology (see Chapter 1). Therefore, the family of this child needs to overcome the initial shock of life-threatening upper airway obstruction and then subsequently face major surgery to repair the palate. Once past these initial problems, the family may think that they are "out of the woods," when all of a sudden a severe myopia is detected. Other problems detected later could include chronic joint pains. Repeated visits to orthopedists may fail

FIGURE 6–2. Three-year-old child with Stickler syndrome. Note the round face, short nose, and anteverted nostrils (*right*) and epiphyseal dysplasia at the ankle (*left*).

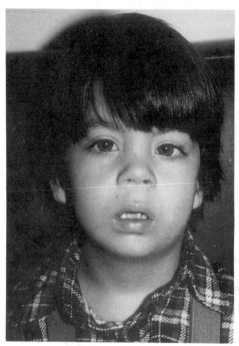 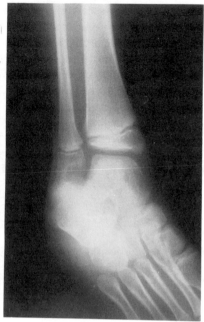

to explain this problem. Eye problems could worsen. A mild to moderate sensory hearing loss may also be detected, as reported by Konigsmark and Gorlin (1976) in some 15 percent of the patients they reviewed.

In other words, at each new turn, the child seems to be developing a new problem, but without adequate explanation from treating doctors as to why. The plastic surgeon who repaired the palate may have given correct counseling about children with cleft palate, the ophthalmologist about children with myopia, the audiologist or otolaryngologist about children with hearing loss, and the orthopedist about children with joint pains, but none of them gave the parents the one piece of information that would have tied everything together—the diagnosis of Stickler syndrome. Had that diagnosis been made, they could have supplied the phenotypic spectrum that includes myopia with possible *vitreoretinal degeneration, epiphyseal dysplasia* resulting in arthritic pain, sensory hearing loss, a narrow airway predisposing the patient to obstructive *apnea,* and both mandibular and maxillary hypoplasia. Knowing that these symptoms are expected parts of the syndrome, the frustration involved in confronting unexplained problems is prevented. Some comfort is taken in the fact that the professionals managing the patient know what is happening and what to anticipate.

The Prevention of Unnecessary or Dangerous Treatments

Knowing the natural history of a disorder, clinicians have the foresight to know which treatments have proven beneficial in the past, which have been futile or dangerous, and the appropriate timing for their application when necessary. In Prader-Willi syndrome, hypotonia is usually present in infancy and childhood. Hypernasality is a common sequela of the hypotonia. However, with increasing age, the hypotonia usually resolves and hypernasality along with it (Foushee 1987; Sadewitz and Shprintzen 1987). Clinicians unaware of the probable resolution of the hypernasality in Prader-Willi syndrome may be likely to refer these patients for pharyngeal flap surgery, which, in most cases, would be totally unnecessary.

Dangerous treatments can also be predicted once a syndrome has been diagnosed. A similar example, cleft palate is a frequent finding in the Treacher Collins syndrome (Figure 6–3). On occasion, following palate repair or as a result of a submucous cleft palate, hypernasality may be present. However, the pharyngeal airway in Treacher Collins syndrome is known to be very small (Shprintzen et al. 1979; Shprintzen 1982), and obstructive apnea is recognized as a frequent complication of this

FIGURE 6–3. Adult male with Treacher Collins syndrome. Note the down-slanting eyes with lower lid defects (*left*) and the micrognathia and extension of hair onto the cheek (*right*).

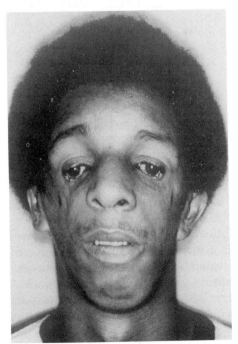
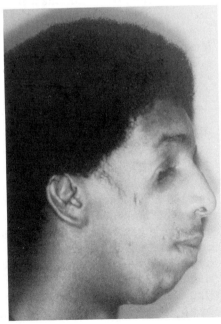

syndrome (Sher, Shprintzen, and Thorpy 1986; Shprintzen et al. 1979). Pharyngeal flap surgery would so severely compromise the airway in Treacher Collins syndrome that postoperative upper airway obstruction and death are possible complications. Pharyngeal flap surgery is, therefore, always contraindicated in Treacher Collins syndrome (Shprintzen 1982).

The Prevention of Missed Opportunities

Knowing the natural history of a syndrome also prevents care providers from missing the opportunity to apply a treatment that could improve the quantity or quality of life. In Crouzon syndrome (Figure 6–4), the majority of affected individuals have *craniosynostosis,* or premature fusion of the cranial sutures. However, in infancy, many patients with Crouzon syndrome have widely patent fontanels. If a widely patent anterior fontanel were palpated, a clinician might mistakenly think that the patient did not have craniosynostosis and therefore not explore the matter further. But X-ray examinations will often reveal the presence of increased intracranial pressure in spite of a patent fontanel. In many patients, the cranium will become gradually more stenotic with time (Smith 1982). If the increased intracranial pressure is not relieved, neurologic complications could arise including increased pressure on the optic nerve, headaches, *ataxia,* and eventual cognitive impairment. If a *craniectomy* is performed early in life (within the first several months after birth), all such complications can be avoided. If left too long, these complications may become permanent. Also, when done early, craniectomy is far easier to do and has fewer complications than when done later in life. Missing the opportunity to do an early craniectomy could turn out to be a mistake causing lifelong regret.

The Prevention of Progression

Understanding the natural history of a syndrome will also tell the clinician when an anomaly could get progressively worse. Therefore, if treatments are available, the progression of the problem can be stopped. Hemifacial microsomia (also known as Goldenhar syndrome, oculo-auriculo-vertebral dysplasia, facio-auriculo-vertebral malformation sequence, first and second branchial arch syndrome) is a relatively common craniofacial disorder (Figure 6–5). The entire mandible tends to be underdeveloped, but one side is generally worse than the other. As the child grows, the more normal side of the mandible grows at a more rapid rate than the more hypoplastic side. Therefore, the face develops a "rotational" abnormality in that the concavity of the more abnormal side becomes progressively worse, thus accentuating the facial asymmetry. This progression can be avoided by applying early surgery to lengthen the mandible on the more deficient

FIGURE 6–4. Three-year-old girl with Crouzon syndrome who did not have early craniectomy. Note the severe exorbitism (*top*), the abnormal skull shape (*center*), and "beaten metal" appearance of the skull indicating the convolutions of the brain being "etched" on the inner surface of the cranium (*bottom*).

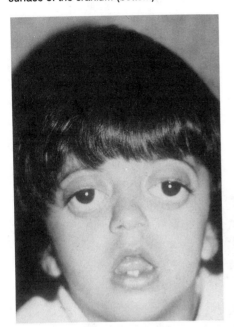

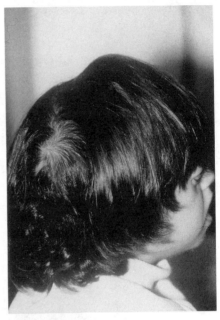

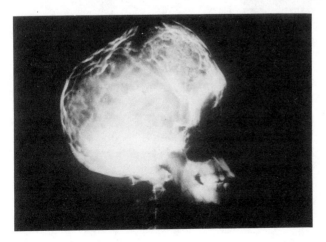

FIGURE 6–5.   Nineteen-year-old male with untreated hemifacial microsomia in frontal (*left*) and both profile (*center* and *right*) views. Note the grade three microtia (*center*).

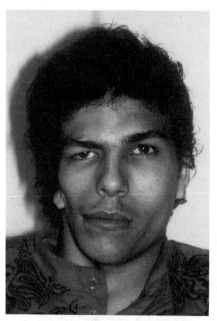

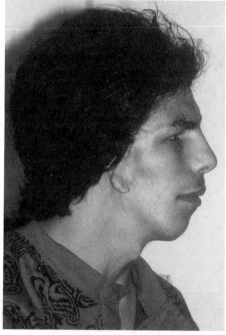

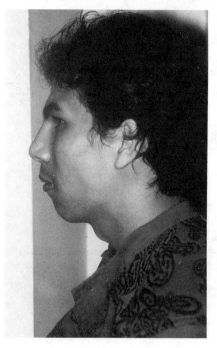

side and orthodontically redirecting future growth. Therefore, progression of some disorders can be prevented by knowing the future course of the syndrome.

The Prevention of Uncertainty

An accurate diagnosis yields an accurate prognosis. Although on occasion a prognosis can be poor, perhaps even dismal, the certainty of an accurate prognosis has been regarded as preferable to uncertainty. On occasion, it may take time for the natural defense mechanism of denial to be resolved, but the predictive value of prognosis, especially when confirmed by actual events, allows parents to get on with the rest of their lives while still realistically attending to the needs of the child. Delivering a prognosis, of course, must be tempered with allowance for clinical variability. It is dangerous for any clinician to make a snap judgment. The clinician must balance the truth with equal parts of candor and kindness.

IS THIS APPLICABLE?

This discussion may seem more akin to a genetic counselor's text than one for specialists in the communicative sciences. However, any professional having a hand in patient care must be able to discuss a patient's condition with clarity. The clinician must also be prepared to refer to other specialists who can provide as much information as is necessary for a complete delineation of the disorder. Is this type of discussion applicable to communicative disorders specialists? Most certainly. There have already been litigations against speech pathologists and audiologists for failing to recognize certain congenital malformations and to refer appropriately. Obviously, if a speech pathologist or audiologist did not know a disorder's phenotypic spectrum, he or she would not even know to whom to refer the patient. Therefore, in the next section, some of the more readily recognized and more common craniofacial multiple anomaly disorders are listed. The phenotypic spectrum is given, along with the natural history, the prognosis, and the communicative consequences. When appropriate, prevention is also detailed.

COMPLEX CRANIOFACIAL MULTIPLE ANOMALY DISORDERS

There are literally hundreds of complex syndromes involving craniofacial anomalies. Describing all of them would far exceed the scope of this chapter and would merit a separate text. There are some excellent catalogs of these syndromes, and three in particular are recommended: Buyse (1988), Cohen, Gorlin, and Levin (1988), and Smith (1982). Described below are 60 categories of disorders, including over 50 specific syndromes. They are described in terms of their etiology, phenotypic spectrum, natural history, and prognosis. Also described are the communicative impairments often found associated with these disorders. Finally, preventive factors are also listed.

Achondroplasia Syndrome (Figure 6-6)

Etiology: Autosomal dominant genetic disorder.

Phenotypic spectrum: Small stature, macrocephaly, constricted foramen magnum occasionally resulting in hydrocephalus, frontal bossing, saddle nose, short anterior cranial base, anterior skeletal open bite, kyphosis and/or lordosis, small hands, anomalous pelvis, and multiple skeletal abnormalities.

Natural history: Disproportionate small stature tends to become progressively worse through adult life; craniofacial growth becomes more abnormal with time, with anterior skeletal open bite becoming progressively worse; obstructive sleep apnea may occur secondary to the severely abnormal skull base and compromised upper airway (Goldstein et al. 1985); chronic serous otitis is common; obesity is relatively common after menses.

FIGURE 6–6.   Eight-year-old girl with achondroplasia syndrome in frontal (*left*) and profile (*right*) views. Note anterior open bite, depressed nasal root, obtuse nasolabial angle, and frontal bossing.

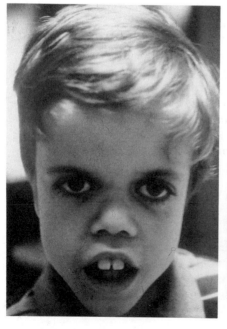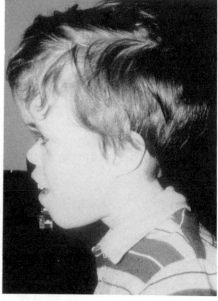

Prognosis: Intellect is usually normal unless hydrocephalus is severe; life span is essentially normal, although complications secondary to apnea, skeletal anomalies, and chronic upper airway compromise may contribute to earlier death.

Communication: Hyponasality, conductive hearing loss, articulatory impairment secondary to anterior skeletal open bite.

Prevention: The facial anomalies are secondary to the very abnormal cranial base and therefore are not easily modified; orthodontia to close the skeletal open bite is strongly contraindicated; constant monitoring for the development of obstructive sleep apnea should be implemented; treatment for increased growth, such as growth hormone, is also strongly contraindicated as individuals with achondroplasia secrete normal amounts of growth hormone; genetic counseling should be offered; shunts for hydrocephalus are typically not indicated; airway obstruction may require tracheostomy or other surgery; ventilating tubes may be applied to prevent conductive hearing loss.

ADAM Sequence (Amniotic Disruptions, Amputations, and Mutilations) (Figure 6–7)

Etiology: Mechanical disruption from amniotic tears and adhesions.

Phenotypic spectrum: Various structural anomalies, especially of the limbs and craniofacial complex, including amputations, clefting of the face, lip, and palate, ringlike constrictions of the limbs, and other tissue disruptions.

Natural history: This is a nonprogressive disorder with the structural anomalies present at birth comprising the entire phenotypic spectrum.

Prognosis: Intellect is normal unless the cranium and brain have been involved; growth and development will be normal with the only affected functions being those related to the structural anomalies caused by disruptions.

Communication: Hypernasality secondary to cleft palate.

Prevention: None known.

Apert Syndrome (Figure 6–8)

Etiology: Autosomal dominant genetic disorder.

Phenotypic spectrum: Craniosynostosis, short anterior cranial base, constriction of foramen magnum, hydrocephalus; cleft palate, soft tissue hypertrophy of hard palate, maxillary hypoplasia, beak nose; *exorbitism, hypertelorism; syndactyly* and *symphalangism* of hands and feet, valgus thumbs, short humerus, radial-humeral *synostosis;* acne vulgaris; chronic middle ear disease with conductive hearing loss; obstructive airway problems and obstructive sleep apnea.

FIGURE 6–7. Newborn with ADAM sequence showing complete facial clefts extending from the orbits through the lip (*top*) and multiple digital amputations (*bottom*).

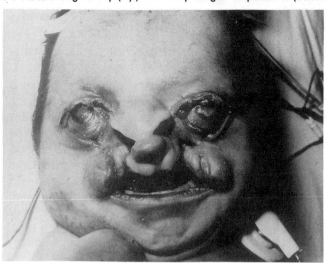

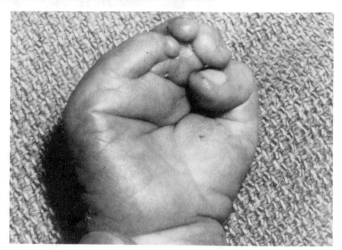

Natural history: The facies at birth are often relatively normal in appearance, but will begin to show evidence of increasing maxillary hypoplasia early in childhood; anterior skeletal open bite may be evident in childhood and gets progressively worse with age; with surgery, digits can be sufficiently separated to allow good manual function; although fontanels may be open in early infancy, craniosynostosis may still be present and usually progresses rapidly after birth, and craniectomies are almost always indicated.

Prognosis: The majority of patients with Apert syndrome probably have some cognitive deficiencies, and many are mentally retarded;

FIGURE 6–8. Seven-year-old child with Apert syndrome. At left, note the hypertelorism, down-slanting eyes, and downturned oral commissures. At right, note the "mitten hand."

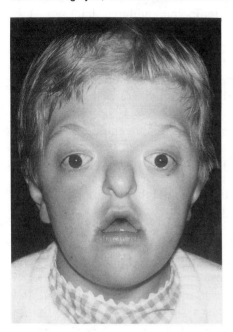 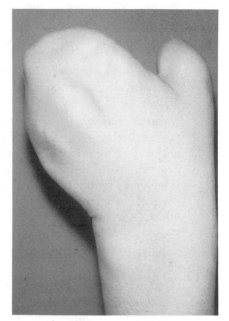

limitations of joint movement and syndactyly may reduce dexterity slightly, but can be overcome with treatment.

Communication: Hyponasality, occasionally (but rarely) hypernasality secondary to cleft palate; language impairment; articulation disorders secondary to anterior skeletal open bite and airway compromise.

Prevention: Early craniectomy and early limb surgery can help provide normal function, and aesthetic surgery can be timed according to the degree of midfacial deficiency to prevent severe degrees of stigmatization; attention should also be turned to the airway very early to avoid chronic hypoxia; although malocclusions are found in essentially all patients with Apert syndrome, they are not orthodontically correctable and require surgery of the facial skeleton for resolution; patients should be carefully monitored for hydrocephalus, and shunting may be necessary in some cases; chronic serous otitis may warrant ventilating tubes to prevent conductive hearing loss.

Arthrogryposis, Isolated Form (Amyoplasia Congenita Sequence)

Etiology: Arthrogryposis, multiple joint contractures present at birth, is a sequence (not a syndrome) and therefore of heterogeneous etiology.

When the contractures occur early in fetal development, a variety of secondary deformations can occur, including cleft palate, reduced mandibular opening caused by temperomandibular joint ankylosis or excessively tight throat and neck muscles, and micrognath.

Phenotypic spectrum: Multiple joint contractures, especially of the limbs, abnormal body position in infancy (such as "arched" back, torticollis, or *talipes equinovarus*), cleft palate, micrognathia, Robin deformation sequence, rounded shoulders, decreased muscle mass, dislocated hips.

Natural history: Decreased intrauterine movement is often reported during pregnancy, and delivery is frequently breech; because of the severe contractures and abnormal muscle forces on the limbs, growth may be deficient; muscle atrophy may progress if movement is severely restricted; motor milestones will be impaired because of restriction of movement, but intellectual milestones are usually within normal limits.

Prognosis: Cognitive prognosis is excellent; physical movement deficiencies remain evident but are variable, depending on the severity of the initial disorder.

Communication: Hypernasal resonance secondary to cleft palate is possible, but more problematic are the cases where mandibular movement is impaired; articulation may be disordered and oral resonance impaired because of limited oral opening; furthermore, palate repair may also be compromised by the inability of patients to open the mouth adequately for surgical or prosthetic treatment of the cleft.

Prevention: Occasionally, uterine or intrauterine abnormalities that cause fetal constriction can be detected prenatally; after birth, the early application of both physical therapy and orthopedic surgery can markedly decrease joint constrictions and thereby improve range of movement, including oral articulation.

BBB (Opitz) Syndrome (Opitz, Smith, and Summitt 1965)

Etiology: Autosomal dominant genetic disorder.

Phenotypic spectrum: Orbital hypertelorism; cleft palate or cleft lip and palate; low set and posteriorly rotated pinnae; hypospadias, cryptorchidism, abdominal hernias; strabismus, occasional cardiac anomalies; mild to moderate mental retardation.

Natural history: All anomalies are present at birth and neither improve nor worsen with age.

Prognosis: Unless cognitive deficiencies are severe, prognosis for habilitation with surgery is good.

Communication: Language impairment secondary to cognitive disorders; resonance and articulation may be impaired if clefting of the lip and/or palate is present.

Prevention: Reconstructive surgery for functional and aesthetic reasons is indicated with consideration for severity of cognitive impairment.

Beckwith-Wiedemann Syndrome (Figure 6–9)

Etiology: Probably an autosomal dominant genetic disorder (McKusick 1986).

Phenotypic spectrum: Overgrowth in childhood; omphalocele; thick subcutaneous tissue; advanced skeletal maturation, mandibular prognathism; macroglossia; metopic ridging; large fontanels, prominent occiput, creases in the earlobes; enlarged kidneys, enlarged pancreas, neonatal polycythemia, infantile hypoglycemia; cryptorchidism; cleft palate, Robin sequence.

Natural history: Robin sequence secondary to tongue enlargement may be present with upper airway obstruction (also related to lingual enlargement); neonatal course may be very difficult because

FIGURE 6–9. Infant with Beckwith-Wiedemann syndrome in frontal (*left*) and profile (*right*) views. Note the protrusive tongue and open mouth posture.

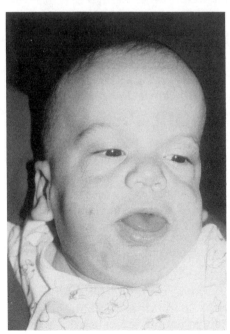
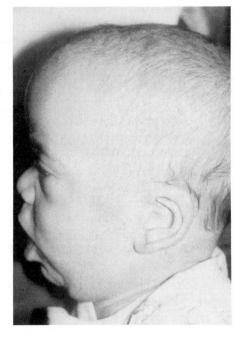

of numerous medical complications such as hypoglycemia and poly-cythemia; later in life, there is an increased risk of abdominal tumors such as Wilms tumor, gonadoblastoma, and adrenal carcinoma; hypotonia is possible in infancy, but improves with age; macrosomia (overgrowth), though often present in early childhood, gradually diminishes and eventual adult height is within normal limits; mandibular prognathism is more severe in early childhood, remains throughout life, but is less pronounced after puberty.

Prognosis: Cognitive prognosis is variable, ranging from normal to moderately impaired; the potential for the development of abdominal tumors warrants special attention; other associated anomalies, such as omphalocele and cleft palate, are surgically correctable.

Communication: Language impairment is evident in those children with cognitive impairment; the large tongue causes articulation problems, and palatal clefts may result in velopharyngeal insufficiency, which may subsequently result in compensatory articulation impairment.

Prevention: Relative to speech, early surgical intervention for the cleft palate and even tongue reduction when macroglossia is severe are indicated; omphalocele can be detected prenatally by ultrasound and also can be surgically repaired; because overgrowth is present only in early childhood, treatment is contraindicated; constant medical attention is essential because of the possibility of the eventual development of surgically removable abdominal tumors; the possibility of infantile hypoglycemia should also be heeded in case early steroid therapy becomes necessary.

Bilateral Femoral Dysgenesis Unusual Facies Syndrome
(Figure 6–10)

Etiology: Unknown, with all cases reported being sporadic, although one apparently autosomal dominant case has been described (Lampert 1980).

Phenotypic spectrum: Bilateral hypoplasia or aplasia of the femurs resulting in small stature; cleft palate, Robin sequence, short nose, up-slanting eyes, narrow alar base; occasional anomalies of the humerus bilaterally resulting in limitation of bend at the elbow, lower spine anomalies; absent labia majora in females, cryptorchidism in males, inguinal hernias, and toe anomalies.

Natural history: Robin sequence may initially result in upper airway obstruction and failure to thrive; cognitive milestones are within normal limits. The majority of patients are ambulatory even though the femurs may be severely hypoplastic or absent.

FIGURE 6–10. One-year-old child with bilateral femoral dysgenesis unusual facies syndrome. At the top, note micrognathia and short nose. At center, note the U-shaped palatal cleft indicative of Robin sequence. At the bottom left, note the absent upper leg and labia majora. At the bottom right, note the absent femurs.

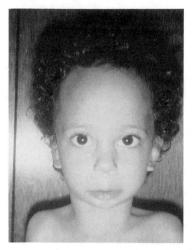
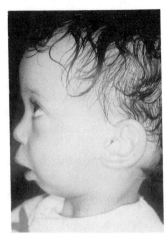
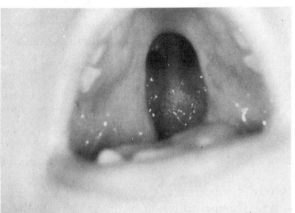
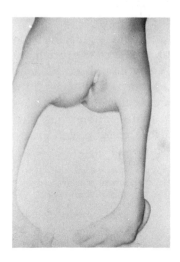
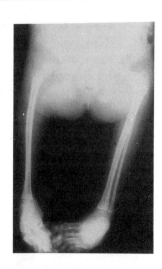

Prognosis: Ambulatory modifications are the major long-term problems associated with this syndrome. Cleft-related disorders are treated as in other patients with clefts.

Communication: Hypernasality secondary to cleft palate, articulation impairment secondary to VPI.

Prevention: Orthopedic surgery to the legs is generally contraindicated because the majority of patients with this syndrome become ambulatory. Physical therapy may be indicated in more severe cases. Palate repair may prevent hypernasality.

Carpenter Syndrome

Etiology: Probably autosomal recessive genetic disorder.

Phenotypic spectrum: Craniosynostosis, brachycephaly, posteriorly sloped forehead, dystopia canthorum, mental retardation, preaxial polydactyly of the feet (duplicated big toe), partial syndactyly of fingers and toes, brachydactyly, occasional congenital heart disease, abdominal hernias.

Natural history: Growth and development are generally impaired. There is usually marked delay of all milestones.

Prognosis: Variable, dependent on degree of cognitive impairment, which has been reported in nearly all cases.

Communication: Language impairment, oral resonance disorders secondary to craniosynostosis and resultant possible airway obstruction.

Prevention: Early craniectomy to relieve increased intracranial pressure. Early hand surgery to increase manual dexterity.

CHARGE Association (see Figure 1–2)

Etiology: Etiologically heterogenous with CHARGE being a nonrandom association that can occur in conjunction with several syndromes of known etiology (Shprintzen 1987).[1]

Phenotypic spectrum: CHARGE is an acronym signifying coloboma, heart disease, atresia of the choanae, retarded growth and development, genital anomalies, and ear anomalies. Specific anomalies include colobomas of the iris and retina, congenital heart defects, choanal atresia, small stature, mental retardation, *holoprosencephaly*, genital hypoplasia in males, anomalous auricles, sensory-neural or conductive hearing loss, cleft lip, cleft palate, micrognathia, and tracheoesophageal fistula.

---

[1]Although most of the literature refers to CHARGE association, some more recent work claims to have established it as a syndrome (Davenport, Hefner, and Mitchell 1986).

Natural history: Many infants with CHARGE association do not survive the neonatal period. Neonatal death has been caused by apnea, hypocalcemia, or congenital heart disease. The majority of patients have been born with a normal birth weight and length but subsequently fail to thrive and fall off the growth curve. Central nervous system anomalies become evident, and cognitive dysfunction is further hampered by both visual and hearing disorders.

Prognosis: Many of the congenital anomalies in CHARGE association may be life-threatening. If the infant survives the newborn period, the prognosis will depend on the severity of the cognitive and sensory defects. In general, prognosis for normal maturation and cognitive development is poor.

Communication: Conductive hearing loss, sensory-neural hearing loss, resonance disorders secondary to cleft palate, severe language impairment and possibly hyponasality secondary to choanal atresia, and articulation impairment secondary to VPI.

Prevention: Many of the defects associated with CHARGE association can be detected in utero by fetal ultrasound. Following birth, the congenital anomalies comprising the CHARGE spectrum must be treated symptomatically. Apnea may be prevented by surgical correction of the choanal atresia, which may also resolve feeding difficulties.

Chromosomal Syndromes (see Chapter 2)

Etiology: Additions or deletions of whole chromosomes or parts of chromosomes in some or all of the cells of the developing fetus. Numerous chromosomal syndromes have been reported and continue to be delineated as karyotyping becomes more sophisticated. Many chromosomal anomalies have been associated with advanced maternal age.

Phenotypic spectrum: Each separate chromosomal syndrome has its own phenotypic spectrum; however, the majority of them have severe anomalies as part of their phenotypic spectrum, including mental retardation, failure to thrive, small stature, and multiple structural anomalies.

Natural history: Each separate chromosomal syndrome has a very characteristic natural history such as Down syndrome (trisomy 21) that includes predictable patterns of developmental milestones, predictable somatic growth, and premature senility.

Prognosis: For many chromosomal syndromes, prognosis is extremely poor for normal life, though several chromosomal syndromes have less severe prognoses.

Communication: Language impairment is a very frequent finding associated with chromosomal syndromes. Cleft palate is similarly a frequent feature leading to resonance imbalance, and conductive or sensory-neural deafness may also occur in many chromosomal syndromes.

Prevention: Chromosomal syndromes can be detected in utero by amniocentesis or chorionic villus sampling. Furthermore, certain chromosomal disorders can be predicted based on karyotypes in the parents. In many chromosomal syndromes, vigorous treatment is contraindicated because of incompatibility with life.

Clefting and Oral Teratoma Syndrome (Figure 6–11)

Etiology: Sporadic disruption syndrome caused by the deforming effects of a *teratoma* inhibiting the fusion of an intrinsically normal embryonic palate.

Phenotypic spectrum: The presence of a teratoma will disrupt the normal fusion patterns of embryonic elements, and, therefore, depending on the location and size of the teratoma, various forms of cleft palate and other oral and cranial anomalies will be observed.

FIGURE 6–11. Cleft palate in a child with clefting and oral teratoma syndrome. Note the irregular shape of the cleft, which is a disruption secondary to the oral teratoma.

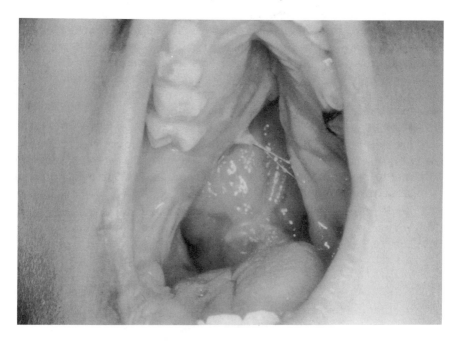

The most common finding is a wide and irregularly shaped cleft of the palate coinciding to the size and shape of the teratoma.

Natural history: Following removal of the teratoma, this presents as a static disorder without progression.

Prognosis: If the teratoma and cleft are treatable, the prognosis is good for normal life span and habilitation of associated structural anomalies.

Communication: Resonance imbalance secondary to cleft palate and possible language impairment secondary to central nervous system anomalies associated with the presence of the teratoma, articulation impairment secondary to VPI. If other portions of the oral cavity are also disrupted or deformed, articulation impairment may also be present.

Prevention: Fetal ultrasound may detect the presence of a large teratoma.

Cleidocranial Dysplasia Syndrome (Figure 6–12)

Etiology: Autosomal dominant genetic disorder.

Phenotypic spectrum: Abnormal cranial shape marked by frontal bossing, midline depressions of the cranium secondary to late closure of the fontanels. Relative to the forehead, the midface will often look deficient. The nasal bridge tends to be depressed. Cleft palate, late eruption of the permanent dentition, and abnormal tooth development; the clavicles may be absent or underdeveloped, and the chest may show decreased diameter. Anomalies of the fingers and fingernails have also been reported. Conductive hearing loss may also occur.

Natural history: Cognitive and motor development are usually normal. The absence of the clavicles generally does not cause any motor development problems, and the general course in this syndrome is benign. However, the fontanels may remain widely patent throughout childhood, and bone development, in general, may be significantly delayed. Communicative disorders and conductive hearing loss are usually mild to moderate.

Prognosis: There are generally normal life span and cognition.

Communication: Hypernasality secondary to cleft palate, articulation impairment secondary to both VPI and/or dental anomalies, conductive hearing loss.

Prevention: Widely patent fontanels through childhood may require protection if there is risk of brain injury. Because of abnormal dental development, vigorous dental hygiene is necessary. Ventilating tubes may be used to prevent conductive hearing loss.

FIGURE 6–12. Four-year-old child with cleidocranial dysplasia syndrome. Note the broad forehead (*top*) and the adduction of the shoulders because of the absent clavicles (*center* and *bottom*).

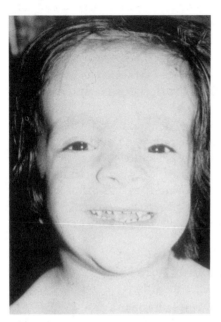

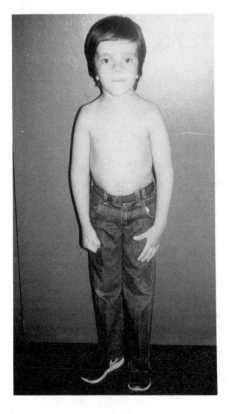

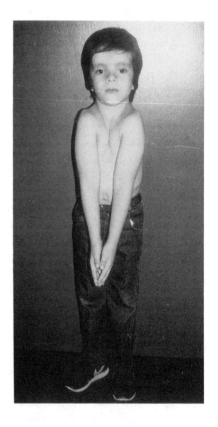

Cornelia de Lange Syndrome (Figure 6–13)

Etiology: Autosomal dominant genetic inheritance has been suggested (McKusick 1986), although most cases are sporadic. Both chromosomal and autosomal recessive etiologies have also been postulated.

Phenotypic spectrum: Short stature, mental retardation, rigid infantile posture, weak cry, microcephaly, abundant eyebrows connected in the midline (synophrys), thick curled eyelashes, short nose with depressed nasal root, hypoplastic alar cartilages, thin upper lip with downturned oral commissures, cleft palate, micrognathia, limb and digital anomalies, contractures of the elbows, genital anomalies,

FIGURE 6–13. Cornelia de Lange syndrome. Note the eyebrows and the microcephaly.

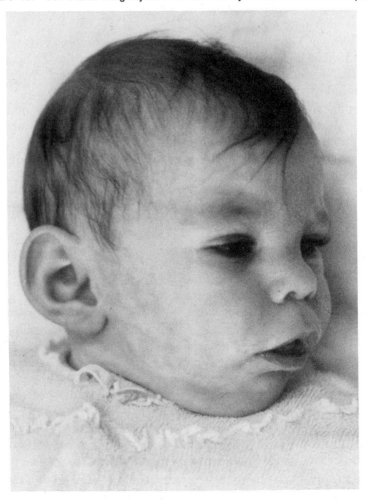

congenital heart anomalies, bowel anomalies, and failure to thrive common in the neonatal period. Cognitive impairment becomes immediately apparent and is very often severe. Chronic illness is common in infancy with apparently poor resistance to infections. Later in life, behavior may be almost autistic in nature, and self-destructive behavior has been observed. A distinctive behavioral profile has been reported.

Natural history: There is both prenatal and postnatal growth deficiency. Failure to thrive in the neonatal period is common, as is possible upper airway obstruction. Motor milestones are generally severely impaired, and behavior may often be very detached and inappropriate to the situation. Patients occasionally engage in self-mutilation. The combination of cognitive impairment and behavioral abnormality makes the quality of their social interactions very poor.

Prognosis: Long-range prognosis for normal quality of life is generally poor. There are frequent neonatal and infant deaths because of chronic illness, and significantly impaired behavior and intellect generally provide a poor prognosis for social interaction.

Communication: Failure to develop useful language or severe language impairment, voice abnormalities, resonance imbalance secondary to cleft palate.

Prevention: Because of the severity of the multiple congenital anomalies in this syndrome, certain treatments may not be indicated. For example, if there is no evidence of language development, palate repair would be contraindicated.

Craniofrontonasal Dysplasia Syndrome (Figure 6–14)
Etiology: Autosomal dominant genetic disorder.

Phenotypic spectrum: Orbital hypertelorism, cleft lip or cleft lip and cleft palate, cleft nose, agenesis of the corpus callosum, and longitudinal grooves in the fingernails. Chronic serous otitis is common.

Natural history: All anomalies, with the possible exception of the grooves in the fingernails, are readily apparent at birth. Unless the brain is significantly involved, both cognitive and motoric development are entirely within normal limits. The severe orbital hyper-telorism may result in eye muscle imbalance problems and strabismus.

Prognosis: The prognosis for normal development is generally favorable. However, in those patients with significant midline defects of the brain, more significant functional anomalies may be present.

Communication: Language impairment may be present if the brain is involved. Otherwise, resonance imbalance and articulation disor-

FIGURE 6–14. Fourteen-year-old girl with craniofrontal dysplasia syndrome

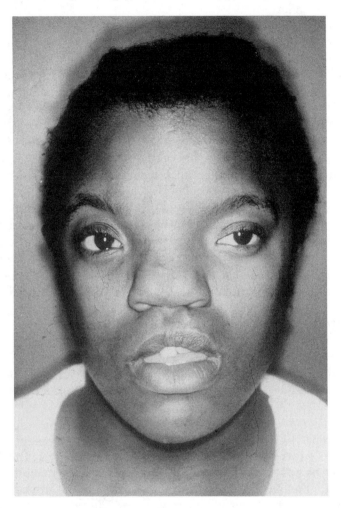

ders may occur secondary to cleft lip and/or cleft palate. Conductive hearing loss may also be present secondary to chronic serous otitis media.

Prevention: Unless cognitive impairment is severe, reconstructive surgery is indicated to prevent severe stigmatization. Ventilating tubes to prevent conductive hearing loss.

Craniometaphyseal Dysplasia

Etiology: There are both autosomal dominant and autosomal recessive genetic types of craniometaphyseal dysplasia. The recessive type is far more severe.

Phenotypic spectrum: Progressive osteosclerosis involving all of the body's bones.

Natural history: The osteosclerosis often first becomes noticed with development of an abnormal facies, including orbital hypertelorism and marked broadening of the root of the nose. Increasing sclerosis of the facial bones will often obstruct the nasal cavity and may also invade the temporal bone and middle ear causing both conductive hearing loss and sensory hearing loss. Less frequently, the osteo-sclerosis may impinge upon the optic nerve or facial nerves causing visual impairment or facial paresis.

Prognosis: The prognosis is poorer for the recessive form than the dominant form. However, in all cases, the disease is always progressive with variable expression.

Communication: Marked hyponasality, conductive hearing loss and sensory hearing loss. Cognitive development is generally within normal limits. There is a chronic open mouth posture secondary to nasal obstruction, which may result in articulatory disorders as well.

Prevention: Because of the progressive nature of this disorder, extensive reconstructive surgery may be contraindicated.

Crouzon Syndrome (Figure 6–4)
Etiology: Autosomal dominant genetic disorder.

Phenotypic spectrum: Cranial synostosis (premature fusion of the cranial sutures), hypoplasia of the midface, exorbitism, class III malocclusion, low set posteriorly rotated ears, and "beak"-shaped nose.

Natural history: Premature fusion of the cranial sutures with increased intracranial pressure may often be present at birth in more severe expressions. In milder expressions, the fontanels may be patent in spite of the fact that craniosynostosis is occurring. Fusion of the cranial sutures will occur in the maxilla as well as in the bones of the calvarium. There is a gradual worsening of an acute cranial base angle, which secondarily frequently leads to obstructive sleep apnea. Hydrocephalus may result secondary to the craniosynostosis and decreased circumference of the foramen magnum, which then causes aqueductal stenosis. The eyes tend to have a divergent *strabismus,* and *papilledema* may be seen from pressure on the optic nerve. If early craniectomies are not performed, skull shape may become severely abnormal, and the increasing intracranial pressure may result in cognitive impairment. Chronic serous otitis is common and conductive hearing loss may also be caused by anomalies of the middle ear space. The mandible tends to grow normally and, in relation to the severely deficient midface, a significant class III malocclusion often develops, which may include an anterior skeletal open bite.

Prognosis: With early treatment, the prognosis for normal development and normal life span is excellent.

Communication: Articulation impairment secondary to anterior skeletal open bite and malocclusion, conductive hearing loss and hyponasality secondary to nasal obstruction caused by a decreased circumference of the upper airway. When increased intracranial pressure is not relieved, language impairment may also result.

Prevention: The numerous secondary problems encountered in Crouzon syndrome can be avoided with early craniectomy. In addition, the physical stigmata of the syndrome can be treated successfully with craniofacial surgery. Chronic serous otitis should be treated with ventilating tubes. Airway compromise should be treated as early as possible in order to avoid chronic hypoventilation. Orthodontic therapy to normalize occlusion should be avoided because the problem is that of a skeletal discrepancy, not a dental one. Dental malocclusions require surgical management.

Diastrophic Dysplasia Syndrome

Etiology: Autosomal recessive genetic disorder.

Phenotypic spectrum: Prenatal and postnatal growth deficiency, limb anomalies, including talipes varus, limited bend of the digits and elbow, and, on occasion, hip or knee dislocation. Spinal curvature anomalies include scoliosis and kyphoscoliosis which may be progressive. Swelling of the auricles is common in infancy, which subsequently develops into hypertrophic ear cartilage. Micrognathia and a cleft palate occur frequently in the syndrome, thus resulting in the association of the Robin sequence. The larynx and trachea may be narrowed in diameter. Middle ear anomalies and chronic serous otitis are also present.

Natural history: Short stature is evident at birth. Frequently, with the Robin sequence associated as well as in combination with lower airway anomalies, respiratory obstruction can occur in the neonatal period and, if not treated immediately, result in death. Limitation of joint mobility and the developing kyphoscoliosis can result in multiple joint limitations and gait abnormalities. Growth continues slowly with a mean adult height of approximately 50 inches.

Prognosis: If patients with this syndrome survive the neonatal period, the prognosis for a normal life span is good, although progressive kyphoscoliosis and other skeletal anomalies of the torso may eventually result in other respiratory complications.

The multiple joint anomalies in this syndrome tend to be rather resistant to orthopedic correction.

Communication: Conductive hearing loss is a common finding; hypernasality secondary to cleft palate, articulation impairment secondary to VPI.

Prevention: Limb anomalies may be identified prenatally with ultrasound imaging. Early airway compromise should be anticipated and treated. Caution should be exercised with anesthesia. Ventilating tubes to prevent conductive hearing loss may be employed. Orthopedic surgery is generally contraindicated, and therefore should be avoided unless true benefit can be demonstrated.

EEC (Ectrodactyly-Ectodermal Dysplasia-Clefting Syndrome) (Figure 6–15)

Etiology: Autosomal dominant genetic disorder.

Phenotypic spectrum: Ectodermal dysplasia; cleft lip, cleft palate, or both; fair thin skin, abnormal thin and sparse hair; dental anomalies, including multiple missing teeth and poor enamel formation; photophobia, lacrimal duct stenosis; maxillary hypoplasia, and "lobster claw" with severely displastic nails.

Natural history: The anomalies are almost always present at birth, although, in milder expressions where the limbs are not severely

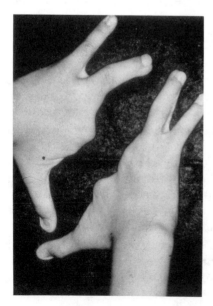

FIGURE 6–15.
Hands of a child with EEC syndrome. The syndactyly between the small finger and ring finger has been surgically repaired.

affected, the patients may present as children with clefts without associated anomalies. Eventual diagnosis of lacrimal duct stenosis and photophobia would give clues to the syndromatic diagnosis. Conductive hearing loss secondary to chronic serous otitis will also generally develop in early childhood. With chronic lacrimal duct stenosis, chronic ophthalmologic disease such as dacryocystitis may develop, resulting in eventual visual impairment.

Prognosis: Intellectual development is usually within normal limits, and manual dexterity can usually be very good because the thumb is unaffected in the majority of cases.

Communication: Hypernasality secondary to cleft palate and articulation disorders secondary to cleft lip and cleft palate and VPI may occur. Conductive hearing loss from chronic serous otitis media is also possible.

Prevention: The limb anomalies may be detected in utero, as could a cleft lip and cleft palate. After birth, surgery for complete habilitation of orofacial clefts is indicated. Separation of syndactylous digits will prevent more severe manual dexterity problems. Other cosmetic approaches can be taken, including cosmetic dentistry, prosthodontics, and the use of wigs. Ventilating tubes for chronic otitis. Lacrimal duct probing and/or surgery may be done to relieve dacryocystitis.

Fetal Alcohol Effects (Figure 6–16; see Chapter 4)

Etiology: Teratogenic (effects of ethanol).

Phenotypic spectrum: The phenotypic spectrum can be quite variable, depending on the timing and amount of alcohol consumed by the mother. Alcohol effects are transmitted maternally only. In its most severe form, fetal alcohol syndrome, the phenotypic spectrum includes low birth weight with prenatal and postnatal growth deficiency, mental retardation, heterotopia of the brain, short palpebral fissures, microcephaly, flattened philtrum with thin upper lip, a short nose, maxillary and mandibular hypoplasia, hypoplastic or missing fingernails, hypoplastic or missing distal phalanges of one or more fingers, characteristic palmar creases, congenital heart disease, and multiple behavioral manifestations, including extreme irritability as an infant and hyperactivity in childhood. Cleft palate is an underreported though common finding in this disorder, especially associated with micrognathia, thus also resulting in the Robin sequence.

Natural history: Failure to thrive in the neonatal period is common. Upper airway obstruction secondary to Robin sequence or

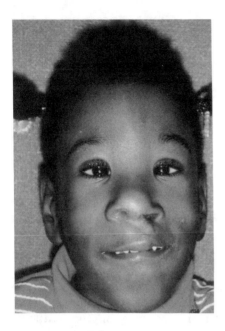

FIGURE 6–16.
Four-year-old child with fetal alcohol syndrome.
Note the short palpebral fissures.

micrognathia without clefting is common. Central apneas caused by severe brain anomalies may also be evident. Extreme irritability makes feeding extremely difficult, especially if care is being provided by an alcoholic mother. Cognitive developmental delay occurs frequently with delayed onset of most motor milestones. Mental retardation occurs in almost all cases of the fetal alcohol syndrome, and less significant cognitive impairment such as learning disability and language impairment can occur in milder fetal alcohol effects.

Prognosis: The abnormalities found are static, and the prognosis depends on the severity of the fetal alcohol effects present at birth.

Communication: Language impairment, hypernasality secondary to cleft palate, articulation disorder secondary to poor motor control, as well as cleft palate or cleft lip and palate. Conductive hearing loss secondary to chronic serous otitis.

Prevention: Avoidance of maternal alcohol consumption. Airway compromise should be anticipated and treated. Palate repair is contraindicated if cognitive dysfunction is severe enough to prevent language development. Chronic upper respiratory illnesses should be anticipated. Ventilating tubes to prevent conductive hearing loss. Special education placement to prevent school failure.

Fetal Hydantoin Effects (see Chapter 4)

Etiology: Teratogenic effect of hydantoin (an anticonvulsant).

Phenotypic spectrum: The phenotypic spectrum of fetal hydantoin syndrome will also be dependent on the dose and timing of delivery of the medication as well as the mother's ability to absorb the medication. In its most severe form, fetal hydantoin syndrome shows both prenatal and postnatal growth deficiency, cognitive impairment, facial anomalies, including a depressed nasal root, short nose, thin upper lip, cleft lip and cleft palate, or cleft palate only, micrognathia, multiple limb anomalies, including hypoplasia of the distal phalanges with small or absent fingernails, especially on the fourth and fifth fingers, occasionally a triphalangeal thumb, esotropia, mild hirsutism, and several other low frequency anomalies, including congenital heart disease, abdominal hernias, pyloric stenosis, and genital anomalies. Occasionally, the combination of cleft palate and micrognathia will prompt the diagnosis of Robin sequence.

Natural history: Following relatively low birth weight, failure to thrive occurs with frequency. This may be related both to upper airway obstruction and central nervous system impairment. Past the newborn period, general health is normal.

Prognosis: The prognosis is dependent on the severity of the effects of fetal exposure to hydantoin. In general, life span is unaffected, and the degree of cognitive deficiency is mild.

Communication: Language impairment, hypernasality secondary to cleft palate, articulation impairment secondary to VPI, mild conductive hearing loss secondary to chronic serous otitis media.

Prevention: Close monitoring of maternal blood levels of hydantoin can reduce risk prenatally. Airway obstruction and failure to thrive may be anticipated and prevented with adequate airway maintenance techniques and modified feeding regimens. Palate repair is indicated. Ventilating tubes for serous otitis. Special class placement to avoid school failure.

Freeman-Sheldon Syndrome (Figure 6–17)

Etiology: Autosomal dominant genetic disorder.

Phenotypic spectrum: Small, puckered mouth, deep-set eyes, long philtrum, cranial base anomalies, cleft palate, Robin sequence, small tongue, camptodactyly (finger contractures) with ulnar deviation of the fingers, and talipes equinovarus.

Natural history: Birth is often in breech presentation. There may be early upper airway obstruction and failure to thrive. Limb contractures may improve slightly with age, but usually remain unchanged. Facial appearance improves with age. Scoliosis may develop in later childhood. Cognitive functioning is usually normal.

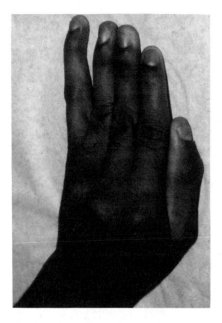

FIGURE 6–17.
Hand of an individual with Freeman-Sheldon syndrome showing the ulnar deviation of the fingers

Prognosis: Life span and cognitive functioning are normal. With surgical intervention, limb use can be greatly improved. Palate repair is indicated, but care should be taken to protect the airway.

Communication: Hypernasality secondary to cleft palate, articulation impairment secondary to VPI, reduced oral resonance secondary to small mouth, chronic serous otitis media and conductive hearing loss, reduced oral articulator mobility.

Prevention: Surgery for contractures should be deferred until there is sufficient growth and time to see if the problem will resolve partially or wholly. Palate repair and ventilating tubes are indicated, as is speech therapy for reduced articulator mobility.

G Syndrome (Opitz-Frias Syndrome) (Figure 6–18)
Etiology: X-linked recessive genetic trait.

Phenotypic spectrum: Hypertelorism, hypospadias, cleft palate or cleft lip-cleft palate, laryngeal cleft, bifid scrotum, cryptorchidism, low set posteriorly rotated ears, pulmonary hypoplasia.

Natural history: Male infants with this syndrome may have dysphagia, aspiration, weak cry, and failure to thrive secondary to laryngeal cleft. Males are more severely affected than female carriers, who show only minor stigmata, such as mild hypertelorism. Dysphagia and respiratory difficulty resolve with age unless the laryngeal cleft is severe. Profound sensory-neural hearing loss has been found in one patient.

FIGURE 6–18. Twelve-year-old boy with severe expression of G (Opitz-Frias) syndrome in frontal (*left*) and profile (*right*) views

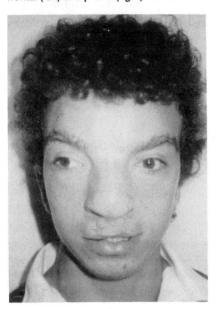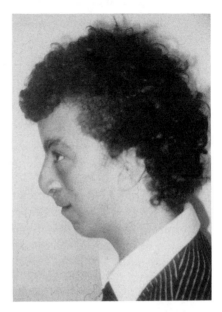

Prognosis: Life expectancy is normal if the infant survives the neonatal period. Several patients have displayed learning disabilities and even mild cognitive impairment.

Communication: Hoarse voice, possible sensory-neural hearing loss, hypernasality secondary to clefting, articulation impairment secondary to VPI, language impairment.

Prevention: Surgical repair of laryngeal cleft will prevent aspiration and voice problems. Cleft repair is indicated if cognitive or hearing impairment is not profound. In female carriers, reconstructive surgery is contraindicated, but in males, the severe hypertelorism may warrant craniofacial reconstruction.

Hemifacial Microsomia (Facioauriculovertebral Malformation Sequence, Goldenhar Syndrome, Oculo-Auriculo-Vertebral Dysplasia) (Figure 6–5)

Etiology: Generally reported to be sporadic, but several familial cases have been reported, including apparent autosomal dominant transmission in a number of cases. This is an etiologically heterogenous sequence, rather than a specific syndrome.

Phenotypic spectrum: Facial asymmetry with one side of the face showing hypoplasia. Occasionally both sides of the face are affected, but asymmetry is almost always present. Microtia, accessory ear tags, preauricular pits, mandibular hypoplasia (generally unilateral, occasionally bilateral), facial palsy, ocular choristomas (dermoid cysts), cleft palate or cleft lip-cleft palate, eyelid clefts, unilateral macrostomia (commissural cleft), conductive hearing loss (usually unilateral), occasional sensory-neural hearing loss, vertebral anomalies (especially of the cervical spine), and occasional microphthalmia or anophthalmia.

Natural history: At birth, facial asymmetry may be difficult to appreciate, but microtia or accessory ear tags may be present. Upper airway obstruction is common secondary to mandibular and pharyngeal anomalies, and failure to thrive may result. With growth, the facial asymmetry becomes increasingly more severe. The affected side of the face shows worsening concavity. Facial palsy may be partial or complete on one side.

Prognosis: If early airway obstruction is resolved, life span is normal and reconstructive surgery can largely resolve the aesthetic and functional problems associated with facial hypoplasia. Though some patients have been reported to be mentally retarded, the majority have normal intellect.

Communication: Conductive hearing loss, occasional sensory-neural hearing loss, hypernasality secondary to pharyngeal asymmetry.

Prevention: Early mandibular surgery can redirect facial growth in a more symmetrical plane. Standard pharyngeal flap surgery should not be performed in this group of patients because of the risk of airway obstruction and because velopharyngeal gaps are usually skewed to the affected side rather than being central in location. Amplification is essential when hearing loss is bilateral.

Holoprosencephaly Sequence (Figures 6–19, 6–20, and 6–21)

Etiology: Etiologically heterogenous malformation sequence with some reported autosomal dominant cases, chromosomally transmitted cases, and teratogenic cases. Holoprosencephaly has been reported in association with trisomy 13, trisomy 4p, 4p-deletion, 13q- deletion, 18p- deletion, velocardiofacial syndrome, and CHARGE association.

Phenotypic spectrum: The facial and CNS anomalies in this disorder can vary significantly from case to case. In general, the disorder is one of abnormal midline cerebral septation and facial development. In its most severe form, cyclopia with total absence of midline brain septation is present. Hypotelorism, nasal anoma-

FIGURE 6–19. Two neonates with holoprosencephaly sequence. The baby at the top has the premaxillary agenesis type. Note the severe hypotelorism and absence of the midline nasal structures. The infant at the bottom has the cebocephaly type with a nostril with only a single opening that ends in a blind pit.

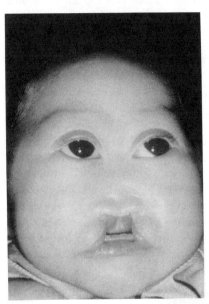

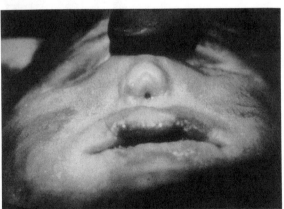

lies (such as a nose with a single nostril), dental anomalies (single central incisor), brain anomalies ranging from a single undifferentiated holosphere to more normal brain development (Figure 6–20) with absence of the corpus callosum and other midline structures, absence of the olfactory tracts or bulbs, anosmia, frontal lobe deficiency, cleft lip, cleft palate, midline cleft lip, microcephaly, pituitary

FIGURE 6–20. The brain of a baby with alobar holoprosencephaly. At the top, the holoprosencephalic brain (left side) is compared to a control specimen from a baby of the same age who did not have holoprosencephaly. Note the absence of a sagittal fissure in the holoprosencephalic brain. At the bottom, the brains shown at left have been sectioned transversely. Note the single central ventricle in holoprosencephalic brain on the left side; the normal brain has normal ventricular differentiation.

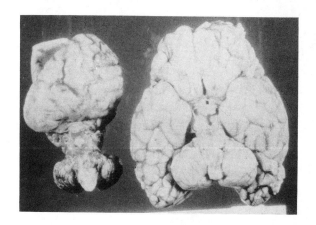

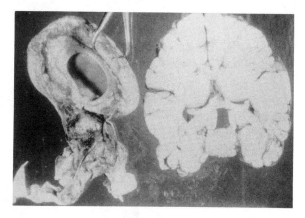

aplasia or hypoplasia, small stature, mental retardation, and ocular colobomas (iris, retina, and optic nerve). Brain anomalies are categorized as alobar, partially lobar, or lobar holoprosencephaly according to the degree of cerebral septation found.

Natural history: When the brain anomaly is severe (as in a lobar or partially lobar holoprosencephaly), survival past the neonatal period is unusual. In patients with lobar holoprosencephaly, development may be relatively normal or be marked by varying degrees of cognitive impairment. The more severe the brain anomaly, the more likely seizures, central apnea, and failure to thrive are to be found.

FIGURE 6–21.   A child with partially lobar holoprosencephaly (*top*) who died of a central apnea at four months of age. The brain at autopsy (bottom) shows an absence of hemispheric differentiation in the frontal lobes.

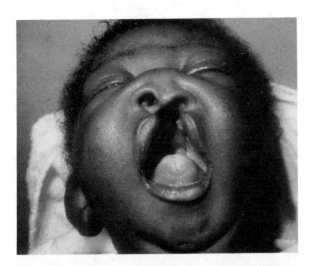

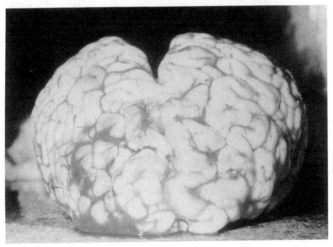

Small stature will occur in those children with pituitary anomalies. A variety of functional anomalies may also accompany the brain's failure to regulate bodily functions, such as poor temperature regulation, disordered metabolic function, and irritability.

Prognosis: In the majority of cases, the prognosis is very poor, and the more severe forms of this disorder are incompatible with life. In mild forms of lobar holoprosencephaly, the prognosis for normal cognitive functioning and life span can be very good.

Communication: In more severe cases, speech and language are never attained and central deafness is common. In milder cases, language impairment should be anticipated. Hypernasality secondary to cleft palate is possible; articulation impairment secondary to VPI.

Prevention: The brain anomalies found in this disorder may be detected on fetal ultrasound. In neonates with more severe brain anomalies and facial clefts, surgery should be avoided because of the poor prognosis for long-term survival.

Hypoglossia-Hypodactyly Syndrome

Etiology: The majority of cases have been sporadic, though this has been described as an autosomal dominant genetic condition (McKusick 1986) and has also been hypothesized to be autosomal recessive (Tuncbilek, Yalcin, and Atasu 1977).

Phenotypic spectrum: Microstomia, micrognathia, hypoglossia or aglossia, hypodontia, cleft palate, facial paresis, probable CNS anomalies resulting in Moebius sequence, adactyly or hypodactyly, and possible syndactyly.

Natural history: There may be neonatal feeding problems secondary to the aglossia or hypoglossia, which can be further complicated by cleft palate and micrognathia. However, intellect is generally within normal limits. Surprisingly, speech can often be acoustically normal.

Prognosis: Life span is normal, and the combination of surgery (hands and orofacial) and speech therapy can dramatically improve the quality of life.

Communication: Articulatory impairment secondary to hypoglossia, hypernasality secondary to cleft palate.

Prevention: In spite of aglossia or hypoglossia, clinicians should not assume that normal speech is out of the question. Many affected individuals have shown the ability to compensate for the absence of a tongue and have been able to have acoustically normal speech.

Kniest Syndrome

Etiology: Autosomal dominant genetic disorder.

Phenotypic spectrum: Disproportionate short-limbed dwarfism secondary to collagen abnormality, cleft palate, short nose, depressed nasal root, myopia, retinal degeneration, chronically enlarged joints, kyphoscoliosis, short clavicles, and abdominal hernias.

Natural history: Affected individuals tend to have limited joint mobility and joint pain. Though intellect is normal, walking is late, as are other limb-related developmental milestones. Adult height ranges between 40 and 55 inches. Chronic serous otitis is a common finding.

Prognosis: Short stature is a certainty and may be aggravated by kyphoscoliosis. Cognitive prognosis is excellent and language development is normal.

Communication: Hypernasality, articulation impairment secondary to velopharyngeal insufficiency, conductive hearing loss secondary to chronic serous otitis.

Prevention: Palate repair is indicated. Growth hormone treatment is contraindicated (short stature is not related to pituitary abnormality). Ventilating tubes for chronic serous otitis to prevent hearing loss.

Larsen Syndrome

Etiology: Autosomal dominant genetic disorder.

Phenotypic spectrum: Joint dislocations of the elbows, hips, and knees, short nose, depressed nasal root, frontal bossing, hypertelorism, cleft palate, Robin sequence, talipes equinovarus.

Natural history: Cognitive development is normal. Motor milestones will be impaired relative to multiple joint anomalies. Chronic serous otitis is common.

Prognosis: Life span is normal, and surgery can restore motor function.

Communication: Hypernasality secondary to cleft palate, articulation impairment secondary to VPI, conductive hearing loss secondary to serous otitis.

Prevention: Palate repair and ventilating tubes are indicated to prevent communicative impairment.

LEOPARD Syndrome

Etiology: Autosomal dominant genetic disorder.

Phenotypic spectrum: LEOPARD is an acronym describing the phenotype of this syndrome and stands for multiple *lentigines,* EKG abnormalities, ocular hypertelorism, pulmonic stenosis, abnormalities of the genitalia (hypogonadism and hypospadias), retarded growth, and deafness (sensory-neural).

Natural history: The lentigines (small, dark, pigmented birthmarks) are present at birth and tend to increase in number as children get older. General development tends to be normal, but cognitive impairment may occur in some cases.

Prognosis: Cardiac anomalies may cause the early prognosis to be guarded. Otherwise, with appropriate treatment, life expectancy and quality of life can be essentially normal.

Communication: Sensory-neural hearing loss, possible language impairment.

Prevention: The administration of appropriate hormone therapy (i.e., testosterone) may prevent hypogonadism. Amplification is indicated to prevent the negative effects of hearing loss and the development of language impairment.

Lysosomal Storage Syndromes (see Chapter 8)

Etiology: There are many types of lysosomal storage disorders, including Hurler syndrome, Hunter syndrome, Morquio syndrome, Scheie syndrome, LeRoy I-Cell syndrome, Tay-Sachs syndrome, and Sanfilippo syndrome. The majority of these syndromes are of autosomal recessive etiology, although X-linked recessive inheritance has been demonstrated in Hunter syndrome.

Phenotypic spectrum: The phenotype of each lysosomal storage syndrome is dependent on the specific metabolic waste product stored within the body's tissues (e.g., specific mucopolysaccharides, mucolipids, mannose, etc.). Each syndrome is caused on the biochemical level by a missing enzyme which results in some type of metabolic failure. In the more severe syndromes, patients have coarse features, chronic mucous congestion, respiratory failure, CNS dysfunction secondary to the storage of metabolic wastes in the brain's tissues, corneal opacities, growth retardation, mental retardation, and early death.

Natural history: In the more severe lysosomal storage syndromes, death occurs in infancy or early childhood. In less severe disorders, there is a slower progression of physical and functional disabilities, including scoliosis, chronic illness, obstructive sleep apnea, joint stiffness, and respiratory failure. In the majority of these syndromes, there is a shortened life span.

Prognosis: Generally poor.

Communication: Lack of language development in the more severe syndromes (such as Tay-Sachs syndrome and Hurler syndrome), or generalized developmental delay with language impairment in the majority of the syndromes. Conductive hearing loss is frequent secondary to chronic serous otitis.

Prevention: In the syndromes with more severe effects, vigorous treatments tend to be contraindicated because of the certainty of negative outcome. In the less severe disorders, symptomatic treatments are of value.

Miller-Diecker Syndrome

Etiology: Autosomal recessive genetic disorder.

Phenotypic spectrum: Lissencephaly, or "smoothbrain," characterized by an absence of cerebral sulci and gyri, microcephaly, micrognathia, cleft palate, Robin sequence, arthrogryposis, and anomalies of the heart, kidneys, and gastrointestinal tract.

Natural history: Death generally occurs in early infancy, although longer survival has been noted in several cases. Even in cases of longer survival, there is severe cognitive impairment.

Prognosis: Very poor.

Communication: There is no speech or language development.

Prevention: Palate repair is strongly contraindicated.

Multiple Synostosis Syndrome

Etiology: Autosomal dominant genetic disorder.

Phenotypic spectrum: Multiple joint fusions, especially of the digits, wrists, elbows, feet, and ankles. The ossicles are also fused to varying degrees, including stapes footplate fixation. Minor vertebral anomalies may be present, and the facies may show minor stigmata, including a narrow base of the nose, slender facies, and prominent nasal root.

Natural history: Conductive hearing loss and limitation of joint movement are present at birth and are nonprogressive.

Prognosis: Surgery can largely restore the function related to the multiple joint abnormalities. Cognition is normal.

Communication: Conductive hearing loss.

Prevention: Early middle ear surgery to normalize hearing can help prevent other secondary communicative impairments.

Nager Syndrome

Etiology: Possibly autosomal recessive, but not confirmed.

Phenotypic spectrum: Craniofacial characteristics very similar to Treacher Collins syndrome, including micrognathia, cleft palate, Robin sequence, malar hypoplasia, zygomatic aplasia or hypoplasia, down-slanting palpebral fissures, microtia, and middle ear anomalies. Limb anomalies are also present, including hypoplasia or aplasia of the thumbs, and anomalies of the radius.

Natural history: Upper airway obstruction and failure to thrive are common in the newborn period. The combination of micrognathia, cleft palate, and upper airway obstruction may present early on as

Robin sequence. With age, however, the mandible continues to be severely hypoplastic. Conductive hearing loss has been evident in essentially all cases to date. Radial anomalies may limit upper limb mobility.

Prognosis: With craniofacial surgery and amplification, the prognosis is good for normal functioning. Hand surgery to policize the index finger can also result in normal manual dexterity.

Communication: Conductive hearing loss, hyponasality, possible hypernasality secondary to cleft palate, and articulation impairment secondary to limited oral opening or VPI.

Prevention: Early hand surgery to prevent problems with manual dexterity, early treatment of airway problems to provide normal ventilation and alimentation. Pharyngeal flap is strongly contraindicated in this syndrome in order to prevent the development of severe obstructive apnea.

Neurofibromatosis (Figure 6–22)
Etiology: Autosomal dominant genetic disorder.

FIGURE 6–22. Cafe au lait spots on the thorax and abdomen of a 14-year-old child with neurofibromatosis (*left*) and a large neurofibroma on the back of an adult with the same syndrome (*right*).

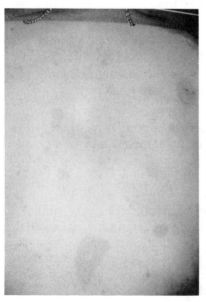
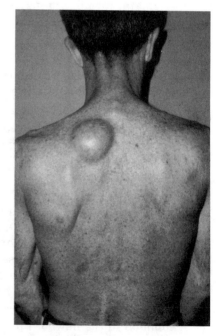

Phenotypic spectrum: There are several different forms of neurofibromatosis (Riccardi and Eichner 1986) with various phenotypes. The most common form presents as multiple cafe' au lait spots on the skin, including axillary freckling. Neurofibromas may also be present, along with other tumors, such as optic gliomas and acoustic neuromas (see Chapter 3). In severe forms, large tumors may be present, especially in the craniofacial complex. Macrencephaly and mild orbital hypertelorism are common, as are learning disabilities and multiple speech and voice disorders.

Natural history: In its milder forms, neurofibromatosis first presents as multiple cafe' au lait spots on the skin, especially in the axillary area and on the torso. With age, more of these pigmented areas appear. Eventually, multiple neurofibromas appear on the skin. Tumors may also appear on peripheral nerves, cranial nerves, and within the central nervous system, including acoustic neuromas and optic gliomas. These lesions are rarely malignant. In more severe cases, children may be born with multiple large neurofibromas, especially on the face, cranium, and other structures of the head and neck. With age, asymmetry of the limbs, torso, and face may become apparent. Macrencephaly is common, and learning disabilities with concomitant attention deficit disorders and coordination problems are common.

Prognosis: In milder forms, the prognosis for remediation of problems associated with neurofibromatosis is excellent. In more severe forms, habilitation is far more problematic. Unless neuromas present in particularly dangerous areas (such as the brain, optic nerve, auditory nerve, and other intracranial locations), the lesions themselves are usually fully treatable.

Communication: Hearing loss, stuttering, language impairment, hypernasality, dysarthria, articulation disorders.

Prevention: The site, location, and extent of neurofibromatosis lesions cannot be anticipated and, therefore, cannot be prevented. Treatment must be palliative.

Noonan Syndrome (see Chapter 3)
Etiology: Most cases have been sporadic, although both autosomal dominant and autosomal recessive etiology have been reported (McKusick 1986).

Phenotypic spectrum: Short stature, webbing of the neck, developmental delay and learning disabilities or mental retardation, mild hypertelorism, eyelid ptosis, anterior skeletal open bite, narrow chest, cubitus valgus, genital anomalies in males, and right-sided congenital heart disease, including pulmonic stenosis.

Natural history: All problems are present at birth, and there is no evidence of progression of any problems.

Prognosis: Once congenital heart disease has been resolved, the prognosis for achievement is commensurate with intellectual capacity.

Communication: Language impairment, delayed speech onset, articulation disorder secondary to anterior skeletal open bite, and sensory-neural hearing loss (infrequent).

Prevention: Neckwebbing and congenital heart disease may be detected in utero. When genital anomalies are present, early treatment may be successful in normalizing genital size.

Oral-Facial-Digital Syndromes (Figure 6–23)

Etiology: There are possibly as many as seven or eight different types of "oral-facial-digital" syndromes. Smith (1982) described two (OFD type I and OFD type II or Mohr syndrome). At present, several other forms are also recognized, and there is clearly etiologic heterogeneity among the different types, ranging from autosomal recessive in Mohr syndrome, to autosomal dominant with male lethality in OFD I, to sporadic (unknown etiology) forms.

Phenotypic spectrum: Clefts of the lip, or lip and palate, including midline "pseudo-clefts" of the lip caused by a short and attenuated

FIGURE 6–23. A three-year-old child with Mohr syndrome (OFD type II) with midline notching of the lip (*left*) and polydactyly (*right*). She is severely retarded.

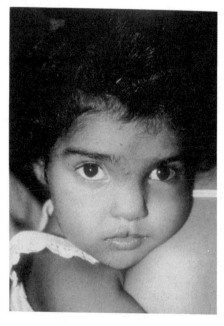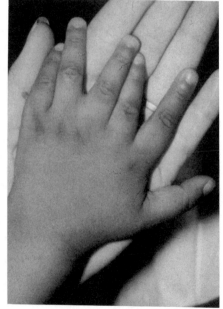

labial frenulum; mental retardation; small stature, digital anomalies, including polydactyly and shortening of digits; missing teeth and hypoplastic enamel, trilobulated tongue; skin abnormalities; ossicularmalformation.

Natural history: Failure to thrive in infancy occurs in several forms of OFD and may be followed by neonatal death. Mental deficiency ranges from mild to severe, including complete absence of intellectual development in some forms.

Prognosis: Poor in the more severe forms, but normal life span with intellectual deficiencies can be anticipated in the milder forms.

Communication: Conductive hearing loss, severe language impairment, or perhaps the total absence of speech and language development, articulation impairment secondary to lingual and oral malformations.

Prevention: Many of the anomalies, including clefting and polydactyly, may be detected in utero. In cases with the most severe cognitive defects, surgery for the correction of clefts or digital anomalies is strongly contraindicated because of the poor prognosis for speech development.

Otopalatodigital Syndrome (Figure 6–24)

Etiology: Either X-linked recessive genetic disorder or autosomal dominant with more severe expression in males.

Phenotypic spectrum: Cleft palate, micrognathia, upper airway obstruction, Robin sequence; small stature, short torso; mental retardation or learning disabilities; conductive hearing loss; frontal bossing, mild hypertelorism, down-slanting palpebral fissures; multiple missing teeth; multiple joint abnormalities, including limited bend at elbow, short hallux (big toe), thickened soft tissues of the distal ends of the fingers and toes.

Natural history: Immediately after birth, failure to thrive, poor feeding, and the development of a pectus excavatum occur secondary to upper airway obstruction. Delayed development may be signaled by late speech onset. Digital anomalies become more pronounced with age.

Prognosis: Commensurate with intellectual development. Other anomalies are not major limitations to progress with the exception of early airway obstruction. Mandibular deficiency does not improve with age.

Communication: Conductive hearing loss, language impairment, delayed speech onset, hypernasality secondary to cleft palate, articulation impairment secondary to malocclusion or VPI.

FIGURE 6–24.   Eight-year-old child with otopalataldigital syndrome in frontal *(top)* and profile *(center)* views showing hypertelorism, down-slanting eyes, and micrognathia.   At the bottom, note the short hallux (great toe) and thickened tips of the other toes.

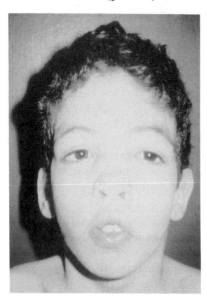

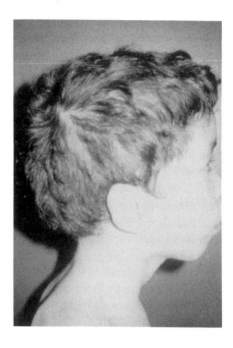

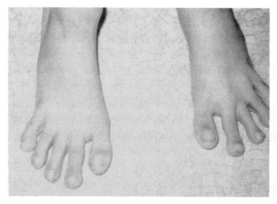

Prevention: Because of predisposition to upper airway obstruction, pharyngeal flap should be carefully considered before implementation if hypernasality is present. Because conductive hearing loss is often present, early use of hearing aids may prevent exacerbation of language impairment.

Pfeiffer Syndrome (Figure 6–25)

Etiology: Autosomal dominant genetic disorder.

Phenotypic spectrum: Essentially the same as for Crouzon syndrome (see above), except that in Pfeiffer syndrome, there is the additional finding of broad thumbs and halluces, and other minor digital and limb anomalies.

Natural history: Neonatal appearance may be relatively normal and craniosynostosis may not be obvious at birth, but craniofacial anomalies become progressively worse with age. Hydrocephalus may occur secondary to aquaductal stenosis. A variety of secondary abnormalities may also occur if early skull anomalies are not treated, including optic nerve compression and worsening stenosis of the nasal cavity. Upper airway obstruction may occur in the neonatal period. Mouth breathing and open mouth posture worsen with time.

FIGURE 6–25. Neonate with Pfeiffer syndrome showing acrocephaly (*left*) and broad hallux (*right*)

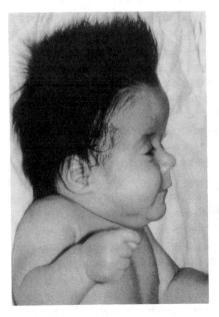
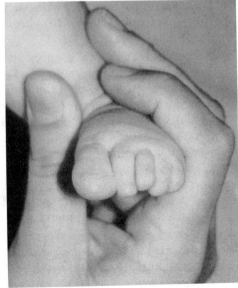

Prognosis: With early craniectomy, prognosis is generally good, although, in some cases, anomalies of the cranial base may be so severe that CNS functioning will be permanently impaired.

Communication: Hyponasality, articulatory impairment secondary to anterior skeletal open bite and airway obstruction; conductive hearing loss; possible language impairment secondary to CNS compression.

Prevention: Compression of the CNS and optic nerve can be avoided with early cranial surgery (craniectomy). Chronic choanal stenosis is secondary to skull base abnormalities. Therefore, surgical treatment of choanal stenosis, although occasionally successful temporarily, will most certainly fail long term.

Popliteal Pterygium Syndrome

Etiology: Autosomal dominant genetic disorder.

Phenotypic spectrum: Cleft palate, or cleft lip and cleft palate, micrognathia, lower lip pits, upper airway obstruction, Robin sequence, webbing of the *popliteal* joint space, lower lip pits, multiple oral frenula, genital anomalies, and anomalous toenails.

Natural history: All anomalies are present at birth and are nonprogressive. If the popliteal webs are very tight, early ambulation may be impeded.

Prognosis: Cognition and life span are normal. With treatment, anomalies can be habilitated to prevent permanent problems.

Communication: Hypernasality secondary to cleft, articulation disorders secondary to VPI, chronic serous otitis may result in mild conductive hearing loss.

Prevention: Palatal surgery and myringotomy and tube surgery are indicated in order to prevent communicative impairments. Surgeons must be aware that the popliteal webs cannot be simply divided because nerves and blood vessels typically follow an abnormal path in the web spaces. Therefore, appropriate radiographic and MRI studies are indicated in order to correct the limb anomalies without prompting surgically induced abnormalities.

Prader-Willi Syndrome

Etiology: Sporadic (unknown etiology), although a small chromosome interstitial deletion has been noted in some cases.

Phenotypic spectrum: Severe obesity, short stature, up-slanting palpebral fissures, mental retardation, infant and childhood hypotonia, small hands and feet, hypogonadism and micropenis.

Natural history: Hypotonia may be very severe in infancy, giving the patients a more "retarded" appearance than is actually the case.

Hypotonia tends to improve with age, especially in adolescence. Hypernasal speech is often evident in early speech, but improves and disappears with improving muscle tone (Foushee 1987; Sadewitz and Shprintzen 1987). Eating habits are often difficult to control, and patients are known to be compulsive binge eaters. Adult height is reduced, but with proper control, weight can be within normal limits. Personality and affect are socially affable. There is an apparent predisposition to diabetes mellitus, which is correlated with the degree of obesity.

Prognosis: Because of social affect, these children often perform better than their IQs might suggest. The prognosis for weight loss is highly dependent on parental or caretaker ability to prevent children from obtaining food.

Communication: Hypernasality, language impairment.

Prevention: Pharyngeal flap or other palatopharyngeal surgery for hypernasality in childhood should be avoided because of the gradual disappearance of the symptom. Obesity can be avoided by using strict behavior modification programs and by keeping food out of reach of children who have little behavioral control.

Provisionally unique syndromes This is a sort of "wastebasket" diagnostic category introduced by Cohen (1981) to describe children who have multiple anomalies that do not seem to fit any other diagnostic category. The term implies that the affected child has multiple anomalies that have a syndromic pattern (i.e., they would all seem to have a common pathogenesis). However, that pattern is not one that the clinician has ever seen before, is not one that has been described previously in the scientific literature, and following consultation with learned colleagues, would seem to be unknown as a specific syndrome to them as well. Therefore, as far as the clinician knows, the child has a unique pattern of malformations that seems to be syndromic in nature. However, the additional label of "provisionally" is added to the diagnosis because:

1. The child may not really be unique. There may be another individual with the same pattern of malformations somewhere about whom the clinician has no knowledge.

2. In the future, a report of the same pattern of malformations may appear in the literature as a new recurrent pattern syndrome.

3. The affected individual may eventually reproduce, or his parents may have more children, and produce a child with the same pattern of anomalies.

This particular grouping of cases may actually represent the largest number of patients seen by clinical geneticists.

Rapp-Hodgkin Syndrome (Figure 6–26)

Etiology: Autosomal dominant genetic disorder.

Phenotypic spectrum: Hypohidrotic ectodermal dysplasia; cleft lip, cleft palate, or cleft lip and cleft palate; sparse hair, dysplastic finger- and toenails; multiple missing and/or malformed teeth; occasional hypospadias.

Natural history: Because of sweating deficiency (hypohidrosis), body temperature control can be faulty, especially in infancy and early childhood. Generally, there is frequent serous otitis media and conjunctivitis.

Prognosis: Longevity and mentation are not affected. With appropriate treatment, prognosis is excellent.

Communication: Hypernasality secondary to clefting, articulation impairment secondary to VPI, conductive hearing loss secondary to chronic otitis, and voice disorders (hoarseness) secondary to ectodermal dysplasia.

Prevention: Knowledge of hypohidrosis can avoid early crises caused by poor temperature regulation. Appropriate prosthodontic treatment can provide normal dentition, and early myringotomy and tube surgery can prevent conductive hearing loss.

FIGURE 6–26. Nine-year-old child with Rapp-Hodgkin syndrome showing thin, sparse scalp hair (*left*) and absent fingernails (*right*).

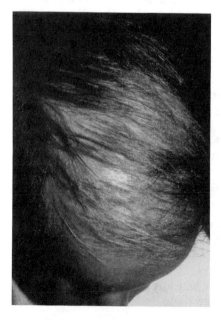
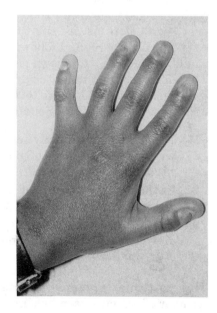

Robin Deformation Sequence (Figure 6–27)

Etiology: Intrauterine constriction caused by uterine anomalies, twinning, or *oligohydramnios.*

Phenotypic spectrum: Micrognathia, U-shaped cleft palate, and upper airway obstruction often presumed to be caused by glossoptosis.

Natural history: The presentation at birth is that of severe mandibular deficiency and persistent apnea, both during sleep and wakeful periods. Though respiratory movements may appear normal, the presence of substernal, suprasternal, and intercostal retractions signals obstruction of the upper airway and a failure to exchange air. Once resolved, growth and development proceed normally. Airway problems also result in failure to thrive and feeding difficulties. Because the mandible is intrinsically normal, growth of the lower jaw after birth is essentially normal, and considerable, if not complete, "catch-up" growth occurs. "Catch-up" growth would not occur if the Robin sequence occurred secondary to a syndrome with intrinsic mandibular hypoplasia as a frequent feature, such as Stickler syndrome or fetal alcohol syndrome. If early airway problems are not resolved, the patient is at risk for sudden death or for hypoxic brain damage.

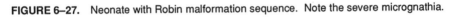

FIGURE 6–27.   Neonate with Robin malformation sequence. Note the severe micrognathia.

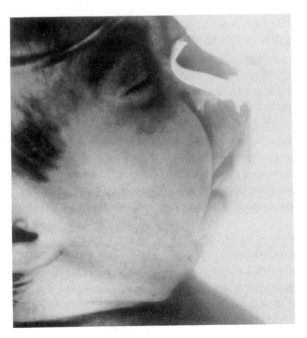

Prognosis: Early infancy can be a particularly dangerous time because of the risk of sudden death caused by airway obstruction. If the apnea can be resolved, life span and cognitive development should be normal.

Communication: Hypernasality secondary to cleft, articulation disorders secondary to VPI. Language impairment could potentially occur secondary to hypoxia.

Prevention: Early recognition and resolution of obstructive apnea is essential to prevent death or chronic hypoxia. Once apnea is resolved, palate repair can prevent the development of abnormal speech. If the mandible is intrinsically normal, early excessive treatment of the mandible should be avoided.

Robinow Syndrome (Figure 6–28)
Etiology: Autosomal dominant genetic disorder.

Phenotypic spectrum: Hypertelorism, wide palpebral fissures, short nose, frontal bossing; cleft lip, cleft palate, or both; limb anomalies, including shortening of the forearms and digits; osteosclerosis, vertebral anomalies, flattened skull base, chronic middle ear disease, and micropenis.

Natural history: All anomalies are present at birth, but the facial dysmorphia tends to become more pronounced with age. Osteosclerosis becomes evident after puberty. Untreated, penile hypoplasia does not improve.

Prognosis: Life span and mentation are normal. With proper treatment, quality of life need not be affected considerably.

Communication: Hyponasality secondary to severely flattened basicranium reducing the size of the nasopharyngeal vault, occasional hypernasality secondary to clefting, articulatory impairment secondary to VPI or malocclusion, conductive hearing loss secondary to chronic serous otitis.

Prevention: With early identification, testosterone therapy can result in increased or normalized penile growth. Myringotomy and tube surgery are indicated to prevent middle ear disease, and reconstructive surgery is indicated to prevent hypernasality and the social stigmata of severely abnormal appearance.

Rubinstein-Taybi Syndrome
Etiology: Unknown; sporadic, although autosomal recessive inheritance has been suggested (McKusick 1986).

Phenotypic spectrum: Small stature, mental retardation, microcephaly, small face with beaked nose, down-slanting palpebral fissures, strabismus; broad thumbs and occasionally other digital

FIGURE 6–28. Father and son with Robinow syndrome. Note the hypertelorism, wide palpebral fissures, frontal bossing, and posteriorly displaced ears.

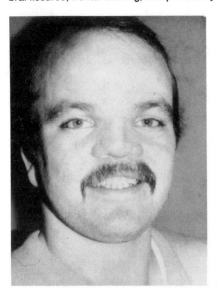
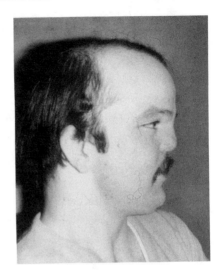
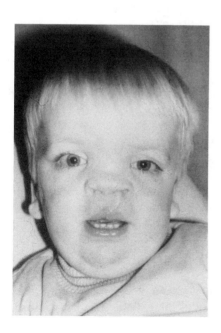
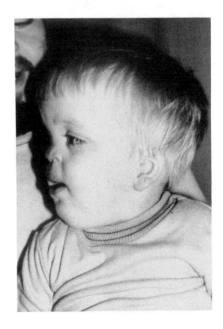

anomalies, cryptorchidism, congenital heart anomalies, and renal disorders.

Natural history: There is early failure to thrive and respiratory obstruction. Later, obstructive sleep apnea may occur. Mental retardation is evident early on and tends to be in the moderate to severe range.

Prognosis: Developmental and cognitive prognosis is poor. The development of multiple health related problems caused by chronic hypoxia or apnea may also occur and reduce life span in some cases.

Communication: Severe language impairment and severe articulatory impairment.

Prevention: None known.

Saethre-Chotzen Syndrome

Etiology: Autosomal dominant genetic disorder.

Phenotypic spectrum: Craniosynostosis, mild facial asymmetry, small ears, eyelid ptosis, conductive hearing loss; soft tissue syndactyly of the fingers and toes, clavicular hypoplasia; occasional mental retardation; occasional cleft palate.

Natural history: Anomalies are present at birth; if untreated, craniosynostosis is progressive and may cause problems secondary to increased intracranial pressure.

Prognosis: Life span and cognition are generally normal, although a small percentage of patients are cognitively impaired, possibly secondary to increased intracranial pressure.

Communication: Hyponasality, articulation impairment secondary to malocclusion, language impairment in some cases, conductive hearing loss.

Prevention: Early cranial surgery can reduce the risks associated with increased intracranial pressure.

Shprintzen-Goldberg I Syndrome (Figure 6–29)

Etiology: Autosomal dominant genetic disorder.

Phenotypic spectrum: Characteristic facies, including dystopia canthorum, downturned oral commissures, unusual eyebrow pattern, and frontal bossing; high pitched voice, hypotonia, learning disabilities, omphalocele or umbilical hernia.

Natural history: The neonatal period can be marked by failure to thrive and respiratory difficulties, presumably related to both hypotonia and laryngeal anomalies. Developmental milestones are mildly delayed and cognitive functioning very mildly impaired. Learning disabilities become evident at school age. Hypotonia improves with age, but is always present.

FIGURE 6–29. Father and two daughters with Shprintzen-Goldberg I syndrome. Note the dystopia canthorum (telecanthus), epicanthi, and down-slanting oral commissures.

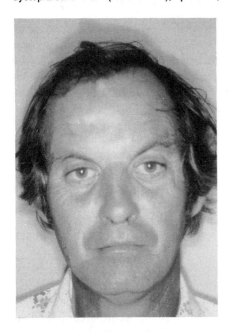

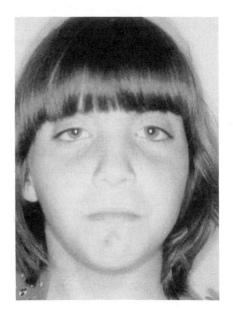

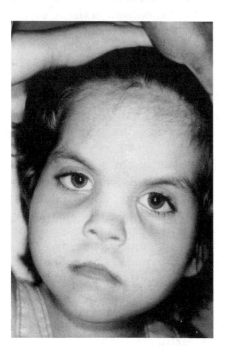

Prognosis: All problems associated with this syndrome can be remediated, including learning disabilities, which have typically been dealt with via special education or resource room help. Life span is normal.

Communication: High pitched voice and language impairment.

Prevention: Infantile respiratory problems should be treated aggressively given the generally favorable outcome of this syndrome. Omphalocele can be detected prenatally by ultrasound.

Shprintzen-Goldberg II Syndrome (Figure 6–30)
Etiology: Unknown, sporadic.

Phenotypic spectrum: Craniosynostosis, micrognathia, midface deficiency, exorbitism, hypertelorism, soft tissue hypertrophy of the hard palate, anterior skeletal open bite, arachnodactyly, joint contractures, multiple abdominal hernias, soft cartilaginous ears, mitral valve prolapse, mental retardation, obstructive apnea, scoliosis, and other spine anomalies.

Natural history: Obstructive apnea is generally present at birth along with craniosynostosis. Developmental milestones are severely delayed, and mental retardation is evident at an early age. Abdominal hernias may continue to appear, even after surgical repair. Almost all of the body's connective tissue seems to be involved, and multiple disorders related to connective tissue can be found with advancing age, such as joint contractures, mitral valve prolapse, and advancing scoliosis. Speech and language development are particularly delayed, and mental retardation tends to be severe.

Prognosis: The outlook for cognitive development is generally poor.

Communication: Severe language impairment, articulation impairment secondary to malocclusion, CNS anomalies, and airway obstruction.

Prevention: The soft tissue hypertrophy of the hard palate, or "pseudo-cleft," may potentially be mistaken for a cleft of the palate. Surgery to the palate obviously should be avoided. Also, the co-occurrence of craniosynostosis and obstructive apnea may lead to the mistaken assumption that the airway problems are secondary to the craniosynostosis. However, the pharynx in this syndrome is severely constricted, and the apnea is purely obstructive in nature and not related to increased intracranial pressure.

Sotos Syndrome
Etiology: Nearly all cases have been sporadic, although autosomal dominant inheritance is speculated (McKusick 1986).

FIGURE 6–30. Patient with Shprintzen-Goldberg II syndrome showing hypertelorism and exorbitism (*top*), arachnodactyly and camptodactyly (*center*), and "pseudo-cleft" of the hard palate (*bottom*)

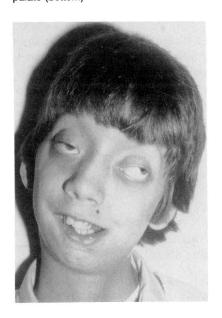

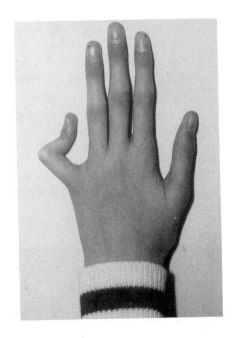

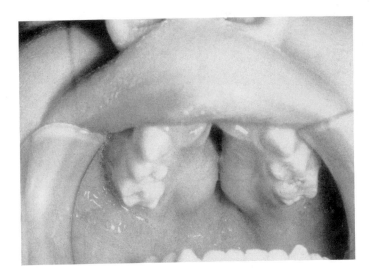

Phenotypic spectrum: Large stature, mental retardation, hypotonia, advanced bone maturation, large head, relative prognathism, and occasional seizures.

Natural history: Though birth size may be only slightly large or within normal limits, growth becomes exceptionally rapid in the first three years of life. Growth rate then decreases so that adult stature is generally large, but within normal limits. Aggressiveness has been noted in some patients later in childhood. Mental retardation is generally in the moderate range.

Prognosis: Prognosis for cognitive development is generally poor and social adaptation is similarly poor.

Communication: Language impairment, articulation disorders.

Prevention: Though early growth is accelerated, there is a decline in growth rate after puberty so that adult stature, although large, is not as disproportionately large as in childhood.

Spondyloepiphyseal Dysplasia Syndrome (Figure 6–31)
Etiology: Autosomal dominant genetic disorder.

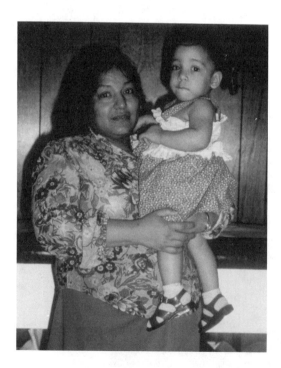

FIGURE 6–31.
Mother and daughter with spondyloepiphyseal dysplasia syndrome. The daughter had Robin sequence.

Phenotypic spectrum: Short stature, micrognathia, cleft palate, Robin sequence, mildly flattened facies; myopia and vitreoretinal degeneration; vertebral anomalies, pectus cavinatum, delayed osseous maturation, reduced joint mobility, hip dislocation, muscle weakness.

Natural history: Small stature is of prenatal onset and is evident at birth. Hypotonia is also evident, and motor milestones are generally delayed. Walking is most severely delayed. Early respiratory obstruction is secondary to Robin sequence (micrognathia), cranial base anomalies, and hypotonia.

Prognosis: Life span is generally normal, and cognition is normal. Patients generally compensate well for skeletal and muscle problems.

Communication: Hypernasality secondary to cleft palate, articulation disorders secondary to VPI, conductive hearing loss secondary to chronic serous otitis.

Prevention: Prenatal diagnosis by ultrasound is possible. Early and regular ophthalmic care should be scheduled to avoid retinal detachment.

Stickler Syndrome (Figure 6–2)

Etiology: Autosomal dominant genetic disorder.

Phenotypic spectrum: Micrognathia, cleft palate, upper airway obstruction, Robin sequence, maxillary hypoplasia; myopia, vitreoretinal degeneration; juvenile arthropathy, epiphyseal dysplasia, spinal anomalies; sensory-neural hearing loss, chronic serous otitis media; round facies, anteverted nostrils, short nose, depressed nasal root, epicanthi, basicranial kyphosis, and talipes equinovarus.

Natural history: It has been reported that one-third of infants with Robin sequence has Stickler syndrome (Herrmann and Opitz 1975; Shprintzen 1988a). The upper airway obstruction may be related more to a congenitally small airway secondary to skull base anomalies rather than glossoptosis (Sadewitz and Shprintzen 1986). Myopia may be present at birth, though in many cases, it does not become apparent until later in childhood. A high percentage of children with Stickler syndrome eventually develop retinal detachments. Though micrognathia is present at birth, hypoplasia of the maxilla may eventually result in relatively normal jaw relationships. Obstructive sleep apnea may develop later in life.

Prognosis: Life span and mentation are typically normal. However, there is a high percentage of severe eye problems, retinal detachment, and partial blindness.

Communication: Hypernasality secondary to cleft palate, articulation problems secondary to VPI or high frequency sensory-neural hearing loss; occasional hyponasality secondary to reduced upper airway size; and both sensory-neural and conductive hearing loss.

Prevention: Severe eye problems can be avoided with preventive ophthalmologic care. The appropriate diagnosis of the specific type of hearing loss (conductive, sensory-neural, or mixed) will result in more effective treatment and a smaller likelihood of language impairment. Resolution of airway problem will prevent chronic hypoxia and the potential for brain damage. It should not be assumed that the upper airway obstruction is caused by glossoptosis.

Steinert Syndrome

Etiology: Autosomal dominant genetic disorder.

Phenotypic spectrum: This syndrome can be expressed at birth, or may not become expressed until the second or third decade of life. It is also known as myotonic dystrophy, one of the muscular dystrophies. When present at birth, there is severe myotonia, lack of facial expression with open mouth posture (myopathic facies), vertically long face, retrognathia, occasionally cleft palate and Robin sequence, upper airway obstruction; cataracts; testicular atrophy in males, amenorrhea in females; cardiac arrhythmias; occasional cognitive impairment, hypernasality, delayed speech onset; and talipes equinovarus. In the late onset form, myotonia, hypernasal speech, male pattern baldness, personality change and mental deterioration, vertical maxillary excess, steep mandibular plane angle, and cataracts. There is the tendency to develop malignant hyperthermia (sudden and severe temperature elevation) when given general anesthetics which could be potentially life-threatening.

Natural history: In the early onset form, essentially all anomalies are present at birth and do not progress dramatically, although some slight deterioration may occur. Many secondary problems occur secondary to the chronic muscle weakness, including progressive facial growth abnormality, malocclusion, and somatic deformity. Often the first detectable symptom, in the late onset form, is the onset of hypernasal speech, usually just after puberty, but possibly later. Male pattern baldness occurs prematurely, and subtle personality changes may occur. Myotonia becomes increasingly worse with time, often limiting manual abilities. Progressive cardiac problems have been known to result in early death in the fifth or sixth decade of life.

Prognosis: Prognosis is poorer for early onset form, though the disorder is generally more progressive in the late onset form.

Communication: Hypernasality; articulation problems secondary to both myotonia and malocclusion.

Prevention: General anesthesia should be avoided unless anesthesiologist is prepared for the use of specific agents to avoid malignant hyperthermia. Pharyngeal flap surgery is contraindicated because of risk of malignant hyperthermia, the risk of airway compromise, and because of the progressive nature of the myotonia. Genetic counseling of affecteds is strongly recommended.

Townes Syndrome

Etiology: Autosomal dominant genetic disorder.

Phenotypic spectrum: Facial asymmetry, commissural cleft, auricular anomalies (usually microtia), accessory ear tags; thumb anomalies (triphalangeal thumb or thumb duplication); imperforate anus, renal anomalies; conductive hearing loss, occasionally sensory-neural hearing loss.

Natural history: All anomalies are present at birth and are not progressive.

Prognosis: With surgical treatment, prognosis for normal life span and remediation of anomalies is good.

Communication: Conductive and/or sensory-neural hearing loss; hypernasality secondary to palatal asymmetry.

Prevention: Early surgery to correct facial asymmetry and improve facial aesthetics is indicated. Genetic counseling is indicated.

Treacher Collins Syndrome (Figure 6–3)

Etiology: Autosomal dominant genetic disorder.

Phenotypic spectrum: All anomalies occur in the craniofacial complex. They include mandibular hypoplasia, cleft palate, upper airway obstruction, Robin sequence, maxillary hypoplasia, pharyngeal airway narrowing; skeletal orbital clefts, zygomatic clefts or aplasia, down-slanting palpebral fissures, absent lashes on the lower eyelid, astigmatism, lower eyelid depressions; absent nasofrontal angle, beak shaped nose, anterior skeletal open bite; microtia, conductive hearing loss, ossicular anomalies, occasional sensory-neural hearing loss; tonguelike projection of hair onto the cheeks.

Natural history: All anomalies are present at birth and often result in upper airway obstruction. Robin sequence is often present and, if the expression of Treacher Collins syndrome is mild, a mistaken diagnosis is possible. Conductive hearing loss may be mild but is almost always present. Upper airway obstruction may be lifelong unless treated, and obstructive sleep apnea later in life has been noted. Abnormal neck posturing and altered sleep patterns are frequent, and numerous instances of sudden death have been noted.

Prognosis: If upper airway obstruction is resolved, life span and mentation are usually normal, and surgical correction of facial anomalies at craniofacial centers is possible.

Communication: Hyponasality, occasional mixed hyper- and hyponasality, conductive hearing loss, occasional sensory-neural hearing loss, articulation impairment secondary to upper airway anomalies and anterior skeletal open bite.

Prevention: Can be detected in utero by diagnostic real-time ultrasound imaging. Hearing should be checked as soon as possible so that amplification can be provided, if necessary. Airway problems should be immediately suspected, even if not obvious, in order to prevent chronic hypoxia. Pharyngeal surgery, such as pharyngeal flap surgery, should be avoided at all costs because of the high risk of obstructive apnea and death after surgery. However, tonsillectomy may be necessary in many cases to relieve upper airway problems. Tracheotomy is often recommended. Early reconstructive surgery may be important to redirect facial growth or relieve apnea. Early eye examinations should be scheduled because of the high risk of astigmatism related to eyelid and eyelash anomalies. Genetic counseling is recommended.

Turner Syndrome (see Chapter 2)

Etiology: Chromosomal anomaly caused by the absence of one sex chromosome in an individual who has one X chromosome only.

Phenotypic spectrum: Small stature; hypoplasia or aplasia of the ovaries and uterus, congenital lymphedema, webbing of the neck, low posterior hairline, broad chest with wide spaced nipples; protuberant auricles; cubitus valgus and other minor skeletal anomalies of the limbs, abnormal fingernails (usually small, very convex, and deep set), numerous nevi; renal anomalies; cardiac anomalies (usually coarctation of the aorta); occasional sensory-neural hearing loss; occasional mental retardation, occasional thyroid disorders; occasional cleft palate, occasional micrognathia, occasional Robin sequence.

Natural history: The lymphedema is one of the more prominent features at birth, but usually subsides shortly after birth. The skin tends to remain very loose for a while after birth. Webbing of the neck, especially associated with lymphedema and other anomalies, should prompt recommendation for a karyotype. Later on, primary amenorrhea occurs. In mosaics for Turner syndrome, all findings are essentially reduced in severity.

Prognosis: Longevity is usually not affected, and quality of life can be relatively normal in many cases.

Communication: Language impairment secondary to cognitive disorders, hypernasality and articulation disorders secondary to cleft palate, sensory-neural hearing loss.

Prevention: Estrogen replacement therapy is often indicated to allow the development of some secondary sexual characteristics and to prevent further stigmatization. All other problems can be treated symptomatically.

Van der Woude Syndrome (Figure 6–32)

Etiology: Autosomal dominant genetic disorder.

Phenotypic spectrum: Cleft lip, cleft palate, or both, congenital fistulae (pits) or mounds of the lower lip, platybasia, congenitally missing premolars, characteristic "gull wing" appearance to the upper lip.

Natural history: At birth, infants with Van der Woude syndrome resemble babies with nonsyndromic clefts with the exception of the presence of pits or mounds of the lower lip. The lower lip anomalies represent communicating tracts to small salivary glands. As a result, these lower lip pits may often extrude saliva, especially when squeezed. If the pits are large, they may become infected because of food particles entering into them. Therefore, when large, when they secrete saliva, or when they present an aesthetic problem, they should be surgically removed at the time of lip or palate repair. Because of platybasia (a flattened skull base), the pharynx tends to be very deep. Therefore, velopharyngeal insufficiency is common in this syndrome, even after palate repair. The facial appearance tends to be characteristic with the alar cartilages of the nose being im-

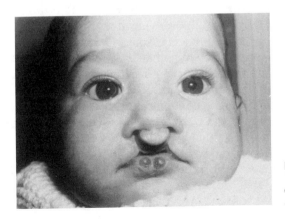

FIGURE 6–32.
Infant with Van der Woude syndrome with bilateral cleft lip and palate and large lower lip pits

planted higher than the columella and the upper lip having a wide cupid's bow with a "gull wing" appearance. With age, facial growth proceeds normally. One or more of the secondary premolars may be absent in many cases.

Prognosis: Life span and intellect are unaffected.

Communication: Hypernasality secondary to cleft palate and platybasial, articulatory disorders secondary to VPI.

Prevention: Lower lip pit infections can be avoided by early surgical removal of the communicating tracts. Genetic counseling is indicated.

Velocardiofacial (Shprintzen) Syndrome (Figure 6–1)

Etiology: Autosomal dominant genetic disorder.

Phenotypic spectrum: Cleft palate (overt, submucous, or occult), congenital heart disease possibly including ventriculoseptal defect, tetralogy of Fallot, right-sided aortic arch, coarctation of the aorta, aberrant subclavian arteries, pulmonic stenosis, patent ductus arteriosis, microcephaly, learning disabilities, mild mental retardation (in approximately 40 percent), relatively small stature, characteristic facies with large nose, narrow, slitlike eyes, downturned oral commissures, masklike face, mild facial asymmetry, flattened malar eminences, retrognathia, upper airway obstruction, Robin sequence, platybasia, pharyngeal hypotonia, minor auricular anomalies, ocular anomalies, thick scalp hair, slender digits, scoliosis, abdominal hernias, medially displaced internal carotid arteries, absent or hypoplastic adenoids, absent thymus, Reynaud's phenomenon.

Natural history: The first anomaly found in many cases is the congenital heart disease, especially if serious. Palatal anomalies are often undetected until after speech development because of a high frequency of submucous or occult submucous clefts. Retrognathia, cleft palate, and pharyngeal hypotonia often combine to result in upper airway obstruction and Robin sequence with early failure to thrive. There may be frequent upper respiratory infections and pneumonia caused by poor immunologic response because of absent thymic hormone and generalized hypoplasia of lymphoid tissue resulting in decreased numbers of T lymphocytes. Developmental milestones are usually within normal limits, though may be mildly delayed. There is a characteristic behavioral profile, including disinhibition, concrete thinking, and flat affect. Hypernasality is usually severe and is often accompanied by articulatory compensations, such as glottal stop substitutions. In early childhood, intellectual testing is usually within normal limits, but with age, the IQ tends to deteriorate because of specific learning disabilities that negatively affect abstract reasoning. Mathematic ability and reading comprehension are most severely affected, but rote reading and counting ability are not impaired. Educational setting usually requires modification, including resource room or special class placement.

Prognosis: Learning disabilities may improve with special education, but they do not fully resolve. Concrete learning patterns remain lifelong. Early failure to thrive may present as significant problems because of generalized hypotonia, but once overcome, general quality of life is good, though special adjustments need to be made for behavioral and learning problems.

Communication: Language impairment, hypernasality secondary to cleft palate, platybasia, and pharyngeal hypotonia, articulation impairment secondary to VPI, conductive hearing loss secondary to chronic serous otitis, occasional sensory hearing loss, and high pitched voice.

Prevention: Early failure to thrive is caused by upper airway obstruction and pharyngeal hypotonia. It is possible to establish normal alimentation with effort, and gastrostomy should be avoided. Failure in school early on can be prevented by withholding children from school for a year to allow additional maturation. MRI or CT scan of the posterior pharyngeal wall and nasopharyngoscopy must be used to site the internal carotids to avoid severing them during pharyngeal flap surgery.

Waardenburg Syndrome

Etiology: Autosomal dominant genetic disorder.

Phenotypic spectrum: Sensory hearing loss, pigment abnormalities of the skin and hair, heterochromia iridium, somatic asymmetry, telecanthus, short palpebral fissures, occasional cleft lip and/or palate, occasional Hirschsprung aganglionic megacolon, synophrys, and hypoplastic alar cartilages (see Figure 3–12).

Natural history: Sensory hearing loss is congenital and when present is usually severe and bilateral. The most common and easily recognized pigmentary change is the presence of a white forelock of hair. However, the entire scalp hair may change to white prematurely and mask the presence of the white forelock.

Prognosis: Life span is normal and intellect is normal.

Communication: Sensory deafness, speech disorders associated with deafness, hypernasality secondary to cleft palate in some cases.

Prevention: Early identification of the hearing loss with ABR is essential and early amplification is strongly indicated when possible.

Weaver Syndrome (Figure 6–33)

Etiology: Unknown, with most cases being sporadic, but autosomal dominant or X-linked recessive etiology has been hypothesized (Ardinger et al. 1986).

Phenotypic spectrum: Macrosomia (large stature), delayed development, abnormal muscle tone (usually hypertonic), broad forehead, flat occiput, mild hypertelorism, large ears, mild retrognathia, small fingernails, limited joint movements at the knees and elbows, metaphyseal splaying of the long bones, minor digital anomalies, occasional cleft palate, mild cutis laxa, umbilical hernia.

Natural history: Excess size is of prenatal onset and is maintained through childhood. Only one adult has been reported in the literature and was found to be abnormally tall. Developmental delay has been noted to be accompanied by mild hypertonicity.

Prognosis: Developmental impairment often subsequently presents as mild cognitive impairment and perhaps mild mental retardation.

Communication: Language impairment, mild hypernasality secondary to cleft palate.

Prevention: None known.

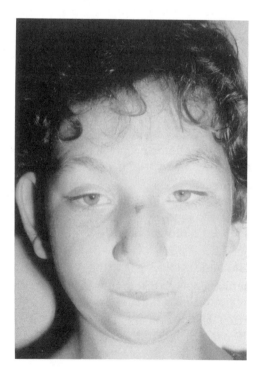

FIGURE 6–33.
Seven-year-old boy with Weaver syndrome

Williams Syndrome (Figure 6–34)

Etiology: Essentially all reported cases to date have been sporadic, but autosomal dominant inheritance has been hypothesized (McKusick 1986).

Phenotypic spectrum: Microcephaly, mental retardation, characteristic behavioral and language profiles, mild growth deficiency, characteristic facies, including prominent lips and large mouth, generally blue eyes with "stellate" pattern in iris, depressed nasal root, long philtrum, soft tissue hyperplasia of the periorbital region, left-sided congenital heart disease, usually including supravalvular aortic stenosis with occasional hypercalcemia, congenitally missing teeth, occasional renal disease.

Natural history: The early neonatal and infantile course is characterized by irritability, possible hypercalcemic seizures, and mild developmental delay. Later in childhood, children with Williams syndrome tend to be very talkative and socially affable. Their language usage is actually very sophisticated and is far in advance of the cognitive skills that usually fall in the educably retarded range, although some cases are more severe. Hyperactivity is common and behavioral control may be difficult. Children with Williams syndrome often relate better to adults than to their peers.

Prognosis: Early infancy may be problematic and the combination of congenital heart lesions and hypercalcemia may be life threatening. If hypercalcemia persists, secondary problems may develop in adulthood. Life span may be shortened as a result. Cognitive impairment and behavioral disorders often prompt recommendations for sheltered environments.

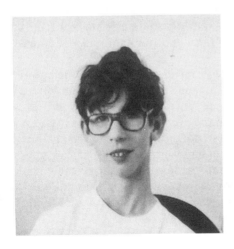

FIGURE 6–34.
Twelve-year-old boy with Williams syndrome

Communication: Characteristic "loquaciousness" and "cocktail party manner" speech and language pattern.

Prevention: None known.

CONCLUSION

Again, there are literally hundreds of unique and identifiable syndromes of congenital anomalies that have or can have adverse consequences for one's ability to communicate. It is essential—sometimes critical—for us to be alert to them. Most of us who are communicative disorders specialists are not syndromologists or dysmorphologists, and we have neither the expertise nor the right to diagnose a syndrome. However, we do have an obligation to know if there is one. This becomes our obligation because we are often the only ones who look at the whole child, the ones who are concerned with speech and language and hearing in one patient. We are the ones who know that the generation of speech is a function of the respiratory system and that the production and perception of language depend on the integrity of the nervous system.

Although it isn't always necessary for us to identify the syndrome, it is essential that we learn if there is one. There are several reasons for this, and they all become secondary prevention. To refer to the dysmorphologist permits us to learn what other behavioral functions may be affected in a given patient and, therefore, to modify our treatment accordingly. Returning to the example given at the beginning of this chapter: If we know that a child has a velocardiofacial syndrome, then we also know that the child will have a learning disability. Knowing that, we may want to modify the treatment used for the resonance difficulties that appear in this syndrome. In some cases, we may want to know that the syndrome is potentially life-threatening, and then we must make proper referrals. The audiologist should know that cafe'-au-lait spots on the skin may be an early warning of acoustic tumor, to take another example. Of course, examples abound.

As clinicians, it is equally important for us to know that our patient does *not* have a syndrome. In such a case, it may be that secondary prevention takes the form of tertiary prevention. However, as indicated above, secondary prevention is available for most of these patients. Primary prevention is a different matter, though. In most cases, primary prevention may have to be in the form of genetic counseling to prevent (or at least to inform) the risk of additional incidents. We must know when to refer to the genetic counselor, to the neurosurgeon, to the maxillofacial plastic surgeon, to the otorhinolaryngologist, to the neurologist, and so on. This is our role in secondary prevention.

GLOSSARY

aglossia: aplasia (absence) or hypoplasia (underdevelopment) of the tongue.

apnea: a cessation of respiration, generally classified as obstructive (caused by an occlusion of the upper or lower airway), central (neurogenically based), or mixed (both central and obstructive components).

arachnodactyly: long, "spidery" fingers and/or toes that are disproportionately long compared to the total length of the hand or foot.

ataxia: abnormality of muscular coordination.

choristoma: congenital presence of normal tissues in abnormal locations, such as ear tags and ocular dermoids (epibulbar dermoids and lipodermoids).

craniectomy: surgical opening of the skull, specifically the calvarium.

craniosynostosis: premature fusion of the cranial bones, which are typically separated by sutural spaces.

dysmorphology(-ist): the study of (one who studies) congenital anomalies for purposes of diagnosis, delineation, and classification (cf. *syndromology*).

dysphagia: abnormality of swallowing.

epiphyseal dysplasia: underdevelopment or abnormality of the extremities of the long bones.

esotropia: convergent *strabismus*.

exorbitism: excessive protrusion of the globe of the eye from its socket.

holosphere: a brain with a single central ventricle and the absence of cerebral hemispheric differentiation.

hypertelorism: excessive distance between the eyes.

lentigines: darkly pigmented flat brown spots on the skin.

lymphedema: swelling originating from the lymphatic system.

oligohydramnios: a deficiency of the amniotic fluid.

omphalocele: congenital herniation of the gut through the abdominal wall.

papilledema: edema of the optic papilla (the optic nerve disc).

popliteal: the space behind the knee.

strabismus: disorder of the convergence of gaze preventing both eyes from focusing on the same point (see *esotropia*).

symphalangism: the joining of two or more digits by a bony fusion of one or more phalanges.

syndactyly: the joining of two or more digits by soft tissue.

syndromology(-ist): the study of (one who studies) the diagnosis and delineation of multiple anomaly syndromes (cf. *dysmorphology*).

synostosis: fusion of two or more normally separated bones.

talipes equinovarus: club foot.

teratoma: a neoplasm (tumor) made up of two or more different types of tissue, none of which normally occurs in the area in which the teratoma is found.

vitreoretinal degeneration: retinal detachment from the vitreous portion of the eye.

REFERENCES

ARDINGER, H. H., et al. 1986. "Further Delineation of Weaver Syndrome," *J. Peds.*, 108, 228–35.

BUYSE, M. L., ed. 1988. *Birth Defects Encyclopedia*. New York: Alan R. Liss.

COHEN, M. MICHAEL, JR. 1981. *The Patient with Multiple Anomalies*. New York: Raven Press.

——ROBERT J. GORLIN, AND S. LEVIN. 1988. *Syndromes of the Head and Neck*, 3rd ed. New York: Raven Press.

CROFT, C. B. et al. 1978. "The Occult Submucous Cleft Palate and the Musculus Uvulae," *Cleft Palate J.*, 15, 150–54.

DAVENPORT, SANDRA L. H., MARGARET A. HEFNER, AND JOYCE A. MITCHELL. 1986. "The Spectrum of Clinical Features in CHARGE Syndrome," *Clin. Gen.*, 29, 298–310.

FOUSHEE, D. 1987. Personal communication.

GOLDING–KUSHNER, K., G. WELLER, AND ROBERT J. SHPRINTZEN. 1985. "Velo-Cardio-Facial Syndrome: Language and Psychological Profiles," *J. Craniofacial Genet. Devel. Biol.*, 5, 259–66.

GOLDSTEIN, S. et al. 1985. "Correction of Deficient Sleep Entrained Growth Hormone Release and Obstructive Sleep Apnea by Tracheostomy in Achondroplasia," *Birth Defects Original Article Series*, 21(2), 85–92.

HERRMANN, J., AND J. M. OPITZ. 1975. "The Stickler Syndrome (Hereditary Arthro-Ophthalmopathy)," Birth Defects Original Article Series, 11(2), 76–103.

KONIGSMARK, BRUCE W., AND ROBERT J. GORLIN. 1976. *Genetic and Metabolic Deafness*. Philadelphia: Saunders.

LAMPERT, R. P. 1980. "Dominant Inheritance of Femoral Hypoplasia-Unusual Facies Syndrome," *Clin. Genet.*, 17, 255–58.

LEWIN, M. L., C. B. CROFT, AND ROBERT J. SHPRINTZEN. 1980. "Velopharyngeal Insufficiency Due to Hypoplasia of the Musculus Uvulae and Occult Submucous Cleft Palate," *Plast. Reconstr. Surg.*, 65, 585–91.

MACKENZIE-STEPNER, K., et al. 1987. "Abnormal Carotid Arteries in the Velocardiofacial Syndrome: A Report of Three Cases," *Plast. Reconstr. Surg.*, 80, 347–51.

MCKUSICK, VICTOR A. 1986. *Mendelian Inheritance in Man*. Baltimore: Johns Hopkins University Press.

OPITZ, J. M., D. W. SMITH, AND R. L. SUMMITT. 1965. "Hypertelorism and Hypospadias," *J. Peds.*, 67, 968.

RICCARDI, V. M., AND J. E. EICHNER. 1986. *Neurofibromatosis: Phenotype, Natural History, and Pathogenesis*. Baltimore: Johns Hopkins University Press.

SADEWITZ, VICKI L., AND ROBERT J. SHPRINTZEN. 1986. *Pierre Robin: A New Look at an Old Disorder.* Video production. March of Dimes, 1986.

——*Syndrome Identification and Communication Impairment.* Video production. March of Dimes, 1987.

SHER, AARON E., ROBERT J. SHPRINTZEN, AND M. J. THORPY. 1986. "Endoscopic Observations of Obstructive Sleep Apnea in Children with Anomalous Upper Airways: Predictive and Therapeutic Value," *Int. J. Pediatr. Otorhinolaryngol.*, 11, 135–46.

SHPRINTZEN, ROBERT J. 1982. "Palatal and Pharyngeal Anomalies in Craniofacial Syndromes," *Birth Defects Original Article Series*, 18(1), 53–78.

——.1987. "Reply from Dr. Shprintzen," *Am. J. Med. Genet.*, 28, 753–55.

——.1988. "Pierre Robin, Micrognathia, and Airway Obstruction: The Dependency of Treatment on Accurate Diagnosis," *Int. Anesthes. Clin.*, 26, 84–91.

——.1988. "Velo-Cardio-Facial Syndrome," in *Birth Defects Encyclopedia*, ed. M. L. Buyse. New York: Alan R. Liss.

——et al. 1978. "A New Syndrome Involving Cleft Palate, Cardiac Anomalies, Typical Facies, and Learning Disabilities: Velo-Cardio-Facial Syndrome," *Cleft Palate J.*, 15, 56–62.

——.1979. "Pharyngeal Hypoplasia in the Treacher Collins Syndrome," *Arch. Otolaryngol.*, 105, 127–31.

——.1981. "The Velo-Cardio-Facial Syndrome: A Clinical and Genetic Analysis," *Peds.*, 67, 167–72.

SMITH, DAVID W. 1982. *Recognizable Patterns of Human Malformation*, 3rd ed. Philadelphia: Saunders.

STICKLER, GUNNAR B., et al. 1965. "Hereditary Progressive Arthro-Ophthalmopathy," *Mayo Clin. Proc.*, 40, 433–35.

TUNCBILEK, E., C. YALCIN, AND M. ATASU. 1977. "Aglossia-Adactylia Syndrome (Special Emphasis on the Inheritance Pattern)," *Clin. Genet.*, 11, 421–23.

WILLIAMS, MICHAEL A., ROBERT J. SHPRINTZEN, AND R. B. GOLDBERG. 1985. "Male-to-Male Transmission of the Velo-Cardio-Facial Syndrome: A Case Report and Review of 60 Cases," *J. Craniofacial. Genet. Devel. Biol.*, 5, 175–80.

7

Respiratory Disorders

In this chapter, we consider those things that interfere with the ability to breathe, or at least to breathe adequately. These generally fall into three categories: (1) problems with neuromotor control of the respiratory system; (2) problems with the respiratory system itself, the airway; and (3) respiratory system disease.

By problems with neuromotor control of respiration is meant those characteristics of respiratory behavior that are affected by the various conditions collectively called cerebral palsy. Persons with such disorders often have poor control of the kind of smooth expiration required for speech production, or they may have particularly shallow breathing, which leaves an inadequate air supply on which to articulate. Diseases of the respiratory nervous system may also be included; muscular dystrophy, multiple sclerosis, and bulbar poliomyelitis may all interfere with one's ability to breathe satisfactorily for speech production or even for life. In this category, one might even include sudden infant death syndrome (SIDS). Moreover, acquired diseases of the respiratory system can influence the ability to produce, and even to perceive, speech. Controversy still exists about the effect of recurrent otitis media—perhaps the most common respiratory disease of children—on learning and language development. Cystic fibrosis—a common, genetic, and eventually fatal disease—also has consequences for communication. Furthermore, some lung diseases, such as pulmonary tuberculosis, are sometimes treated with ototoxic drugs (e.g., streptomycin), an additional hazard.

We consider in particular those disorders that interfere with respiratory function at birth, respiratory distress syndrome, and its potential sequelae. The chapter also includes problems with the airway itself, some of them life-threatening, and consequences for articulation and phonation. And we examine difficulties that persist into later life or that manifest later in life.

RESPIRATORY DISTRESS SYNDROME

Respiratory distress syndrome is, above all, a threat to life in the early neonatal period. It is found particularly in preterm infants, those born with immature respiratory systems. This immaturity may result in hyaline membrane disease and its frequent consequence, bronchopulmonary dysplasia. Indeed, there are other forms of respiratory distress, but these two stand out. Hence, when discussing respiratory distress syndrome, we must also consider the baby born too soon and/or too small.

The Joint Committee on Infant Hearing (1982) cited low birth weight as a major cause of congenital or early onset deafness; and, in fact, it has been shown to be the second most common cause of such deafness (Mencher, Baldursson, and Mencher 1981; Robertson and Whyte 1983). Furthermore, there is a strong relationship between intrauterine growth retardation and congenital malformations. Khoury et al. (1988) reported that "the frequency of intrauterine growth retardation among malformed infants was 22.3%."

Inability to breathe adequately at birth has long been established as a cause of some of those conditions functionally described as cerebral palsy; it has been reported to account for 75 to 80 percent of the incidence (Jilek, Travnickova, and Trojan 1970). Respiratory distress is responsible, therefore, for the intellectual, phonologic, and linguistic deficits usually found in such patients; and cerebral palsy is the most common motor disability in children (Accardo 1984). Moreover, neonatal asphyxia has been implicated in developmental language disability, whether or not accompanied by hearing impairment (Gerber 1980; Gerber, Wile, and Hamai 1985). This, too, is not news. Myklebust, as long ago as 1954, pointed to *anoxia* as a source of aphasia and mental retardation in children. At that time, neonatal asphyxia appeared in 13.8 of 1,000 live births.

Hyaline Membrane Disease

Hyaline (sometimes spelled hyalin) is a clear, homogeneous substance found in the walls of some small blood vessels and in the fetal lung. In the human lung is a substance called *surfactant*. It is surfactant that prevents the alveoli of the lungs from collapsing when we exhale. As fetuses mature in prenatal life, surfactant supplants the hyaline. An infant born too soon, therefore, has too much hyaline or, more importantly, too little surfactant to breathe adequately. If surfactant is lacking, the result is alveolar collapse and eventual *hypoxemia,* which, in turn, may lead to *acidosis.*

The data relating hyaline membrane disease to birth weight are shown in Table 7–1; notice that the peak is not in the smallest babies. Table 7–2, from the same source, displays these data as a function of gestational age; again, the peak is not found in the youngest group. This shift of the maximum from the smallest and youngest probably reflects the totality of problems of these infants.

Certain other infants, even though born at term (37 to 42 weeks gestational age), may have hyaline membrane disease. There is increased risk of hyaline membrane disease in babies born to diabetic mothers (see Chapter 4), those at risk for Rh-related problems, and those delivered in nonnormal ways such as breech or cesarean (Naeye 1973).[1] Naeye reported that the disease occurs significantly more often in white males than in either females or nonwhite infants and in later (i.e., >3) pregnancies. He found the incidence of hyaline membrane disease to diminish among those born to mothers who had had low calorie diets. On the other hand, there is increased risk of preterm delivery in cases of malnutrition in pregnancy (Catanzarite and Aisenbrey 1988).

One must be cautious in reading the literature on this topic. Frequently, the terms "respiratory distress syndrome" and "hyaline membrane disease" are used synonymously. There are good reasons for this, in spite of the fact that an infant may be in respiratory distress from some other cause. First, it is often (even usually) difficult to determine why an infant is in respiratory distress at birth. Second, hyaline membrane disease is the most common form of respiratory distress in the human newborn; it leads to as many as 10,000 deaths per year in the United States (Todres 1983).

TABLE 7–1. Distribution of Hyaline Membrane Disease among Weight Groups

Birth Weight (grams)	Percentage of HMD Cases
500–999	18
1,000–1,499	29
1,500–1,999	26
2,000–2,499	13
2,500 and over	14

SOURCE: Shirley G. Driscoll and Stella B. Yen, "Neonatal Pulmonary Hyaline Membrane Disease: Some Pathologic and Epidemiologic Aspects," in D. B. Villee et al., eds., *Respiratory Distress Syndrome* (New York: Academic Press, 1973), p. 167.

[1] Curiously, according to Naeye, hyaline membrane disease does not occur in preterm infants born to heroin addicts; this fact remains unexplained.

**TABLE 7–2. Distribution of Hyaline Membrane Disease as a Function
of Gestational Age**

Gestational Age (weeks)	Percentage of HMD Cases
less than 28	9.18
28–30	22.45
31–33	19.39
34–36	34.69
37–39	14.29

SOURCE: Shirley G. Driscoll and Stella B. Yen, "Neonatal Pulmonary Hyaline Membrane Disease: Some Pathologic and Epidemiologic Aspects," in D. B. Villee et al., eds., *Respiratory Distress Syndrome* (New York: Academic Press, 1973), p. 165.

An infant with hyaline membrane disease exhibits rapid respiration, retractions, and an audible grunt. The infant may also be cyanotic. The baby deteriorates, and symptoms peak usually at 48 hours of life. The condition is often complicated by *hypovolemia,* a diminution of blood volume. Clearly, then, the first order of attention is the saving of life by respiratory support. This is done by the provision of oxygen, even by an endotracheal tube if necessary. This, in turn, may lead to bronchopulmonary dysplasia.

The primary goal of early therapy is to relieve the hypoxemia and thereby to avert the risk of acidosis. Simultaneously, the hypovolemia requires attention. Artificial ventilation is mandatory, and this has its own risks, among them, *pneumothorax.* In any case, although today most infants do recover from hyaline membrane disease, some (especially those who have suffered a pneumothorax) later develop bronchopulmonary dysplasia. Remember, too, that the typical infant with hyaline membrane disease was born too small. In these infants, intraventricular hemorrhage is "frequently a lethal complication" (Todres 1983).

Asphyxia

The high-risk register of the Joint Committee on Infant Hearing cites among its risk factors "severe asphyxia which may include infants with Apgar scores of 0–3 who fail to institute spontaneous respiration by 10 minutes and those with hypotonia persisting to two hours of age." Although the term "asphyxia" has the specific meaning of a failure to achieve adequate exchange of respiratory gases, it has also been used to include any oxygen failure (see discussion below). The important point here is that some infants do not breathe spontaneously at birth and thereby suffer some kind or amount of respiratory distress. There are also those who suffer periods of *apnea* later in infancy, and they, too, are at risk for communicative handicap.

Asphyxia is the most frequent cause of brain damage in the perinatal period; it appears in more than 1 percent of all live births. The problem was stated nicely some years ago by Longo and Power (1975): "Fetal tissues, in particular the brain and central nervous tissue, are exquisitely sensitive to oxygen deprivation." It is, moreover, in the very earliest time of life that "the CNS is exposed to an unusually high danger of hypoxic damage" (Jilek, Travnickova, and Trojan 1970).

Why do infants not breathe spontaneously? Southall (1988) has described three mechanisms responsible for the apnea of infancy. First is the absence of inspiratory efforts, which is probably due to a "primary failure of the central inspiratory generator in the brainstem." The second is airway obstruction, a subject discussed below. And the third is prolonged expiratory apnea resulting in hypoxemia in response to crying or feeding or during sleep.

The Consequences of Respiratory Distress

We know that auditory-evoked potentials differ from normal in asphyxiated babies (Kileny, Connelly, and Robertson 1980; Mendelson and Salamy 1981). We know, too, as mentioned earlier, that perinatal asphyxia is one of the most common causes of congenital deafness and also of cerebral palsy. And Ehrlich et al. (1973) found that "significant communicative dysfunction" was found primarily in hypoxics among high-risk children.

The terms "asphyxia", "anoxia", and "hypoxia" have been used interchangeably in the literature. This fact often makes it difficult to tell which children are suffering from what, or what was an actual or suspected etiology in a given patient. They are not synonyms: "Asphyxia is defined as impaired or absent exchange of the respiratory gases (oxygen and carbon dioxide). Hypoxia refers to the diminished availability of oxygen, and anoxia alludes to a total lack of oxygen" (Pappas 1985). Moreover, what may be most relevant is not the oxygen deprivation, per se, but the hypoxic encephalopathy, which may be suggested by acidosis. In 1978, Gerber and Mencher observed that a specified level of acidosis is not necessarily an indicator of subsequent handicap; on the other hand, pH levels under 7.5 appearing with hypoxia have been associated with sensory hearing impairment (Pappas 1983). Sheftel, Perelman, and Farrell (1982) noted that the "relationship of acidosis, apnea, asphyxia, and HMD to later adverse auditory and central nervous system sequelae" is apparent.

And that isn't all. Table 7–3 lists 21 different possible sequelae of hyaline membrane disease; some of these are iatrogenic—that is, they are produced by the treatment of respiratory distress (Sheftel, Perelman, and

TABLE 7–3. Possible Long-Term Consequences of Hyaline Membrane Disease

General Abnormalities

Growth retardation
Hypertension
Hepatic dysfunction
Shortened lower extremity from emboli
Scars of the thorax, abdomen, heels, and elsewhere
Head molding
Nasal septal necrosis
Palatal clefts
Defective dentition
Parenting disorders (child abuse, nonorganic failure to thrive)
Risk of sudden infant death syndrome

Neurologic Disturbances

Neuromotor deficits (cerebral palsy)
Mental retardation and learning disabilities
Speech and language delay
Hydrocephalus—usually due to intraventricular hemorrhage
Decreased visual acuity (RLF, strabismus, myopia)
Impaired auditory function

Cardiopulmonary Disturbances

Upper airway obstruction—laryngeal or tracheal stenosis
Lower respiratory tract infections
Bronchopulmonary dysplasia, possibly accompanied by cor pulmonale
Patent ductus arteriosus

SOURCE: David N. Sheftel, Robert H. Perelman, and Philip M. Farrell, "Long-Term Consequences of Hyaline Membrane Disease," in Philip M. Farrell, ed., *Lung Development: Biological and Clinical Perspectives,* Vol. II: *Neonatal Respiratory Distress* (New York: Academic Press, 1982), p. 136.

Farrell 1982). Most generally, there is evidence that learning disorders, especially of reading and behavior, are the more common sequelae of neonatal respiratory distress. However, Fisch (1985) claimed that, although abnormal development was more frequent in children who had had respiratory distress than in matched controls, the incidence of speech and language disorders was not significantly different at eight years of age. Rather, he observed, the most significant factor was socioeconomic status. However, he failed to add that low birth weight appears more often in lower than in higher socioeconomic groups. Furthermore, it is just those relatively disadvantaged children surviving respiratory distress who get poorer postdischarge care. It should be evident, therefore, that the interaction among economic welfare, access to prenatal and postnatal care, and appearance of respiratory distress is what exacerbates sequelae.

Similarly, Fisch found no increased incidence of hearing impairment among survivors with respect to controls. This is especially interesting in light of the fact that most other research does show a significantly increased incidence. Robertson (1978), for example, found that 3 of her 27 deaf patients had a history of preterm delivery with asphyxia. One does not suppose that one-ninth of nonasphyxiated children would be deaf. The fact is, though, that Fisch reviewed only nine publications to draw this conclusion; eight of them did not appear in the speech-language pathology and/or audiology literature, and the ninth was a chapter that he wrote. Perhaps he missed something.

Our own research (Gerber 1980), admittedly retrospective, has found reports of some kind of neonatal respiratory distress in 10 percent of children who had speech and/or language problems persisting until at least the age of five. Neonatal respiratory distress, of any kind, appears in about 1 percent of births (Schultz 1984), but in 10 percent of those with language difficulties. Moreover, we found that children whose congenital deafness may have been produced by neonatal respiratory distress were linguistically different from (and usually poorer than) age-matched congenitally deaf children with different etiologies (Gerber, Wile,and Hamai 1985). Janowsky and Nass (1987) were able to discriminate between asphyxiated preterm infants with intraventricular hemorrhage (IVH) and those without. They found that the two groups of infants did not differ from each other in the rate at which they fail one or more subscales of the ELM Scale. However, the IVH babies were poorer on the expressive, but not the receptive, subscales of the ELM.

Goldson (1984) found that very low birth weight (<1,500 g) infants who had had bronchopulmonary dysplasia had lower Bayley scores at two years of age than children matched for birth weight who did not have bronchopulmonary dysplasia. Such differences may not be apparent in the earliest time of life. Towbin (1987) observed that infants whose brain lesions are subacute may appear to have good neurologic function for the first few months; later, findings of motor and intellectual dysfunction may become manifest. In fact, Krynski et al. (1973), among their patients, found that 7.4 percent of survivors "developed signs of cerebral lesions a year later."

In the United States, 30 percent of neonatal deaths are due to hyaline membrane disease, and it accounts for 50 to 70 percent of the mortality among preterm infants (Rosetti 1986). Sahu (1984) expected that data on neonatal morbidity would be the same as the data for neonatal mortality vis-a-vis birth weight and gestational age. They are and they aren't. Shapiro et al. (1983) found that decreases in neonatal mortality were not accompanied by corresponding decreases in the incidence of birth defects. One might expect (contrary to Sahu) that a diminution in neonatal mortality would result in an increase in the number of survivors, but that survivors would display an array of defects. However, in a survey by Shapiro et al., it turned out that there was a decrease in the number of one-year-old children with mild defects but not in the number with moderate or severe defects; and this is what caused the actual decrease in the morbidity rate. Moreover, while the rate of infant mortality in the United States continues to diminish, it now declines much more gradually than in the past (Wegman 1987). One might expect to see, over a period of years, a continuing increase in the number of survivors with severe handicaps and a decrease of the number of survivors with mild defects. In other words, the neonatologists' art may save more babies (90 percent survive now) and, in some sense, cure those with lesser problems. Those of us who are secondary or tertiary care providers, then, may see a shift in our caseloads toward a more handicapped population. We must also be alert to the apparent fact that "these infants later on face an increased incidence of behavioral abnormalities, abuse and neglect, developmental delay, educational difficulties, and deficient parent-infant bonding and relationships" (Rosetti 1986).

Table 7–4 lists sequelae that actually did appear in 41 (62 percent) of 66 children with bronchopulmonary dysplasia reported by Daily (1987). All of these infants were discharged from the hospital to continue oxygen therapy at home. It is interesting, especially in light of the comments made above, that 27 percent of her babies had transient neuromotor abnormalities, whereas 15 percent had overt cerebral palsy. Seventeen percent were eventually shown to be hearing impaired, with another 12 percent whose auditory function or dysfunction was unknown. However, of the seven infants with hearing impairments, six had a conductive component.

TABLE 7–4. Development in 41 Infants with Bronchopulmonary Dysplasia Receiving Home Oxygen Therapy

	Yes	No	Unknown
Retinopathy of prematurity	29 (71%)	12 (29%)	
Visual impairment	4 (10%)	35 (85%)	2 (5%)
Brainstem auditory evoked response-pass by criteria	22 (54%)	15 (36%)	4 (10%)
Hearing impairment	7 (17%)	29 (71%)	5 (12%)
Transient neuromotor abnormalities	11 (27%)		
Cerebral palsy	6 (15%)		
Developmental testing	21 (53%)		
Mean corrected developmental quotient	71.6 (range 50–100)		

SOURCE: Donna K. Daily, "Home Oxygen Therapy for Infants with Bronchopulmonary Dysplasia," *Perinatology/Neonatology,* 11 (1987), p. 30.

Goldson (1983), in his ongoing study of the development of survivors of neonatal respiratory distress, concluded that "none of these low birth weight infants were completely normal at 2 years of age." Field, Dempsey, and Shuman (1983) found that some developmental failures were still present at the age of entry into school, in particular, motor delays and problems with social interaction.

Is primary prevention of respiratory distress syndrome possible? In some ways it is. Farrell (1982) pointed out that one would want to (and sometimes can) delay delivery of the infant as long as possible. And we continue to hope for advances in the obstetricians' art that will make this attainable. The fact is, though, that the rate of low birth weight deliveries has not diminished significantly in recent years in spite of decreases in infant mortality (Figure 7–1).

Some procedures do seem to work. Kwong and Egan (1986) were able to delay delivery in cases where premature labor was evident. The incidence of hyaline membrane disease in this treated group was 28 percent as compared to 68 percent in a matched group without this treatment. The ability to increase birth weight should be expected to diminish the extent of the handicap. Figure 7–2 shows that IQ at three years of age correlates with birth weight. The lower the birth weight, the lower the IQ.

We must still find other means to prevent respiratory distress. Farrell goes on to say that it is possible to accelerate development of the fetal lung by the use of corticosteroid hormones, but, of course, this has its own risks. Glucocorticoids administered to the mother have been shown to increase the production of surfactant in the fetus and to increase

FIGURE 7–1.   Infant mortality and low birth weight rates

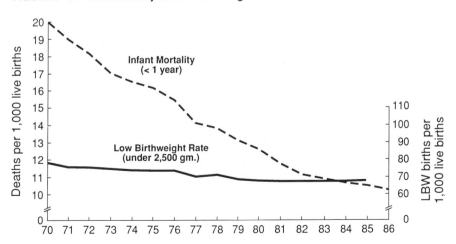

FIGURE 7–2. Intelligence of preterm AGA (Adequate for Gestational Age) infants (1,500 g is upper limit of very low birth weight; IQ = 100 is average)

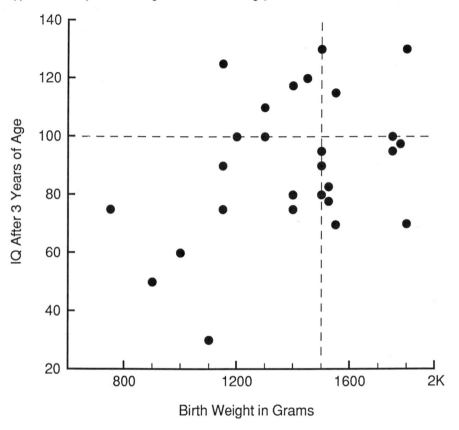

Birth Weight in Grams

the rate of maturation of the fetal lung (Harrison, Golbus, and Filly 1984). In cases where hyaline membrane disease presents as a consequence of maternal diabetes, it is possible to alleviate (i.e., to control) the diabetes; this has been known to be effective. Similarly, the risk that accompanies cases of Rh incompatibility may be diminished with a corresponding diminution of respiratory distress.

The picture for secondary prevention has improved greatly with the ability to synthesize surfactant. Gitlin et al. (1987) treated 41 low birth weight infants with surfactant within eight hours after birth. Significant improvement in respiratory function appeared within four hours. There was concomitant decrease in the incidence of pneumothoraces and in the need for ventilatory support. One supposes, therefore, that the survivors developed with fewer sequelae than those treated by other means.

The other kind of secondary prevention is early identification and therapeutic intervention. There is evidence even from neuroanatomical studies that early intervention in cases of sensory deprivation does take advantage of the neural plasticity that still exists in early life (Greenough 1975). The human brain continues to grow and develop even up to the eighteenth month post-term. Table 7–5 shows the effect of early enrichment of the environment *in the intensive care nursery* on Bayley scores six months later. The scores are all statistically significant. What happens later?

Korner (1987) did a thorough review of the effects of what she called preventive intervention. She found that all studies agreed that preterm infants benefited in some way from intervention but that the effects often do not persist: "When one considers the odds against finding persistent effects of early intervention in terms of the multitude of other variables impinging on the development of infants, it is indeed surprising that the implicit expectation of long-range effects is so widespread." She shared neither the surprise nor the disappointment of other reviewers: "Such intervention may prevent current functioning from getting worse, may forestall specific developmental arrests, may facilitate coping better with new developmental tasks, and, in effect, may put the infants developmentally more on track than might have been possible without such intervention."

Bricker (1978) proposed that we should consider what is an acceptable rate of progress for the child before us. What should be expected from that child? Finally, consider again our discussion in Chapter 6 of the prevention of frustration, of unnecessary treatment, of missed opportunities, of progression, of uncertainty. Intervention on behalf of the handicapped child is not a temporary thing; it continues throughout life. It is both secondary and tertiary.

TABLE 7–5. **Group Comparison of Bayley Scales of Infant Development at Six Month Follow-up**

	Developmental Index Mean Score	
	Control Group	Treatment Group (p.001)
Bayley Mental		
Uncorrected for gestational age	76.50	98.93
Corrected for gestational age	105.21	125.36
Bayley Motor		
Uncorrected for gestational age	78.86	97.86
Corrected for gestational age	104.93	121.86

SOURCE: Louis H. Rosetti, *High Risk Infants: Identification, Assessment, and Intervention* (Boston: College-Hill Press, 1986), p. 153. Copyright 1986.

UPPER AIRWAY AND LARYNGEAL PROBLEMS

For our purposes, the upper airway is defined as everything from the larynx to the nose. It starts at the glottis and ends at the nares. Chapter 6 described many craniofacial disorders; recall that virtually all of them include problems of the upper airway. Also, recall that Chapter 5 gives descriptions of injuries to the face and neck. In this section, we consider congenital and/or progressive disorders of the airway that can affect respiration and, therefore, articulation and phonation.

Laryngomalacia

Cotton and Reilly (1983) defined laryngomalacia as a congenital flaccid larynx the etiology of which "remains enigmatic." It is a condition in which *stridor* is produced by inadequate tension on the supraglottic tissues so that they collapse into the laryngeal inlet. According to L. Holinger (1980), laryngeal anomalies account for 60 percent of laryngeal problems that appear in the newborn, and laryngomalacia produces nearly 60 percent of those. However, the elder Holinger had earlier reported an incidence of 75 percent among infants who present for laryngoscopy (Holinger and Brown 1967). Hirschberg and Szende (1982) reported laryngomalacia to be the most common cause of stridor, and a "cackling" quality to be pathognomonic.

Laryngomalacia results from immaturity of laryngeal cartilage (Wood 1983); hence, it may be still another difficulty found in the preterm infant, a point made also by Cotton and Richardson (1981). There is a decrease in stridor when an infant with laryngomalacia lies prone with neck extended. Even then, the stridor may not be evident until the baby is a couple of months old; in fact, Hirschberg and Szende claimed that stridor increases for the first few months of life. Cotton and Richardson emphasized that the diagnosis requires endoscopy to be confirmed, as there are other possible reasons for a newborn to be stridorous. Among the laryngeal anomalies observed by Holinger (1980) are subglottic stenosis and paralysis of one or both vocal folds.

The clinical description of laryngolomalacia offered by Cotton and Richardson is succinct and appropriate:

> The glottis is usually small, with a long narrow epiglottis that may be omega shaped; the aryepiglottic folds are long and floppy with prominent arytenoids and a deep interarytenoid cleft. In inspiration, these supraglottic structures collapse toward each other, leaving a slitlike opening; if some tension is exerted by the laryngoscope blade to stretch the aryepiglottic folds, the arytenoid cartilages medially infold over the glottis and flutter, thus imparting the fluttering sound to the stridor. During expiration the positive pressure of air blows the tissues apart.

Laryngomalacia is a disorder that should disappear with time as the cartilages of the larynx mature. Ferguson (1972) referred to it as "merely a retardation of normal development" and not a pathology of the larynx, and considered it to be a "temporary physiologic dysfunction which subsides with time and further growth." That, of course, is true if the laryngolomalacia is not associated with something else. For example, it is often not noticed until after a respiratory infection. Solomons and Prescott (1987) found a "number" of children whose laryngolomalacia was associated with neuromuscular disorders preventing maintenance of a patent airway. Such children, obviously, are at still greater risk.

The problem for us, as secondary or tertiary care specialists, is to know when to treat and when not. If, in fact, laryngomalacia is the rare case of "the child will outgrow it," then we should permit our patient to do so. If, on the other hand, a laryngomalacia appears as a property of or as a result of some more serious problem, then early intervention may indeed be appropriate. As long as laryngomalacia continues to be a disorder with an etiology that is "enigmatic," primary prevention will elude us.

Papilloma

The most common of all laryngeal tumors are the *papilloma*. In children, these are usually multiple and recur. Typically, they appear on the vocal folds but are sometimes found on the walls of the pharynx and even the palate and uvula. They may sometimes extend into the subglottal area. Seid and Cotton (1983) claimed that the etiology is unknown but may be viral; in any case, there is no primary prevention of this most common laryngeal disorder in children. Secondary prevention takes the form of surgery, unfortunately, as these tumors must be removed from the larynx to avoid airway compromise. They are not amenable to the skills of the voice therapist in spite of the fact that such a child is always dysphonic and may be aphonic.

Other Problems

There are large numbers and varieties of airway obstructions that could and should come to the attention of communication disorders specialists in addition to those discussed above. For example, choanal atresia could be life-threatening, and is an outstanding example of supraglottal disorders. Especially important is to note that choanal atresia is often associated with other anomalies, and those may turn out to be more significant. For example, Leclerc and Fearon (1987) noted 38 of their 130 patients had at least some of the features of CHARGE association, and 57 of the 130 had anomalies of systems other than the airway. Pertinent to the discussion of Chapter 6, they found three cases with Down syndrome, three with Treacher Collins syndrome, and four with other craniofacial anomalies that have consequences for speech, hearing, and language. Cotton and Reilly (1983) also observed that supraglottic atresias have "a high frequency" of associated anomalies, and expressed the fear that "many children are not properly diagnosed ante-mortem."

Around the level of the larynx, other problems may appear. These could include laryngocele, hemangioma, supraglottic web, laryngeal web, vocal fold paralysis, neurofibromatoses, and clefts of the larynx itself. In addition, many of the identifiable syndromes discussed in Chapter 6 present with respiratory system anomalies. These patients often have shortened anteroposterior length of the oral cavity and oropharyngeal space, as in Down syndrome. They have anomalies of the skull base such that upper airway obstruction can or does appear as in Apert syndrome or Treacher Collins syndrome.

Also, below the larynx there are sometimes problems, but these are less likely to come to the attention of a communication disorders specialist. The assorted stenoses, webs, hemangiomas, and the like that can appear above the glottis can also appear below it. Occasionally, a tracheostenosis can arise due to a constriction from a misplaced innominate artery.

Southall, in his 1988 review, observed that partial or complete airway obstruction may be a source of apnea. These obstructions can be associated with the conglomerate called Pierre Robin and may arise from laryngeal trauma or from disease such as croup. The 180 patients described by Hirschberg and Szende (1982) were divided for study purposes into those whose disorders were of (1) the nose, oral cavity, and pharynx, (2) the larynx, including supraglottic, glottic, and subglottic spaces, (3) the trachea, and (4) the bronchi and lungs. Their descriptions of the resulting stridors are listed in Table 7–6. Note that most of the descriptors that they employed are perceptual acoustic properties of the sounds of stridor. The significance of this is discussed below.

PREVENTION

We have already considered the fact that primary prevention is not usually available for respiratory disorders that arise congenitally or very early in life. There are some general exceptions, however. For example, when the respiratory problems are aspects of heritable disorders, genetic counseling can become a type of primary prevention, or if hyaline membrane disease may appear as a consequence of maternal diabetes, the diabetes may often be brought under control. The problem, frequently stated above, is that the etiology of respiratory distress—even clearly diagnosable respiratory distress—is described as unknown or enigmatic.

TABLE 7–6. Types of Stridor, as Defined by Hirschberg and Szende

Interrupted pharyngeal stridors
  Sawing (buzzing) stridor
  Rasping stridor
  Croaky stridor
  Snoring (snorting, stertorous, grunting) stridor
  Bubbling (gurgling) stridor
  Divided pharyngeal stridor
Lump-in-the-throat stridor
Supraglottic stridor (high, sharp, and loud inspiration and expiration)
Cackling (clucking) stridor
Hissing (whistling, sibilant) stridor
Stridor-phonation
Crowing stridor
Stridor of subglottic character
Deep-hollow stridor
Hollow stridor
Tracheal stridor
Spastic expiratory stridor

SOURCE: Based on data from J. Hirschberg and T. Szende, *Pathological Cry, Stridor, and Cough in Infants,* trans. L. Elias (Budapest: Akademiai Klado, 1982).

Secondary prevention, however, may be more optimistic. Hyaline membrane disease may now be treated with surfactant, for instance. Laryngomalacia can be visualized with endoscopy, and a good diagnostician should be able to determine if it has appeared in isolation and predict that it is a self-curing condition. Papilloma can be removed; and papillomatosis, too, is a self-curing condition eventually. It is possible to learn if choanal atresia is or is not part of a larger syndrome.

There is another and potentially powerful means of secondary prevention, the study of infant cry. Lester (1984) observed that there are two diagnostic uses of cry analysis: as a sign of abnormality and as a sign of risk of abnormality. He reported finding distinctive cries in infants with various respiratory problems, low birth weight, neonatal asphyxia, bacterial meningitis, and hyperbilirubinemia. A clear example of the diagnostic significance of infant cry is Cri du chat syndrome, that is, 5p– (discussed in Chapter 2). The latency of cry in response to a painful stimulus has been investigated as indicative of nervous system impairment. Lester (1987) also found that certain acoustic properties of infants' cries predicted developmental outcome at 18 months and 5 years of age in both normal and preterm infants. Moreover, chronic hoarseness seems to be a property of congestive heart failure in infancy (Condon et al. 1985).

In our clinic, we have shown that the cries of normal, healthy, full-term newborns are very similar to one another (Gerber 1985). Indeed, they should be, and inflicting pain should not be influential except in the instance of cry latency. A given infant, after all, uses the same vocal tract to cry for pain or hunger or discomfort or annoyance. The baby does not change vocal tracts for different purposes (Figure 7–3). Thus, we concluded that "non-cry vocalizations and cry vocalizations do not differ very much from each other." Gray et al. (1985) also found that cries of any one baby do not differ much from time to time. The point is that, if a cry does differ from that of the normal baby, one should and can be suspicious.

The state of the art is such that rather sophisticated analyses are required to determine in what way an odd-sounding cry is pathological. The list of terms in Table 7–6 can be quantized, and, indeed, Hirschberg and Szende (1982) did sonographic analyses. Other, more elegant and detailed analyses may be Fourier analyses (e.g., Gray et al. 1985), power

FIGURE 7–3.   Spectrally nearly identical noncry and cry vocalizations

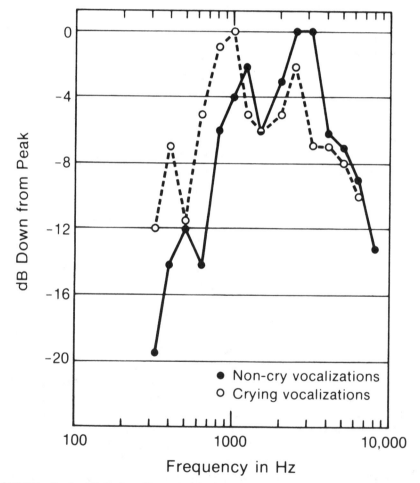

SOURCE: Sanford E. Gerber, "Acoustical Analyses of Neonates' Vocalizations," *International Journal of Pediatric Otorhinolaryngology,* 13 (1987), 5. Reprinted with permission of Elsevier Science Publishers.

spectral density functions (Leiberman, Cohen, and Tal 1986), or three dimensional log magnitude spectrograms (Gerber, Lynch, and Gibson 1987). This last is shown in Figure 7–4 which compares the cry of a normal infant and that of an infant with a unilateral vocal fold paralysis.

If the analysis of infant cry can be made to be diagnostic, or made to be a significant part of the diagnostic armamentarium, a considerable advance can be made in the secondary prevention of respiratory disorders.

FIGURE 7-4. Three-dimensional log magnitude spectra of the cry of a normal infant and the cry of an infant with a paralyzed vocal fold

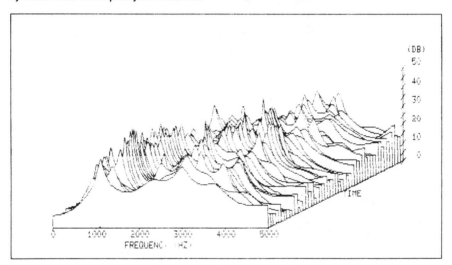

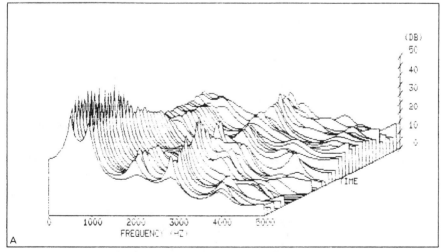

SOURCE: Sanford E. Gerber, Constance J. Lynch, and William S. Gibson, Jr., "The Acoustic Characteristics of the Cry of an Infant with Unilateral Vocal Fold Paralysis, *International Journal of Pediatric Otorhinolaryngology,* 13 (1987), 7, 8. Reprinted by permission of Elsevier Science Publishers.

CONCLUSION

Respiratory disorders of the newly born constitute a major source of mortality (in fact, at least half) among infants. Morbidity appears among survivors in a multitude of ways all of which are the professional concern of communication disorders specialists. The audiologist must be alert to the auditory consequences of failure to breathe at birth; neonatal asphyxia is a common cause of early onset sensory deafness. The speech-language pathologist must attend to the consequences of glottal and supraglottal abnormalities and must be concerned with the effects of long-term tracheotomies on the development of speech and language. We must all take heed of the potential neuromotor, neurosensory, and cognitive consequences of respiratory distress in all its forms.

GLOSSARY

acidosis: a decrease of alkali relative to acid in body fluids leading to a disturbance of tissue function especially of the central nervous system.
apnea: absence of respiration.
hypovolemia: a decrease in the volume of blood.
hypoxemia: blood oxygen less than normal.
papilloma: wartlike growths (i.e., benign tumors) that may appear over a large surface of the vocal folds, resulting in various degrees of dysphonia, even including aphonia.
pneumothorax: the presence of air in the pleural cavity.
stridor: noisy respiration; therefore, a sign of respiratory obstruction.
surfactant: a chemical agent that forms a layer over the alveolar surfaces of the lungs; it alters the relationship between surface tension and surface area, thereby preventing lung collapse upon expiration.

REFERENCES

ACCARDO, PASQUALE J. 1984. "Associated Deficits: The Ecology of Developmental Disabilities in Infants," *J. Dev. Beh. Peds.*, 5, 216–17.
BRICKER, DIANE. 1978. "Early Intervention: The Criteria of Success," *Allied Health and Beh.Sci.*, 1, 567–82.
CATANZARITE, VALERIAN A., AND GARY A. AISENBREY. 1988. "Severe Malnutrition in Pregnancy: Diagnosis, Evaluation, and Management," *Perinat./Neonat.*, 12, 11–12, 14–17.
CONDON, LAWRENCE M., et al. 1985. "Cardiovocal Syndrome in Infancy," *Peds.*, 76, 22–25.
COTTON, ROBIN T,. AND JAMES S. REILLY. 1983. "Congenital Malformations of the Larynx," in *Pediatric Otolaryngology*, Vol. II, ed. Charles D. Bluestone and Sylvan E. Stool. Philadelphia: Saunders.
COTTON, ROBIN T., AND MARK A. RICHARDSON. 1981. "Congenital Laryngeal Anomalies," *Otolaryngol. Clin. N. Amer.*, 14, 203–18.
DAILY, DONNA K. 1987. "Home Oxygen Therapy for Infants with Bronchopulmonary Dysplasia," *Perinatol./Neonatol.*, 11(3), 26, 28, 30, 32, 35–36.
DRISCOLL, SHIRLEY G., AND STELLA B. YEN. 1973. "Neonatal Pulmonary Hyaline Membrane Disease: Some Pathologic and Epidemiologic Aspects," in *Respiratory Distress Syndrome*, ed. Claude A. Villee, Dorothy B. Villee, and James Zuckerman. New York: Academic Press.

EHRLICH, CAROL H. et al. 1973. "Communication Skills in Five-Year-Old Children with High-Risk Neonatal Histories, *J. Speech Hear. Res.*, 16, 522–29.

FARRELL, PHILIP M. 1982. "Introduction to the Preventative Approach to Perinatal Care," in *Lung Development: Biological and Clinical Perspectives*, Vol. II, *Neonatal Respiratory Distress.*, ed. Philip M.Farrell. New York: Academic Press.

FERGUSON, CHARLES F. 1972. "Congenital Malformations," in *Pediatric Otolaryngology.*, Vol. II, *Disorders of the Respiratory Tract in Children*, ed. Charles F. Ferguson and Edwin L. Kendig, Jr. Philadelphia: Saunders.

FIELD, TIFFANY, JEAN DEMPSEY, AND H. H. SHUMAN. 1983. "Five-Year Follow-Up of Preterm Respiratory Distress Syndrome and Post-Term Postmaturity Syndrome Infants," in *Infants Born at Risk*, ed. Tiffany Field and Anita Sostek. New York: Grune & Stratton.

FISCH, ROBERT O. 1985. "Long-Term Consequences of Survivors of Respiratory Distress Syndrome," in *Pulmonary Development: Transition from Intrauterine to Extrauterine Life*, ed. George H. Nelson. New York: Marcel Dekker.

GERBER, SANFORD E. 1980. "Asphyxia Neonatorum and Subsequent Communicative Disorders," paper presented to the XVth International Congress of Audiology, Krakow, Poland.

——.1985. "Acoustical Analyses of Neonates' Vocalizations," Intl. J. Ped. Otorhino-laryngol., 10, 1–8.

——, CONSTANCE J. LYNCH, AND WILLIAM S. GIBSON, JR. 1987. "The Acoustic Characteristics of the Cry of an Infant with Unilateral Vocal Fold Paralysis," *Intl. J. Ped. Otorhinolaryngol.*, 13, 1–9.

——, AND GEORGE T. MENCHER, eds. 1978. *Early Diagnosis of Hearing Loss*. New York: Grune & Stratton.

——, ELIZABETH WILE, AND NANCY T. HAMAI. 1985. "Central Auditory Dysfunction in Deaf Children," *Human Communication Canada*, 9, 39–44.

GITLIN, JONATHAN D. et al. 1987. "Randomized Controlled Trial of Exogenous Surfactant for the Treatment of Hyaline Membrane Disease," *Peds.*, 79, 31–37.

GOLDSON, EDWARD. 1983. "Bronchopulmonary Dysplasia: Its Relation to Two-Year Developmental Functioning in the Very Low Birth Weight Infants," in *Infants Born at Risk*, ed. Tiffany Field and Anita Sostek. New York: Grune & Stratton.

——. 1984. "Severe Bronchopulmonary Dysplasia in the Very Low Birth Weight Infant: Its Relationship to Developmental Outcome," *J. Dev. Beh. Peds.*, 5, 165–68.

GRAY, LINCOLN, et al. 1985. "Fourier Analysis of Infantile Stridor," *Intl. J. Ped. Otorhinolaryngol.*, 10, 191–99.

GREENOUGH, WILLIAM T. 1975. "Experiential Modification of the Developing Brain," *Amer. Sci.*, 63, 37–46.

HARRISON, MICHAEL R., MITCHELL S. GOLBUS, AND ROY A. FILLY. 1984. *The Unborn Patient*. Orlando, FL: Grune & Stratton.

HIRSCHBERG, J., AND T. SZENDE. 1982. *Pathological Cry, Stridor, and Cough in Infants*, trans. L. Elias. Budapest: Akademiai Klado.

HOLINGER, LAUREN D. 1980. "Etiology of Stridor in the Neonate, Infant and Child," *Ann. Otol. Rhinol. Laryngol.*, 89, 397–400.

HOLINGER, PAUL H., AND W. T. BROWN. 1967. "Congenital Webs, Cysts, Laryngoceles and Other Anomalies of the Larynx," *Ann. Otol. Rhinol. Laryngol.*, 76, 744.

JANOWSKY, JERI S., AND RUTH NASS. 1987. "Early Language Development in Infants with Cortical and Subcortical Perinatal Brain Injury," *J. Dev. Beh. Peds.*, 8, 3–7.

JILEK, L., E. TRAVNICKOVA, AND S. TROJAN. 1970. "Characteristic Metabolic and Functional Responses to Oxygen Deficiency in the Central Nervous System," in *Physiology of the Perinatal Period*, Vol. 2., ed. Uwe Stave. New York: Appleton-Century-Crofts.

JOINT COMMITTEE ON INFANT HEARING. 1982. "Position Statement 1982," *Peds.*, 70, 496–97.

KHOURY, MUIN J., et al. 1988. "Congenital Malformations and Intrauterine Growth Retardation: A Population Study," *Peds.*, 82, 83–89.

KILENY, P., C. CONNELLY, AND C. ROBERTSON. 1980. "Auditory Brainstem Responses in Perinatal Asphyxia," *Intl. J. Ped. Otorhinolaryngol.*, 2, 147–59.

KORNER, ANNELIESE F. 1987. "Preventive Intervention with High-Risk Newborns: Theoretical, Conceptual, and Methodological Perspectives," in *Handbook of Infant Development*, 2nd ed., ed. Joy Doniger Osofsky. New York: John Wiley.

KRYNSKI, S., et al. 1973. "Perinatal Anoxia and Mental Retardation," *Acta Paedopsychiatrica*, 39, 347–55.

KWONG, MELINDA S., AND EDMUND A. EGAN. 1986. "Reduced Incidence of Hyaline Membrane Disease in Extremely Premature Infants following Delay of Delivery in Mother with Preterm Labor: Use of Ritodrine and Betamethasone," *Peds.,* 78, 767–74.

LECLERC, JACQUES E., AND BLAIR FEARON. 1987. "Choanal Atresia and Associated Anomalies," *Intl. J. Ped. Otorhinolaryngol.,* 13, 265–72.

LEIBERMAN, ALBERTO, ARNON COHEN, AND ASHER TAL. 1986. "Digital Signal Processing of Stridor and Snoring in Children," *Intl. J. Ped. Otorhinolaryngol.,* 12, 173–85.

LESTER, BARRY M. 1984. "A Biosocial Model of Infant Crying," in *Advances in Infancy Research,* ed. L. Lipsett. New York: Ablex.

———. 1987. "Developmental Outcome Prediction from Acoustic Cry Analysis in Term and Preterm Infants," *Peds.,* 80, 529–34.

LONGO, L. D., AND G. G. POWER. 1975. "Fetal Physiology: A Primer for the 70s," *Doctor,* 3, 10–14.

MENCHER, GEORGE T., GYLFI BALDURSSON, AND LENORE S. MENCHER. 1981. "Prologue: The Way We Were," in *Early Management of Hearing Loss,* ed. George T. Mencher and Sanford E. Gerber. New York: Grune & Stratton.

MENDELSON, TERRIE, AND ALAN SALAMY. 1981. "Maturational Effects on the Middle Components of the Averaged Electroencephalic Response," *J. Speech Hear. Res.,* 24, 140–144.

MYKLEBUST, HELMER R. 1954. Auditory Disorders in Children. New York: Grune & Stratton.

NAEYE, RICHARD L. 1973. "Epidemiology of Hyaline Membrane Disease. Selective Aspects," in *Respiratory Distress Syndrome,* ed. Claude A. Villee, Dorothy B. Villee, and James Zuckerman. New York: Academic Press.

PAPPAS, DENNIS G. 1983. "A Study of the High-Risk Registry for Sensorineural Hearing Impairment," *Otolaryngology— Head and Neck Surgery,* 91, 41–440.

———. 1985. *Diagnosis and Treatment of Hearing Impairment in Children.* San Diego, CA: College-Hill Press.

ROBERTSON, CHARLENE. 1978. "Pediatric Assessment of the Infant at Risk for Deafness," in *Early Diagnosis of Hearing Loss,* ed. Sanford E. Gerber and George T. Mencher. New York: Grune & Stratton.

———, AND LILLIAN WHYTE. 1983. "Prospective Identification of Infants with Hearing Loss and Multiple Handicaps: The Role of the Neonatal Follow-Up Clinic," in *The Multiply Handicapped Hearing Impaired Child,* ed. George T. Mencher and Sanford E. Gerber. New York: Grune & Stratton.

ROSETTI, LOUIS M. 1986. *High-Risk Infants: Identification, Assessment, and Intervention.* Boston: Little, Brown.

SAHU, S. 1984. "Birth weight, Gestational Age, and Neonatal Risks," *Perinat. / Neonat.,* 8(1), 28–30, 32–33, 36.

SCHULTZ, FREDERICK R. 1984. "Respiratory Distress Syndrome," in *Medical Aspects of Developmental Disabilities in Children Birth to Three,* ed. James A. Blackman. Rockville, MD: Aspen.

SEID, ALLAN B., AND ROBIN COTTON. 1983. "Tumors of the Larynx, Trachea, and Bronchi," in *Pediatric Otolaryngology,* ed. Charles D. Bluestone and Sylvan E. Stool. Philadelphia: Saunders.

SHAPIRO, SAM, et al. 1983. "Changes in Infant Morbidity Associated with Decreases in Neonatal Mortality," *Peds.,* 72, 408–15.

SHEFTEL, DAVID N., ROBERT H. PERELMAN, AND PHILIP M. FARRELL. 1982. "Long-Term Consequences of Hyaline Membrane Disease," in *Lung Development: Biological and Clinical Perspectives,* Vol. II, *Neonatal Respiratory Distress,* ed. Philip M. Farrell. New York: Academic Press.

SOLOMONS, N. B., AND C. A. J. PRESCOTT. 1987. "Laryngomalacia. A Review and the Surgical Management for Severe Cases," *Intl. J. Ped. Otorhinolaryngol.,* 13, 31–39.

SOUTHALL, D. P. 1988. "Role of Apnea in the Sudden Infant Death Syndrome," *Peds.,* 80, 73–84.

TODRES, I. DAVID. 1983. "Respiratory Disorders of the Newborn," in *Pediatric Otolaryngology,* Vol. 2, ed. Charles D. Bluestone and Sylvan E. Stool. Philadelphia: Saunders.

TOWBIN, ABRAHAM. 1987. "The Depressed Newborn: Pathogenesis and Neurologic Sequels," *Perinat. / Neonat.,* 11, no. 3, 16–18.

WEGMAN, MYRON E. 1987. "Annual Summary of Vital Statistics—1986," *Peds.,* 80, 817–27.

WOOD, ROBERT E. 1983. "Physiology of the Larynx, Airways, and Lungs," in *Pediatric Otolaryngology,* Vol. II, ed. Charles D. Bluestone and Sylvan E. Stool. Philadelphia: Saunders.

8

Metabolic Disorders

Metabolism is the total exchange of energy and chemical matter of any living cell. In general, then, it is the process by which an animal digests food and converts it to energy. The main metabolite of neural tissue is glucose, and the oxidation of glucose accounts for most of the oxygen utilized by the brain. The metabolic rate of the brain is very high in terms of total body rates; but, in children, brain metabolic rates are lower than in adults. Placental transfer of thyroid hormones is rather limited, and this has interesting implications for prenatal development of thyroid disorders. Nevertheless, "thyroid hormone is essential for early brain development; without it, permanent and irreparable brain damage occurs" (Rovet, Sorbara, and Ehrlich 1986). Hypothyroidism is a treatable disorder, but treatment must begin in the first three months of life.

It is evident that environmental events—whether endogenous or exogenous—will influence brain metabolism and, therefore, brain (and communicative) function. Some of these phenomena have been discussed in previous chapters because they are or could be teratogens. For example, we referred to the infants of diabetic mothers and mentioned Pendred syndrome and cretinism. Some of these metabolic problems are present at birth in some form and some do not appear until later; and some that are present at birth have no effects until later. Some are amenable to primary or secondary prevention.

This chapter considers three categories of metabolic disorders that have significance for communication: thyroid disorders, the mucopolysaccharidoses, and diabetes. There are more than three categories of metabolic disorders, but these are more common and/or more serious than others. All of them may have sequelae in the domains of speech, language, and hearing, in neuromotor and/or neurosensory function, and in cognitive development.

THYROID DISORDERS

As speech-language pathologists, we are familiar with the function of the thyroid cartilage in phonation, its shape and size and its location. But recall that an important purpose of the thyroid cartilage is to protect the thyroid gland, which it houses. In adult humans, the thyroid gland is one of the largest, weighing nearly three-quarters of an ounce. Its blood supply has been described as copious, and in the average adult nearly 5 quarts of blood pass through it every hour which has a major influence on thyroid activity. The specific function of the thyroid gland is to convert (i.e., metabolize) the materials brought to it by the blood into *thyroxine* and *triiodothyronine,* hormones that are necessary for growth and development. Its general purpose, then, is to stimulate metabolism of many other cells and to manage growth. In fact, Fisher and Burrow (1975) stated that the role of thyroid hormones is "crucial" in the development of the organism.

Thyroid function refers to the gland's ability to convert iodine (which the gastrointestinal system releases into the blood as iodide) into thyroxin and triiodothyrine and to release them as needed. Hence, hypothyroidism means that the thyroid gland does a relatively poor job of iodide conversion; hyperthyroidism refers to the release of excessive amounts of the two hormones. Normally, the rate of release is governed by the pituitary gland—the so-called master gland—which discharges *thyrotrophic* hormone as needed by sensing the rate of release of the thyroid hormones. Thus, one influences the other. In addition to hypothyroidism and hyperthyroidism, the thyroid gland is subject to viral and bacterial diseases and can also become cancerous.

Congenital Hypothyroidism

Congenital hypothyroidism occurs in at least 1 in 10,000 births and perhaps in as many as 1 in 5,000. Historically, it had been one of the primary causes of mental retardation. It can appear in the form of cretinism, which is characterized by a distinctive appearance, severe mental retardation, and auditory impairment (see Figure 4–7). One serious problem is that an infant who could become a cretin may appear normal at birth and only gradually develop the relevant clinical signs. Moreover, the time in prenatal life when hypothyroidism first appears has a profound influence on the postnatal sequelae. Stanbury (1982) described the damage as "spotty but generalized" but still "related to severity and timing of hormonal deficiency." The earlier and more severe the deficiency, the greater the intellectual and other nervous system deficits.

The classical endemic cretin still appears in many parts of the world, usually mountainous, notably in Papua New Guinea and in parts of South America. Hetzel (1972) distinguished this type from sporadic cretinism, which, by definition, appears from time to time and place to place. This latter is a state of hypothyroidism accompanied by retarded mental and physical development with or without goiter. Although this is a disorder that arises in prenatal life, the variability of its expression and the typical delay in its appearance make it a disorder of seemingly postnatal onset. Moreover, a given patient may not be a true cretin; so a more contemporary term for this class of disorders is congenital hypothyroidism. Smith (1982) characterized congenital hypothyroidism by "postnatal onset of slow growth, sluggish activity, myxedema, and lag of developmental progression." Furthermore, patients with lesser degrees of congenital hypothyroidism may not have *myxedema,* and the lag of development may not be easily apparent in early life.

What are the consequences of congenital hypothyroidism? Figure 8–1 shows the language delay measured at three years of age in a group of 109 hypothyroid children compared to a control group consisting largely of their siblings (Rovet, Ehrlich, and Sorbara 1987a). Additional study of

FIGURE 8–1. Reynell language test results at three years of age among children with hypothyroidism (CH)

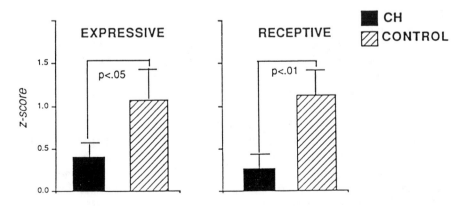

SOURCE: Joanne F. Rovet, Robert M. Ehrlich, and Donna-Lee Sorbara, "Outcome in Neonatally Identified Thyroid Hormone Deficient Children: Persistent Deficits and Associated Risk Factors." Paper presented at the fifth Annual Meeting of the Society for Behavioral Pediatrics, Anaheim, California, 1987. Reprinted by permission of Joanne F. Rovet.

80 children showed that those with delayed physical development (as measured by bone age) had lower developmental scores up to the age of five (the limit of the study) than a group of hypothyroid children without bone age retardation (Rovet, Ehrlich, and Sorbara 1987b). Clearly, then, there is a link between physical development and mental development. Moreover, the scores on tests of cognitive development still fall largely within the range of normal, but the scores on specific language tests do not. Thus, given that these children are treated and do not suffer severe consequences, they still have language retardation, and many of them are hearing impaired.

The issue of auditory dysfunction in hypothyroidism is significant for differential diagnosis and, therefore, for prevention. Bargman and Gardner (1972) observed deafness to be a common defect in association with endemic cretinism in certain parts of the world. Debruyne, Vanderschueren-Lodeweyckx, and Bastijns (1983) concluded that "substantial deafness" appears in about 10 percent of cases of congenital hypothyroidism. This association is not Pendred syndrome.

Pendred Syndrome

Fraser (1976) noted that the association between deafness and goiter has long been studied, having appeared in the literature in the sixteenth century, but the study of what came to be called Pendred syndrome did not appear until the nineteenth century—in fact, in 1896, when Pendred's one-page paper was published.

The essential point for diagnosis, treatment, and prevention is that Pendred syndrome is a genetic disorder, recessively inherited. It is characterized by congenital profound hearing impairment caused by a defect of thyroid metabolism, specifically an inborn error of thyroxine synthesis. It is this error that could account also for the occasional instance of mental retardation in this syndrome. According to Dublin (1976), the inner ear of such a patient would show a Mondini abnormality, and this is consistent with the monograph of Lindsay (1973). Figure 8–2 is a typical audiogram associated with Pendred syndrome. A goiter appears, on the average, by the age of eight (Bordley, Brookhouser, and Tucker 1986), and certainly by adolescence. The goiter is treatable, but its treatment does not influence the hearing loss.

The review of Konigsmark and Gorlin (1976) found that Pendred syndrome had been reported to account for as many as 10 percent of all cases of congenital deafness. Fraser's (1976) surveys came up with somewhat smaller prevalence figures: 4.3 percent in Denmark, 2 percent in the United States, 2.5 percent in the Netherlands, and 4.4 percent in Sweden, and virtually never among Jews. His own data, though, found 7.8 percent in the British Isles.

In any case, Pendred syndrome accounts for a sizable portion of the congenitally hearing impaired population. The differential diagnosis

FIGURE 8–2. Audiogram of a typical patient with Pendred syndrome

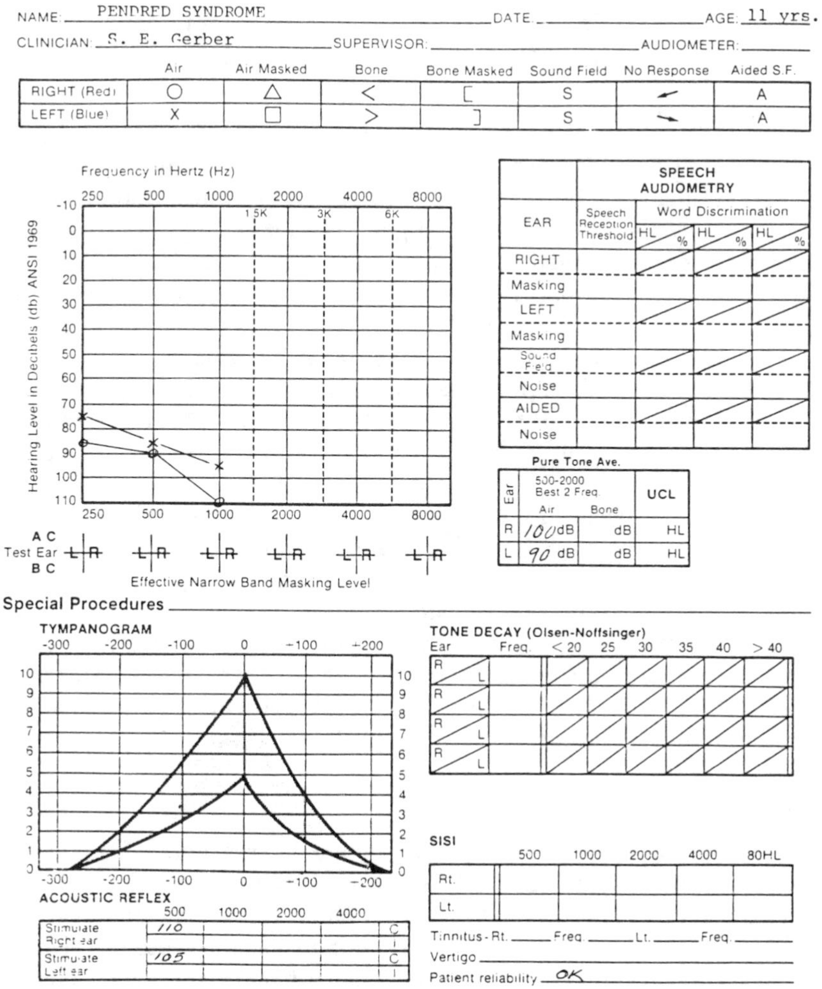

depends on findings of the family history, the fact that the hearing impairment is present at birth,[1] and the presence of the goiter. Failing all three of these, plus some laboratory tests, a patient may have deafness and hypothyroidism but not have Pendred syndrome. Because this disorder is heritable, genetic counseling can become primary prevention. Secondary prevention rests strongly on the differential diagnosis because

[1]However, Fraser observed that the deafness may not be present at birth but be rapidly progressive in the first few weeks of life.

the hearing impairment of Pendred syndrome will be unaffected by the thyroid treatment from which other thyroid-induced losses may benefit. Early identification of and intervention for the hearing impairment (i.e., amplification) are always relevant.

Other Thyroid Disorders

There are other disorders of thyroid metabolism in children that can affect communication, but they are now relatively uncommon. One of these is a syndrome described by Konigsmark and Gorlin (1976) as goiter and sensory-neural deafness accompanied by birdlike facies and skeletal alterations of the thoracic region. This, too, seems to be autosomal recessive.

Myelination of brain tissue can be retarded by neonatal hypothyroidism (Rosman 1972), although it has been known that brain growth is not usually as retarded as total body growth. Nevertheless, in cases of early onset hypothyroidism, brain mass decreases and cell density increases (Brasel and Boyd 1975).

There is also, according to Aronson (1985), a characteristic dysphonia that accompanies hypothyroidism. This is due to the increased mass in the thyroid area and loading of the vocal folds; it is distinguished by hoarseness and excessively low voice fundamental frequency. On the other hand, Aronson reported breathiness with hyperthyroidism. Additionally, the tongue may be infiltrated in cases of thyroid enlargement (Brown 1985), and this could contribute to dysarthria. Brown observed that undiagnosed hypothyroidism also can lead to ataxia syndromes.

Prevention

Hypothyroidism appearing in a gravida is treatable. Man (1975) assessed the offspring of such women by measuring the infants' IQs at four and seven years of age. She found that IQs in 35 percent of the children born to mothers whose hypothyroidism was untreated were more than one standard deviation below those born to *euthyroid* (i.e., normal) mothers. More importantly for our purpose, she found that 20 percent of the babies of treated mothers were that low. It seems, therefore, that treatment works, but not always. It is interesting, too, that some of these untreated mothers did receive treatment before and during subsequent pregnancies, and these infants had a better outcome than their older siblings. Thus, treatment of thyroid disorders in mothers can be a form of primary prevention.

Secondary prevention, as always, depends on sufficiently early identification and intervention. For example, prior to the introduction of mandatory screening in California, as many as 2 percent of state hospital residents were diagnosed as affected by congenital hypothyroidism. In cases of Pendred syndrome, one hopes that the family history is known so that early amplification may be provided. In cases of congenital hypothyroidism, the diagnosis may be delayed to the extent that the onset of symptoms is delayed. Still, introduction of thyroid therapy in the first few months of life is beneficial and essential because of the risk of developmental delay. Reinwein (1982) reviewed the effects of early intervention and found that the mean IQ of children whose hypothyroidism was treated before three months of age was higher than those treated later.

THE MUCOPOLYSACCHARIDOSES

The mucopolysaccharidoses (MPSs) constitute a family of genetic diseases all of which are characterized by *lysosomal* storage disorders. They are distinguished by degeneration of both mental and physical abilities and, sometimes, by early death. It is typical for such a patient to be born without the symptoms of MPS, but the progressive involvement soon becomes evident. Smith (1982) believed the "deceleration of developmental and mental progress" becomes evident late in the first year of life.

A lysosome is a vacuole, a space in the substance of a cell, which carries certain enzymes. Kelly (1986) called lysosomes the garbage disposal system of the cells. The acid mucopolysaccharides are normal parts of many body tissues, and they are constantly being broken down enzymatically. They are large polymers with a protein core and many polysaccharide branches. In MPS, the protein portion has been hydrolyzed (i.e., a process of cell cleavage), but the polysaccharide portion only partly hydrolyzed. Hence, products of this breakdown are stored in lysosomes. When the genetic abnormality called MPS (or sometimes glycosaminoglycans) emerges, there is an enzyme deficiency that leads to incomplete degeneration of mucopolysaccharides.

Six or seven different mucopolysaccharidoses have been described, depending on who is doing the describing. The most important (because they are the most common) are MPS-I (Hurler syndrome; see Figure 8–3) and MPS-II (Hunter Syndrome). The differential diagnosis of Hunter syndrome is essential, as it is X-linked recessively inherited and all the others are of the autosomal recessive type. Genetic and family counseling depend heavily on this distinction because X-linked disorders are characterized by female offspring who are carriers and do not express the disease; autosomal recessive inheritance depends on the parents. The risk of recurrence is 25 percent (Kelly 1986). Fraser (1976) suggested that some of these disorders could be polygenic. MPSs are rather uncommon. They have been estimated to appear no more often than 1 in 16,000 births and perhaps as rarely as 1 in 30,000; this amounts to about 125 cases per year in the United States.

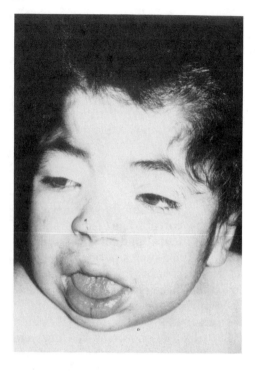

FIGURE 8–3.
Hurler Syndrome
SOURCE: Sanford E. Gerber and George
T. Mencher, *Auditory Dysfunction* (Hous-
ton, TX: College-Hill Press, 1980), p. 91.
Copyright 1980.   Reprinted with permis-
sion.

Hurler Syndrome

Konigsmark and Gorlin (1976) considered Hurler syndrome to be

the classic prototype of the mucopolysaccharidoses. It has the following
cardinal features: growth failure after infancy, marked mental retardation,
progressive coarsening of facial features beginning toward the end of the
first year of life, corneal clouding, chronic nasal discharge and repeated
upper respiratory infections, hernias, progressive lack of mobility of joints
resulting, for example, in clawhand deformity, hepatosplenomegaly,
marked somatic and mental retardation, and biochemical evidence of
intracellular storage and excessive urinary excretion of acid mucopolysaccharides. Death usually occurs before 10 years of age from pneumonia
and/or cardiac failure.

Children with Hurler syndrome have mild to moderate sensory-neural
hearing impairments. Some writers have reported conductive losses in
Hurler syndrome patients, probably due to recurrent upper respiratory
infections with otitis media. Kelmen (1966) studied temporal bones of two
patients with Hurler syndrome. He concluded that "lesions to the middle
ear structures dwarfed further changes" and therefore that "they alone were
sufficient to explain any congenital hearing defect." However, both children
had had a history of recurrent otitis media. In his 1971 nosology, Konigsmark reported that there are "many" cases of Hurler syndrome.

In addition to the intellectual, motor, and auditory deficits that these children present, there can be specific language difficulties and also faulty articulation due to intraoral manifestations. Smith (1982) described such patients as having small malaligned teeth and an enlarged tongue. They appear to be macrocephalic. Corneal clouding, a frequent finding, adds still another handicap to this distressing constellation.

As clinicians, we are frustrated by things like Hurler syndrome because these children will degenerate. At the same time, the fact of degeneration does not give us an excuse to withhold either secondary or tertiary prevention efforts. First, it may be possible to predict degeneration by genetic and/or biochemical studies before it becomes apparent. Second, early intervention still helps; it should minimize the effects of the rate of degeneration.

Hunter Syndrome

The first of the mucopolysaccharidoses to appear in the literature was MPS-II (Hunter 1917). It is distinguished from all the other MPSs by the fact that its mode of inheritance is X-linked; hence, it is never expressed in heterozygous females. The characteristics of Hunter syndrome have been listed as "moderate dwarfing, skeletal anomalies, enlarged head, mental deficiency, abdominal hernias, distinctive coarse facial features, heart disease, and ENT disorders" (Peck 1982). The onset of symptoms in Hunter syndrome is later than in Hurler syndrome; Smith (1982) claimed from two to four years of age. There are two types of this disease: Type A is mild, and patients survive into adulthood; type B is severe and leads to death before adolescence. Correspondingly, type A patients do not display the rapid deterioration of psychomotor function that characterizes type B patients. In either type, one does not find the corneal clouding observed in MPS-I. Both types can appear in the same family.

Hunter type B patients have been noted to be severely mentally retarded and also to display hyperactive, even aggressive, behavior. The rate of bodily growth declines rapidly between the second and sixth years of life, leading to an eventual height of as little as 120 cm. In both types, deafness is usually evident by three years of age, sometimes earlier. Konigsmark and Gorlin (1976) believed that the loss is usually not severe and appears in about half of the cases, some of whom have mixed losses. Anomalies of the round window and other middle ear disturbances have been reported. There may also be reduced vestibular function. According to Kelemen (1966), Hunter himself had noted the hearing impairment. Peck (1982) listed the otorhinolaryngologic manifestations of MPS-II: "upper and lower respiratory infections, narrow nasal passages, hypertrophied adenoids, mucopurulent rhinorrhea and noisy breathing."

There is an audiometric problem with MPS patients. The severity of the intellectual deficit and the seriousness of the motor disabilities can interfere with obtaining a satisfactory audiogram. Electrophysiologic techniques can be brought to bear, of course, but one must be alert to their shortcomings in such a severely multiply handicapped child. Still, Leroy and Crocker (1966) reported impaired hearing in 32 percent of their patients, and Hayes, Babin, and Platz (1980) found that 42 percent of their MPS patients had hearing impairment.

Other Mucopolysaccharidoses

The other MPS syndromes have similar effects. The visual deficits that appear in MPS-I have been reported also in MPS-III, IV, V, and VI. The joint difficulties noted in Hurler syndrome have been seen in MPS-IV, V, and VI. It seems, though, that deafness is reported less often in MPS-III (Sanfilippo syndrome) than in I or II. Mixed hearing losses are found in Morquio syndrome (MPS-IV), and Kelemen (1977) did a temporal bone study that revealed the pathologies of the middle ear. Riedner and Levin (1977) concluded that most MPS-IV patients would have mixed or sensory-neural hearing losses by the end of the first decade of life. Conductive impairments have been seen more often in Maroteaux-Lamy syndrome (MPS-VI). At the time of Konigsmark and Gorlin's compilation (1976), there had been no audiometric studies of MPS-V (Scheie syndrome); later, Smith (1982) did report hearing loss as an occasional abnormality.

In our clinic, we have had the opportunity to study a child with MPS-VII (Figure 8–4). Very few such cases have been reported in the scientific literature, and many of these died within the first three years of life. Our patient was seen at birth to have unusual facies, "puffy" hands and feet, and bilateral inguinal hernias. The preliminary diagnosis was Noonan syndrome with retardation and deafness. At six weeks of age, the diagnosis of Noonan syndrome continued to be preliminary and the possibility of MPS was suggested. At two months of age, urine samples were found to be positive for MPS but the tentative diagnosis of Noonan syndrome continued. At nearly five months of age, the diagnosis of MPS-VII was made.

When he was about ten months old, he had his first episode of otitis media, and recurrent otitis media continues to this writing, when he is nearly eight years old. At 22 months, his language was described as minimal. He had had repeated otitis media, and an increase was noted in his *gibbus,* a spinal deformity. As he approached the age of seven years, he began to complain of not hearing well, and a month later an audiometric evaluation was done that revealed a flat loss of some 25 dB in one ear and nearly 50 dB in the other. Tympanostomy tubes were placed shortly

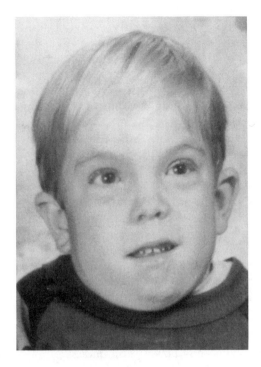

FIGURE 8-4.
Mucopolysaccharidosis–VII

afterward. Within a few weeks he was fitted with a hearing aid, but he does not use it consistently. He was then beginning to show corneal clouding. Also, at that time, the pediatrician geneticist who cares for him reported "no seizures, cerebellar signs, focal findings or involuntary movements." She observed that he had a wide gait and a tendency to stand on one foot, but that this is probably due to orthopedic (rather than neurologic) problems. Hip surgery was suggested but not done. Concern was expressed over sleep apnea.

His initial evaluation at our clinic revealed a child as described above who had articulation errors especially on stops. In fact, 15 percent of his utterances were unintelligible. One of the characteristics of MPS-VII is overabundance of oral and nasal mucus. It was our impression that this contributed to his difficulty with the articulation of plosives; /k/ and /g/ were unstimulable. In addition, his receptive language behavior was portrayed as failing to respond correctly to verbal stimuli. One wonders, of course, if this is due to cognitive, linguistic, or auditory deficits; it is probably all three. His expressive language revealed few personal or social functions; this has improved considerably. His language use at intake was assessed at the second percentile on a standard test. At a chronological age of 6:5, his language age was measured at 3:10. His nonverbal intelligence was found to be at the fifth percentile. In other words, he was delayed in both receptive and expressive language and continued to be unable to articulate most plosives. By the age of seven, he had made considerable progress in improving his receptive language skills.

Given that so few cases of MPS-VII have been reported, it is difficult to say if this child is typical. One might suppose that he is, and therefore to conclude that there are benefits of therapy. The various surgeries—myringotomy, adenoidectomy, hip repair—may all be considered to be secondary prevention. A review of the sparse literature revealed only one child who had lived longer than our patient. We would like to believe that his relative longevity is due to secondary prevention efforts. We would also like to believe that his success (however minimal) in school and in the speech and language clinic has been due to our tertiary efforts. Primary prevention might have been in the form of genetic counseling, but the family reports no knowledge of a history. This often happens in cases of autosomal recessive inheritance. His secondary prevention was that he was diagnosed early, at two months of age.

Prevention

Prevention of mucopolysaccharidoses is largely summarized in the previous paragraph. All seven MPSs are genetically based, one being X–linked. Primary prevention rests entirely on a family having sufficient and appropriate information—not a simple task. Autosomal recessive disorders may not appear for generations; hence, a family may be unaware that there is such a problem until it presents itself. If they are aware, they have difficult and distressing decisions to make. If they are not, we can only hope for the most prompt secondary prevention efforts—early identification and diagnosis. The MPSs are not repairable; they cannot be cured. Yet, as our patient illustrates, prompt and efficacious treatment can make the life of such a child as normal as possible.

DIABETES

In Chapter 4, we observed that diabetic women have a high incidence of malformed or handicapped babies. We concluded that the metabolic swings (from hyperglycemia to hypoglycemia and back) that sometimes occur in diabetics inhibit adequate development. Furthermore, it seems that this frequently results in craniofacial anomalies. There is also some evidence that the neuropathies that may accompany diabetes can arise in prenatal life. For example, O'Loughlin and Lillystone (1983) reported a combination of ear anomalies, deafness, and facial nerve palsy in two unrelated children born to diabetic mothers. One has a sensory-neural impairment in the presence of an anomaly of the petrous bone; the other has an evidently complete microtia and atresia on one side. O'Loughlin and Lillystone postulated that these resulted from poor metabolic control during the first two months of pregnancy. A similar case was reported by Soler, Walsh, and Malins in 1976.

The Diabetic Child

In a sense, diabetes may be teratogenic. Are there effects on communication expressed by the diabetic patient? It must be noted, first, that diabetes is a heterogenous disorder, usually described as "juvenile onset" and "maturity onset" diabetes; and the latter also appears in the form of gestational diabetes. The distinction is important for our purpose, being limited to children, as hearing loss is rare in diabetics under the age of 24 (Rosen and Davis 1971). However, hearing loss is more frequent and more severe as the diabetic patient gets older, presumably because of the continuing changes in vascular supply, which leads to many of the deleterious effects of diabetes.

Insulin-dependent diabetes mellitus (IDDM) is an autoimmune disorder with a genetically based susceptibility. It is thought that there may be two genes that lead to such susceptibility, but IDDM can appear exogenously from certain viruses, some toxins, and from malnutrition (Rosenbloom 1987). Probably the greatest risk of juvenile IDDM is early death, at least among those in whom the disease appears before the age of ten. In fact, the risk of dying at any given age in this population is seven times the risk in the nondiabetic population of the same age. The principal nonlethal effects of juvenile diabetes are in the visual system, but neuropathies also appear. Diabetic retinopathy is the leading cause of blindness in the United States; only about 30 percent of diabetes patients under the age of 30 were found to be free of retinopathy (Klein et al. 1985). Figure 8–5 shows the rapidly increasing percentage of diabetes patients with retinopathy as the duration of the disease increases. Note that it levels off after about 15 years.

There are other consequences to the diabetic child, and these are generally in the psychosocial area. Such children are typically on special diets, are dependent on medication (often by injection), and may have limited joint mobility. Young children with very early onset of IDDM have lower IQs on the WISC-R, although still within the range of normal. They also may have impairments of memory and of reading. Reduced central conduction velocity has been proposed as a manifestation of neuropathy, and has been seen as prolonged ABR latencies. Autonomic reflexes seem

FIGURE 8–5.   Frequency of retinopathy by duration of diabetes

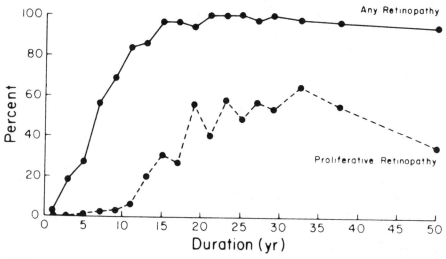

SOURCE: Ronald Klein et al., "The Wisconsin Epidemiological Study of Diabetic Retinopathy, II, Prevalence and Risk of Retinopathy when Age at Diagnosis Is Less than 30 Years," *Archives of Ophthalmology*, 102(1984), 522. Copyright 1988, American Medical Association.

to be suppressed in some patients, but Hosking (1987) commented that "such involvement is very patchy."

Gestational Diabetes

Another expression of diabetes that concerns us is gestational diabetes. This disorder presents complications in two to three percent of pregnancies, but diagnosis is rarely made before the second half of the pregnancy (Kuhl and Molsted-Pedersen 1987). This expression is distinguished by the fact that it does not appear (or is not recognized) prior to pregnancy, and in general its cause is unknown. The consequences for fetal cerebral development are debated, although the effects of gestational diabetes do lead to a decrease of fetal oxygen content. In any case, the fetus carried by a diabetic gravida is at risk whether the diabetes has been present for some time or appears with the pregnancy.

The problem is that the "role of insulin in the CNS is unknown," although insulin receptors have been found in all areas of the mammalian brain (Havrankova, Brownstein, and Roth 1981). Similarly, the role of fetal metabolism as influenced by diabetes in pregnancy remains unclear, but the effects are somewhat more transparent. We must iterate the comment of Myrianthopoulos (1980) that "overt maternal diabetes more than doubles the frequency of malformations across the board including clefts."

Prevention

Finally, though, we must recall that diabetes is treatable. Those who are not insulin dependent may often be treated by diet alone, but many of these later become dependent on insulin. The frequency of islet—and even the entire pancreas—transplants has increased, and the success rate continues to climb. Insulin treatment of IDDM in pregnancy has been shown to postpone delivery closer to term, but the rate of facial malformations still does not diminish. Nevertheless, the treatment of diabetes can be secondary prevention both for the gravid woman and for the patient. Tertiary prevention is, but shouldn't be, more difficult. Tattersall and Peacock (1987) found that fully half of the diabetic children failed to report truthfully about their test results and, regardless, failed to act on the results.

Treatment, of course, is both secondary and tertiary prevention of the adverse consequences of diabetes. Is primary prevention possible? In some ways it is. First, it is clear that the susceptibility to diabetes is genetically based, and it may also be the case that some diabetes gene predisposes patients to prenatal viral disease. Thus, as with any genetic disorder, genetic counseling may be in order. Also, health maintenance is literally critical for the diabetes patient, and all the properties of good health can be secondary prevention. Diabetes, if one considers its seriousness, is a common disease, appearing in at least 60 or as many as 120 among 100,000 children under the age of 16 years in the United States (Mimura 1985). There are clear exogenous factors also. Mimura noted that the incidence of juvenile diabetes among Americans of Japanese descent (43 per 100,000) is much greater than among Japanese (5 per 100,000). It may be indeed a Western disease.

OTHER METABOLIC DISORDERS

The effects of metabolic disorders are so widespread that one should expect communicative sequelae. For example, kidney dysfunction is related to hearing impairment. Thomsen, Bech, and Szpirt (1976) found sensory-neural hearing losses in 10 percent of patients with renal insufficiency, but ototoxic drugs interact with kidney problems in such populations. Bergstrom and Thompson (1983) found hearing loss in 47 percent of 151 pediatric renal patients, a percentage similar to that found in renal patients of any age, but a smaller proportion of the children had unknown etiology. The point is that otic pathology peculiar to renal disease is not easily distinguishable from other sensory-neural losses except in a statistical way—in other words, other causes are not evident (Bergstrom et al. 1973).

Phenylketonuria (PKU) is a genetic disorder in which patients lack an enzyme necessary to process phenylalanine, a substance found in meat and dairy products. Although PKU occurs in only about 1 in 20,000 births, PKU screening is mandated in virtually every state. Why? Because PKU screening may be the best example of secondary prevention. Paine, as long ago as 1964, averred that PKU patients "form perhaps the largest treatable group of cases of mental retardation." The fact is that PKU can be identified by chemical test in the first hours of life. Given that the diagnosis is made, a special diet is introduced that inhibits (even prohibits) the intellectual deficit that would otherwise result.

There are other such examples. Galactosemia may cause death, but can cause severe mental retardation. It originates because of the congenital absence of the enzyme to metabolize galactose, a substance present in all dairy products. Again, it is rare—about 1 in 80,000 births—but totally amenable to secondary prevention by diet.

Seizures, incoordination, hearing loss, and mental retardation have all been noted to result from biotinidase deficiency. This disorder occurs due to a shortage of the catalyst needed to separate a B vitamin, biotin, for normal recycling. It is treatable, and therefore preventable, with regular doses of biotin. Biotinidase deficiency appears in 1 of some 40,000 births.

CONCLUSION

Metabolic disorders are common, and many are treatable. Hypothyroidism and diabetes are controllable, and this is at least a good form of tertiary prevention. The various enzymatic deficiencies with risks for cognitive development are all subject to secondary prevention. Genetic disorders, including MPSs, may come for genetic counseling. As clinicians we cannot withhold preventive efforts even of those disorders that we know to be universally fatal. The quality of life matters, and we can do something about it.

GLOSSARY

euthyroid: the state of normal thyroid function.
gibbus: a spinal defect; hunchback.
hydrolysis: a chemical reaction with water.
lysosome: a membrane-bound particle that contains hydrolyzing enzymes.
myxedema: the extreme of hypothyroidism.
thyrotrophic hormone: a hormone secreted by the anterior lobe of the pituitary that stimulates secretory activity in the thyroid gland.
thyroxin: an amino acid, secreted by the thyroid gland, that contains iodine.
triiodothyronine: an iodide with three atoms of iodine, secreted by the thyroid gland.
vacuole: a fluid-filled space within a cell.

REFERENCES

ARONSON, ARNOLD E. 1985. *Clinical Voice Disorders,* 2nd ed. New York: Thieme.

BARGMAN, GERALD J., AND LYTT I. GARDNER. 1972. "Experimental Production of Otic Lesions with Antithyroid Drugs," in *Human Development and the Thyroid Gland: Relation to Endemic Cretinism,* ed. John B. Stanbury and Robert L. Kroc. New York: Plenum Press.

BERGSTROM, LAVONNE, et al. 1973. "Hearing Loss in Renal Disease: Clinical and Pathological Studies," *Ann. Otol., Rhinol., Laryngol.,* 82, 555–77.

———, AND PATRICIA THOMPSON. 1983. "Hearing Loss in Pediatric Renal Patients," *Intl. J. Ped. Otorhinolaryngol.,* 5, 227–34.

BORDLEY, JOHN E., PATRICK E. BROOKHOUSER, AND GABRIEL F. TUCKER, JR. *Ear, Nose & Throat Disorders in Children.* New York: Raven Press.

BRASEL, JO ANNE, AND D. BARRY BOYD. 1975. "Influence of Thyroid Hormone on Fetal Brain Growth and Development," in *Perinatal Thyroid Physiology and Disease,* ed. Delbert A. Fisher and Gerard N. Burrow. New York: Raven Press.

BROWN, J. KEITH. 1985. "Dysarthria in Children: Neurologic Perspective," in *Speech and Language Evaluation in Neurology: Childhood Disorders,* ed. John K. Darby. Orlando, FL: Grune & Stratton.

DEBRUYNE, F., M. VANDERSCHUEREN-LODEWEYCKX, AND P. BASTIJNS. 1983. "Hearing in Congenital Hypothyroidism," *Audiology,* 22, 404–409.

DUBLIN, WILLIAM B. 1976. *Fundamentals of Sensorineural Auditory Pathology.* Springfield, IL: Chas. C Thomas.

FISHER, DELBERT A., AND GERARD N. BURROW, eds. 1975. *Perinatal Thyroid Physiology and Disease.* New York: Raven Press.

FRASER, GEORGE R. 1976. *The Causes of Profound Deafness in Childhood.* Baltimore: Johns Hopkins University Press.

HAVRANKOVA, JANA, M. BROWNSTEIN, AND J. ROTH. 1981. "Insulin and Insulin Receptors in Rodent Brain," *Diabetologia,* 20, 268–73.

HAYES, ELIZABETH, RICHARD BABIN, AND CHARLES PLATZ. 1980. "The Otologic Manifestations of Mucopolysaccharidoses," *Am. J. Otology,* 2, 65–69.

HETZEL, BASIL S. 1972. "Similarities and Differences between Sporadic and Endemic Cretinism," in *Human Development and the Thyroid Gland: Relation to Endemic Cretinism,* ed. John B. Stanbury and Robert L. Kroc. New York: Plenum Press.

HOSKING, D. J. 1987. "Autonomic Neuropathy," in *The Diabetes Annual/3,* ed. K. G. M. M. Alberti and L. P. Krall. Amsterdam: Elsevier.

HUNTER, C. 1917. "A Rare Disease in Two Brothers," *Proc. R. Soc. Med.,* 10, 104.

KELEMEN, GEORGE. 1966. "Hurler's Syndrome and the Hearing Organ," *J. Laryngol. Otol.,* 80, 791–803.

———.1977. "Morquio's Disease and the Hearing Organ," *ORL,* 39, 233–40.

KELLY, THADDEUS E. 1986. *Clinical Genetics and Genetic Counseling,* 2nd ed. Chicago: Year Book Medical Publishers.

KLEIN, RONALD, et al. 1984. "The Wisconsin Epidemiological Study of Diabetic Retinopathy. II. Prevalence and Risk of Diabetic Retinopathy When Age at Diagnosis is Less Than 30 Years," *Arch. Ophthalmol.,* 102, 520–526.

———.1985. "An Epidemiologic Study of Diabetic Retinopathy in Younger Insulin-Taking Patients," in *Childhood and Juvenile Diabetes Mellitus,* ed. Goro Mimura. Amsterdam: Excerpta Medica.

KONIGSMARK, BRUCE W. 1971. "Hereditary Congenital Severe Deafness Syndromes," in *The Clinical Delineation of Birth Defects,* Part IX, *Ear,* ed. D. Bergsma. Baltimore: Williams & Wilkins.

———, AND ROBERT J. GORLIN. 1976. *Genetic and Metabolic Deafness.* Philadelphia: Saunders.

KUHL, CLAUS, AND LARS MOLSTED-PEDERSON. 1987. "Pregnancy and Diabetes: Gestational Diabetes," in *The Diabetes Annual/3,* ed. K. G. M. M. Alberti and L. P. Krall. Amsterdam: Elsevier.

LEROY, JEWEL G., AND ALAN C. CROCKER. 1966. "Clinical Definition of the Hurler-Hunter Phenotypes, A Review of 50 Patients," *Am. J. Dis. Child.,* 112, 518–530.

LINDSAY, JOHN R. 1973. "Profound Childhood Deafness: Inner Ear Pathology," *Ann. Otol., Rhinol. Laryngol.,* 82, Suppl. 5.

MAN, EVELYN B. 1975. "Maternal Hypothyroxinemia: Development of 4-and 7-Year-Old Offspring," in *Perinatal Thyroid Physiology and Disease,* ed. Delbert A. Fisher and Gerard N. Burrow. New York: Raven Press.

MIMURA, GORO. 1985. "The Present Status of Immunogenetic Research in Japan," in *Childhood and Juvenile Diabetes Mellitus,* ed. Goro Mimura. Amsterdam: Excerpta Medica.

MYRIANTHOPOULOS, NTINOS C. 1980. "The Human Population Data: Critique II," in *Progress in Clinical and Biological Research.* Vol.46, *Etiology of Cleft Lip and Cleft Palate.,* ed. Michael Melnick, David Bixler, and Edward D.Shields. New York: Alan R. Liss.

O'LOUGHLIN, E. V., AND D. LILLYSTONE. 1983. "Ear Anomalies, Deafness and Facial Nerve Palsy in Infants of Diabetic Mothers," *Aust. Ped. J.,* 19, (1983), 109–11.

PAINE, RICHMOND S. 1964. "Phenylketonuria," *Clin. Proc.,* 20, 143–52.

PECK, JAMES E. 1982. "Hearing Loss in Hunter Syndrome—MPS II," paper given at the annual meeting of the American Auditory Society.

REINWEIN, D. 1982. "Treatment of Diminished Thyroid Hormone Formation," in *Diminished Thyroid Hormone Formation: Possible Causes and Clinical Aspects,* ed. D. Reinwein and E. Klein. Stuttgart: Schattauer Verlag.

RIEDNER, ERWIN D., AND STEFAN LEVIN. 1977. "Hearing Patterns in Morquio's Syndrome (Mucopolysaccharidosis IV)," *Arch. Otolaryngol.,* 103, 518–20.

ROSEN, ZVI, AND ELI DAVIS. 1971. "Microangiopathy in Diabetics with Hearing Disorders," *EENT Monthly,* 50, 31, 33–35.

ROSENBLOOM, ARLAN L. 1987. "Diabetes in Children," in *The Diabetes Annual/3,* ed. K. G. M. M. Alberti and L. P. Krall. Amsterdam: Elsevier.

ROSMAN, N. PAUL. 1972. "The Neuropathology of Congenital Hypothyroidism," in *Human Development and the Thyroid Gland: Relation to Endemic Cretinism,* ed. John B. Stanbury and Robert L. Kroc. New York: Plenum Press.

ROVET, JOANNE F., ROBERT M. EHRLICH, AND DONNA-LEE SORBARA. 1987a. "Outcome in Neonatally-Identified Thyroid Hormone Deficient Children: Persistent Deficits and Associated Risk Factors," paper presented at the Fifth Annual Meeting of the Society for Behavioral Pediatrics, Anaheim.

————.1987b. "Intellectual Outcome in Children with Fetal Hypothyroidism," *J. Peds.,* 110, 700–704.

————, DONNA-LEE SORBARA, AND ROBERT M. EHRLICH. 1986. "The Intellectual and Behavioral Characteristics of Children with Congenital Hypothyroidism Identified by Neonatal Screening in Ontario. The Toronto Prospective Study," in *Genetic Disease: Screening and Management,* ed. T. D. Carter and A. M. Witty. New York: Alan R. Liss.

SMITH, DAVID W. 1982. *Recognizable Patterns of Human Malformation,* 3rd ed. Philadelphia: Saunders.

SOLER, N. G., C. H. WALSH, AND J. M. MALINS. 1976. "Congenital Malformations in Infants of Diabetic Mothers," *Q. J. Med.,* 45, 303–13.

STANBURY, JOHN B. 1982. "The Pathogenesis of Endemic Retardation Associated with Endemic Goiter," in *Diminished Thyroid Hormone Formation: Possible Causes and Clinical Aspects,* ed. D. Reinwein and E. Klein. Stuttgart: Schattauer Verlag.

TATTERSALL, ROBERT, AND IAN PEACOCK. 1987. "Assessment of Diabetic Control," in *The Diabetes Annual/3,* ed. K. G. M. M. Alberti and L. P. Krall. Amsterdam: Elsevier.

THOMSEN, J., P. BECH, AND W. SZPIRT. 1976. "Otologic Symptoms in Chronic Renal Failure," *Arch. Oto-Rhino-Laryngol.,* 214, 71–79.

9

Prevention Programs

Prevention is something one *does,* not what one hopes and expects someone else to do. In a draft statement, the Prevention Committee of the American Speech–Language–Hearing Association asserted this principle by reminding us that those of us "who are active in improving prevention of communication disorders will find their efforts more effective if they incorporate communicative wellness practices into their own lives."

In this last chapter, we review some of the things already mentioned, but in a different manner. First, we consider primary prevention of the disorders discussed; second, we present issues for secondary prevention of those same disorders. Finally, we describe some prevention programs and policies, and then conclude with appendixes intended to be helpful to the reader.

We use the word "prevention" in its literal sense. It means the inhibition of development of any disease and/or disorder. To prevent means to obstruct, to interfere, to hinder, to block, to impede, to interrupt. Inherent in this list, however, is a distinction between primary and secondary prevention. To hinder or block is primary prevention; to impede or interrupt is secondary prevention.

PRIMARY PREVENTION

Primary prevention is not inhibition, it is prohibition. It results in the total avoidance of a disease, disorder, or handicapping condition; the disease doesn't happen in the first place. Epidemiologists set out two kinds of primary prevention: the promotion of good health and specific protective measures. The first of these, promoting and maintaining good health practices, is clearly necessary but not sufficient. The specific measures are equally necessary. The fact that I don't smoke doesn't excuse me from wearing my seat belt, for example. The best form of primary prevention, of both kinds, is education. For example, it is actually a contemporary understanding that we have about the teratogenicity of alcohol; it was thought that alcohol ingestion in pregnancy is innocuous. Modern science—and, consequently, education—has shown us that it isn't.

Disorders of Chromosomal Origin

In Chapter 2 we described chromosomes and the chromosomal system. We observed that chromosomal disorders are generally of two kinds: disorders of number and disorders of structure. These include the familiar trisomies (13, 18, and especially 21) and some of the deletion syndromes (e.g., 5p– and 9p–). We also described aberrations of number or structure of sex chromosomes. All of these chromosomal aberration syndromes are distinguished by the fact that most of them aren't viable; they spontaneously abort. In a sense, then, spontaneous abortion is primary prevention. Those few who survive are distinguished by disorders of communication, cognition, and/or behavior—usually all of them.

Chapter 2 also described some forms of early warning that could potentially become primary prevention. Ultrasonography and amniocentesis can become means to primary prevention for those persons who would opt for clinical abortion. Some persons, in fact, may elect to avoid conception because of past history in the immediate family or elsewhere in the family or because of an understanding of the effects of maternal age. A woman who is subjected to therapeutic doses of X-radiation should choose to avoid conceiving. Adoption is a wonderful option for families that know or learn that they are at risk.

Disorders of Genetic Origin

In Chapter 3 we described genes, the genetic system, and the forms of genetic transmission. We observed that many communicative disorders are inherited, but that many of those are polygenic and multifactorial. The communicative disorders that may be the most important ones in this context are familial deafness and stuttering, but clearly there are many others.

Genetic disorders may be the most important example of education as primary prevention. How could one know about the risk of a genetic disorder? The answer is if it has happened before in other children or close relatives, or if there is consanguinity. The obvious problem, of course, is that one may not know that it has happened before in the family or be unaware of consanguinity. If known, though, genetic counseling prior to conception is the best form of primary prevention. Again, a given couple may choose adoption; that is, they may elect not to conceive.

Another problem is that many incidents of genetic disorders are new mutations. By definition, then, they are not predictable and, therefore, not amenable to primary prevention. Still another problem, but one of which one could become aware, are those disorders of delayed onset; the primary example is otosclerosis. A much more worrisome example is von Recklinghausen neurofibromatosis, a potentially fatal disorder; the same is true of cystic fibrosis. It is essential, sometimes critical, for the communicative disorders specialist to be alert to such things for referral to the genetic counselor.

Teratogens, Mutagens, and Iatrogens

The topic of Chapter 4 constitutes the bright spot in primary prevention. Communicable diseases can be and have been eliminated in the populace and/or prevented in a given child. In Chapter 4 we talked about the risk of prenatal viral disease, and also mentioned some of those same diseases when acquired later. Many viral diseases have become uncommon; some (such as smallpox) have disappeared. Measles, mumps, rubella, poliomyelitis, and (soon) varicella are markedly diminished in incidence. Primary prevention of cytomegalovirus is still to be accomplished, and now we must confront the threat of AIDS.

Nevertheless, the incidence of communicative disorders that result from prenatal disease has become quite small when compared to what it was, say, the middle of this century. Bacterial diseases are treatable in a gravida, and such treatment can be primary prevention. The same is true, with varying degrees of success, of chronic maternal diseases such as diabetes or hypothyroidism.

The primary prevention picture is less optimistic when we look at environmental toxins. The U.S. Centers for Disease Control (1985) reported that "excessive absorption of lead is one of the most prevalent and preventable childhood health problems in the United States. Children are particularly susceptible to its toxic effect." It is distressing to learn that lead poisoning is both prevalent and preventable. Education as primary prevention: The CDC recommended that communities "should be informed at every available opportunity" to have children screened for lead poisoning. All children between the ages of nine months and six years should be screened.

One way to lower the incidence of environmental teratogens is to find them, record them, and then attack the source of the problem in a community. These teratogens "include exposure to radiation, drugs, diet, personal habits, and agents encountered in the workplace, in communities, and in the natural environment" (California Birth Defects Monitoring Program 1987). With respect to those in communities, the CBDMP investigated 61 purported clusters of birth defects from April 1981 through June 1987. In 39 of them, there was no evidence of an excess; that is, the incidence was no higher than would be expected based on long-term statistics. Some of the others have undergone continued investigation, and these include purported increases of Down syndrome, cleft lip, trisomy 18, neural tube defects, and many others discussed here. This program is an excellent example of how an entire state—in fact, the largest—can educate itself and its communities about environmental teratogens. Moreover, during that same time period, CBDMP made several hundred responses to inquiries. These inquiries have "expressed concerns about a wide range of issues, including working with solvents, living near freeways, and drinking contaminated water" (CBDMP 1987).

Chapter 4 considered petroleum and petroleum products, pesticides and other chemicals, and foods and food additives. We observed there that the primary issue is to prevent abuse, not use. It is incorrect or excessive use of substances intended to be beneficial that usually creates the risk. Certainly, incorrect or excessive use should be preventable. Abuse extends also to iatrogens. We observed that there are persons who choose to abuse drugs of all kinds—alcohol, heroin, cocaine, and medicines. Then there are those who must take certain medicinal drugs, do not abuse them, and are nevertheless at risk. We mentioned, for example, hydantoin and Accutane.

In sum, though, the area of teratogenicity is one that is subject to primary prevention efforts. Moreover, these efforts have been very successful in many, many instances. Additionally, public health agencies are actively involved.

Trauma

Traumatic communicative disorders are usually preventable. Chapter 5 observed that mechanical trauma is very often incurred in or with automobiles, and that the use of seat belts is effective primary prevention. Similarly, we know that the use of helmets by motorcycle or bicycle riders has diminished the incidence of head injury and its consequences. The larger community, however, has failed to address adequately the issue of child abuse. Many cases of trauma are in that tragic category.

Chemical and thermal injuries are widespread. These include the effects of those same substances just discussed as teratogens and also accidents that happen to children. Programs to educate families about having safer homes, especially with respect to poisons, have demonstrated their effectiveness.

Complex Craniofacial Disorders

These disorders are, in the main, genetic. They are subject to the same kinds of programs recommended for any genetic disorder. In addition, Chapter 6 raised some other primary prevention issues. We do, indeed, want to prevent frustration, unnecessary or dangerous treatments, missed opportunities, progression, and uncertainty. In fact, these are prevention issues—often secondary prevention—for all the things discussed in this book.

Respiratory Disorders

Perinatal respiratory distress presently accounts for a little more than 20 percent of developmentally delayed children reported to appropriate agencies in California. It also accounts for nearly 30 percent of the incidence of congenital or early onset deafness. It is typically associated with low birth weight and preterm delivery, but Chapter 7 noted that the low birth weight rate has barely diminished.

The neonatologists' art is rescuing more and more of the very small and very young babies; consequently, the neonatal mortality rate has dropped remarkably. Moreover, it is possible to increase the birth weight in an entire community—indeed, over a long period—by "an informative policy directed toward all women at risk" (Papiernik et al. 1985). But more survivors also means more very impaired children who deserve our attention. It appears that the infants who would have survived with minor handicaps get better; it also appears that the infants who would have died survive with severe handicaps. This is an issue for secondary prevention. Primary prevention seems to elude us; if anything, it gets worse. Ever increasing numbers of very small babies are being born to very young mothers. We must introduce education programs no later than the sixth grade, and continuing through high school, to prevent birth defects by preventing births. Our young people are not adequately educated. A program to help in this area is presented in Appendix A.

Airway problems are less easily prevented at the primary level. Many of them are in the categories discussed in Chapters 3 and 6 and subject to those concerns. Again, these are often matters for secondary prevention.

Metabolic Disorders

Chapter 8 contains examinations of disorders that may be teratogenic and may have consequences later as well. Thyroid system dysfunction is a familiar example. Endemic cretinism has ceased to be a problem in many parts of the world by the simple process of treating drinking water, but this is still not universal. Hypothyroidism in a gravida can be treated to the benefit of her baby. Pendred syndrome, on the other hand, is a genetic affliction; it is not treatable for prevention, but genetic counseling can be applied.

Similarly, diabetes is controllable, and the baby of the diabetic mother may be placed at reduced risk. The diabetic child, however, suffers a social risk by virtue of being ill, of needing treatment, of needing to avoid certain activities. The matter of the diabetic patient who is lax about self-care is a serious one; again, education can be primary prevention of the sequelae of diabetes.

The mucopolysaccharidoses, on the other hand, are universally fatal. As genetic diseases, they can be brought to the attention of the genetic counselor, and prenatal diagnosis may be possible.

SECONDARY PREVENTION

Secondary prevention means early identification for purposes of early intervention. Mausner and Bahn (1974) held that "with early detection and prompt treatment of disease, it is sometimes possible to either cure disease at the earliest stage possible or slow its progression, prevent complications, limit disability," and so on. This is secondary prevention.

A given disorder may not be totally preventable, but often it is possible to prevent its effects or minimize its consequences. For example, it is known that brain growth continues throughout the fetal period and for several months after birth. This early development is distinguished by neural plasticity, and one may take therapeutic advantage of neural plasticity to stimulate more normal outcomes than would have happened otherwise (Greenough 1975). Early intervention programs are known to have positive effects on the mental development of preterm infants (Resnick, Armstrong, and Carter 1988). And primary care providers must learn to refer early and appropriately (Allen, Rapin, and Wiznitzer 1988).

Certainly those among us who treat hearing impaired infants are aware of the benefits of early amplification (Figure 9–1); and we can become aware of expected risks by the use of high-risk registers. Table 9–1 is a widely used high-risk register intended to detect congenital deafness. The fact is that it predicts a considerable array of communicative disorders.

Disorders of Chromosomal Origin

Many chromosomal aberrations are observable at birth or even before birth. Amniocentesis, ultrasonography, and karyotyping can predict or identify chromosomal disorders. This process of identification

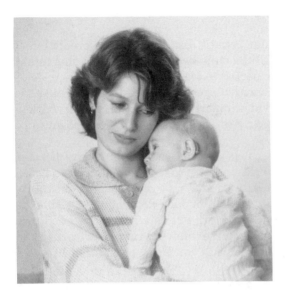

FIGURE 9–1.
Early amplification
SOURCE: Reprinted with the permission of Phonic Ear, Inc.

allows the development of early intervention programs. The issue was summarized nicely by Rossetti (1986): "Children are able to learn and benefit from stimulation provided at an early age." We can provide that stimulation with early identification. Especially notable are the successes achieved with Down syndrome patients whose verbal and social skills have been improved, and this has been known for many years. We can employ therapeutic programs to take advantage of the relative strengths and weaknesses of verbal competence among infants with Turner syndrome, for example, if the diagnosis is made at a very early age.

TABLE 9–1. Factors that Identify Infants at Risk for Hearing Impairment

1. A family history of childhood hearing impairment.
2. Congenital perinatal infection (e.g., cytomegalovirus, rubella, herpes, toxoplasmosis, syphilis).
3. Anatomic malformations involving the head or neck (e.g. dysmorphic appearance including syndromal and nonsyndromal abnormalities, overt or submucous cleft palate, morphologic abnormalities of the pinna.
4. Birthweight less than 1500 grams.
5. Hyperbilirubinemia at level exceeding indications for exchange transfusion.
6. Bacterial meningitis, especially H. influenza.
7. Severe asphyxia which may include infants with Apgar scores of 0–3 who fail to institute spontaneous respiration by 10 minutes and those with hypotonia persisting to two hours of age.

SOURCE: Joint Committee on Infant Hearing, "Position Statement 1982," *Peds.*, 70, (1982), 496. Reprinted by permission.

Disorders of Genetic Origin

Identification of a particular genetic disorder permits prediction of sequelae. Is the child deaf? Will the child become deaf? Does this infant have a syndrome that can be expected to lead to learning or language or reading disabilities? Is this disorder degenerative? Again, learning the answers to such questions provides opportunities for early intervention. And, as above, the benefits of early intervention have been shown to be worthwhile.

Secondary prevention in cases of genetic disorders may become primary prevention in others. Having diagnosed a genetic dysfunction in a given patient alerts a family to the risk of the same disability appearing in later pregnancies. First, the odds don't change with each succeeding pregnancy. Second, however, a couple may have been previously unaware of any risk, as they were unaware that the disorder had ever appeared in the family. As a result, primary prevention becomes possible.

Another form of secondary prevention is in the area of preventing progression. Early identification and early intervention may prevent a disability from getting worse, or, at least, it may slow the rate of degeneration. A patent example is the treatment of disease. Again, the disease may not be curable, but it may be controllable. Examples include diabetes and other metabolic disorders for which a genetic predisposition exists.

Teratogens, Mutagens, and Iatrogens

We just mentioned that diseases can be treated, sometimes cured. Identification of prenatal viral disease (see Table 3–1) alerts practitioners to the possibility of treatment, at least of acute problems, and to the necessity for monitoring potential sequelae. We know, for example, that the deafness that may result from prenatal cytomegalovirus is progressive, and, therefore, it is essential to examine auditory function over the first several months of life. But the diagnosis must be made first; then secondary prevention becomes available. We know, furthermore, that bacterial diseases are treatable, and the potential for communicative sequelae is related in some way to the underlying organism.

Toxins may be brought under control. It is clear that the elimination of alcohol consumption during pregnancy improves chances for success. The social milieu of street drugs can be prevented, and usually is, by removing the infant who is born addicted from that environment. Iatrogens, also, are sometimes susceptible; switch from hydantoin to valproic acid if possible.

Trauma

One might suppose that secondary prevention would not apply to cases of trauma (Chapter 5), but indeed it does. Counseling abusive parents may prevent further abuse of those children. Advice about poisons found in the home will reduce the probability of further incidents. Removal, in the proper manner, of environmental toxins in a community would reduce the incidence of additional cases and thereby diminish the prevalence in the community. A system like that of the California Birth Defects Monitoring Program, which responds to community concerns arising from actual cases (i.e., therefore, secondary prevention), leads to identification and additional (i.e., primary) prevention.

Complex Craniofacial Disorders

Chapter 6 contains wise advice on the prevention of additional problems in children born with these anomalies. The prevention of unnecessary treatment, for example, is certainly a boon to a child and family confronted with such a multitude of difficulties. Correct identification of any given syndrome is essential to planning what to do and what to avoid. This is secondary prevention at its best.

Respiratory Disorders

The ability to synthesize surfactant has led to a decreased incidence of the sequelae of hyaline membrane disease. This, in turn, has led to a diminution of the incidence of bronchopulmonary dysplasia, pneumothorax, and like disorders. The next step is the reduced prevalence of children who are learning disabled as a consequence. This, too, is secondary prevention at its best.

Planning for the infant who is at risk for deafness and/or nervous system sequelae due to perinatal asphyxia depends on continued monitoring. Laryngeal papillomata can and must be removed. Laryngomalacia is, if you will, self curing. Secondary prevention in both these examples requires assurance that the papillomata or the laryngomalacia is not part of a more general syndrome. Then conservative treatment is indicated until the child is older. Other airway problems may require surgical intervention, especially lower airway. Anomalies of the innominate artery sometimes lead to stenosis of the lower trachea. Inspiratory stridor results, and is an early warning sign. This problem can be surgically corrected. And there has been an instance of teaching sign language to a child with a laryngeal web (English and Prutting 1975).

Metabolic Disorders

Hypothyroidism is treatable, and its consequences for phonation, articulation, and even mentation can be minimized. Diabetes is controllable, thereby controlling its sequelae. The mucopolysaccharidoses, unfortunately, are another story. These are degenerative diseases. Our hope in secondary prevention is to impede the consequences of degeneration, to make a short life as communicative as possible, and to contribute to a child's education while it is possible. We have the opportunity to study a child with MPS–VII (see Chapter 8). That study has shown us that his language skills and his auditory function have gotten poorer over the time we have seen him. We would like to believe that they would have been poorer still without our intervention.

PUBLIC EDUCATION ACTIVITIES

At the outset of this chapter, we mentioned our belief that the best form of prevention is education. And the best place for education is in the junior and senior high schools. It can be done, and it is being done. In one five-year period, a prevention education program was presented to 368,000 teenagers attending 737 secondary schools in 23 states (Rhine 1983). This number continues to increase. In our own relatively small community, we have spoken to some 1,500 teenagers in a similar program (see Appendix A).

Similar programs exist in an assortment of public and private agencies. California was the first state to have a prevention task force, an office of prevention, and a statewide prevention program. It is housed, appropriately, in the Department of Developmental Services but interacts with the genetic disease branch of the health department, the birth defects monitoring program mentioned above, the maternal and child health professionals, and so on. This task force has produced a plan "to reduce the incidence and severity of birth defects and developmental disabilities" (Hickman et al. 1984). The plan covers perinatal care services, early intervention, genetic services, environmental hazards, prevention education, public and professional education, and management information systems. The plan has a single goal: "To ensure that all infants born in California are able to develop to their full potential and to the extent possible are free of birth defects or other developmental disabilities."

Another example is found in the state of Illinois. Its department of Alcoholism and Substance Abuse operates a Prevention Resource Center. This center has a quarterly publication and sponsors conferences, and its staff engages in community activities. The state of Oregon has produced a health curriculum for high schools that deals with the causes and prevention of mental retardation (Plumridge and Hylton 1987). There are many programs of this kind in all states.

PROFESSIONAL SOCIETIES

It is important to observe, as we did at the opening of the book, that the American Speech–Language–Hearing Association (ASHA) has an active prevention committee. Its concerns are not limited to children, of course; it does deal with, for example, noise-induced hearing losses, the effects of stroke, the consequences of cancer. Its policies constitute Appendix B.

Other professional societies—notably the American Academy of Pediatrics (AAP)—have prevention and/or prevention education programs. Throughout this volume, the reader has been referred to policy statements of the academy, for example, on lead poisoning, meningitis, and varicella.

Cooperation among professionals is exemplified by the Joint Committee on Infant Hearing. Begun in 1969 as the Joint Committee on Newborn Hearing Screening, it now incorporates several societies, including ASHA, AAP, American Academy of Otolaryngology—Head and Neck Surgery, and American Nurses Association. A similar committee exists in Canada and has become a government task force. Its constituents are Canadian Association of Speech–Language Pathologists and Audiologists (CASLPA), Canadian Pediatric Society, Canadian Educators of the Hearing Impaired, College of Family Physicians of Canada, and Canadian Society of Otolaryngology—Head and Neck Surgery. This task force has published an outstanding monograph with a strong emphasis on prevention (Shea et al. 1984). There are many others, and certainly not only in North America. In fact, the World Health Organization has endorsed the International Agency for the Prevention of Deafness.

Another example is the National Coalition on Prevention of Mental Retardation. Its members are AAP, American Association of University Affiliated Programs for Persons with Developmental Disabilities, American Association on Mental Deficiency, Association for Retarded Citizens—United States, and President's Committee on Mental Retardation. From time to time, this organization publishes *Prevention Update*.

VOLUNTARY ORGANIZATIONS

High on the list of organizations of volunteers are the Associations for Retarded Citizens (ARC) of the United States. Speakers, publications, and legislative efforts at all levels are carried on by these associations. The program operated by Rhine (1983) is conducted by an ARC in Indianapolis. Ours is sponsored by the Association for Retarded Citizens—Santa Barbara Council. The ARC—California has an outstanding prevention committee that is heavily engaged in legislative and educational activities. It publishes a prevention newsletter and releases prevention fact sheets from time to time. ARC—New Mexico has released an excellent videotape and published an outstanding brochure. ARC—United States engages in similar activities. It publishes *ARC Facts* to inform the public. It has published an excellent brochure on what one should do to initiate prevention activities (Neman 1984).

There are others: Epilepsy Foundation, National Society for Autistic Children, United Cerebral Palsy Association. There is now a national Healthy Mothers, Healthy Babies coalition that through grass-roots efforts promotes and ensures early and regular prenatal care.

In sum and in conclusion, this is an appeal to you, the reader, to get out there and *do* prevention. Mao Tse-tung reminded us that a trip of a thousand miles begins with a single step. And Rabbi Tarfon taught us that we are not required to finish the task, but we must not desist from beginning it.

REFERENCES

ALLEN, DORIS A., ISABELLE RAPIN, AND MAX WIZNITZER. 1988. "Communication Disorders of Preschool Children: The Physician's Responsibility," *J. Dev. Beh. Peds.*, 9, 164–70.

CALIFORNIA BIRTH DEFECTS MONITORING PROGRAM. 1987. CBDMP Progress Report PR#2 (87). Sacramento: California Birth Defects Monitoring Program.

CENTERS FOR DISEASE CONTROL. 1985. *Preventing Lead Poisoning in Young Children.* Atlanta, GA: Centers for Disease Control, Center for Environmental Health, Chronic Diseases Division.

ENGLISH, SUSAN, AND CAROL A. PRUTTING. 1975. "Teaching American Sign Language to a Normally Hearing Infant with Tracheostenosis," *Clin. Peds.*, 14, 1141, 1145.

GREENOUGH, WILLIAM T. 1975. "Experiential Modification of the Developing Brain," *Amer. Scient.*, 63, 37–46.

HICKMAN, MARY LU, et al. 1984. *Prevention 1990: California's Future.* Sacramento: State of California, Health and Welfare Agency, Department of Developmental Services.

JOINT COMMITTEE ON INFANT HEARING. 1982. "Position Statement 1982," *Peds.*, 70, 496–497.

MAUSNER, JUDITH S., AND ANITA K. BAHN. 1974. *Epidemiology, An Introductory Text.* Philadelphia: Saunders.

NEMAN, RONALD. 1984. *Prevention: If Not You, Who? If Not Now, When?* Arlington, TX: Association for Retarded Citizens.

PAPIERNIK, E., et al. 1985. "Prevention of Preterm Births: A Perinatal Study in Haguenik, France," *Peds.*, 76, 154–58.

PLUMRIDGE, DIANE, AND JUDITH HYLTON. 1987. *Smooth Sailing into the Next Generation.* Clackamas County, OR: Association for Retarded Citizens.

RESNICK, MICHAEL B., SUSAN ARMSTRONG, AND RANDY L. CARTER. 1988. "Developmental Intervention Program for High-Risk Premature Infants: Effects on Development and Parent-Infant Interactions," *J. Dev. Beh. Peds.*, 9, 73–78.

RHINE, SAMUEL A. 1983. "The Most Important Nine Months," *The Science Teacher,* October, 46–51.

ROSETTI, LOUIS M. 1986. *High-Risk Infants: Identification, Assessment, and Intervention.* Boston: Little, Brown.

SHEA, ROBERT D. et al., 1984. *Childhood Hearing Impairment.* Ottawa: Health Services Directorate, Health Services and Promotion Branch.

Appendix A

Preventing Mental Retardation: A Slide Presentation

The program includes:

- 42 color slides
- 24 page narrative

The slides include graphics and actual photographs of chromosomal and genetic disorders and the results of disease and trauma. The narrative description that accompanies the slides begins with a statement of the program, gives examples of cause and effect, and finishes with six easy steps to prevent mental retardation and birth defects.

A Cautionary Note: The slides of actual abnormalities and defects are graphic and explicit as they are designed to engage the attention of the viewer.

The slide presentation and written narrative is approximately 40 minutes in length.

Equipment required: slide projector and viewing screen.

The Association for Retarded Citizens-Santa Barbara Council has developed an effective community education program on the prevention of mental retardation and birth defects.

This slide presentation illustrates that at least fifty percent of mental retardation and birth defects can be prevented by education.

We are now making available to our sister organizations our successful prevention package.

Reprinted by permission from ARC-Santa Barbara Council, 629A. Firestone Road, Goleta, CA 93117.

This package has been designed for and enthusiastically received by secondary school teachers and students, community service organizations, as well as ARC parents and friends.

This program has been used at the secondary level in conjunction with

- health education
- drug prevention
- family life skills
- nutrition programs

In conjunction with community organizations, this slide presentation has

- promoted visibility of the ARC and its efforts
- increased awareness of and sensitivity to mental retardation

This prevention program was designed by Sanford E. Gerber, Ph.D. He is a professor at the University of California, Santa Barbara and has received a Fulbright Fellowship to pursue his continued commitment to research and education in the field of mental retardation and birth defects.

This program has been developed in conjunction with members of the ARC-SBC Prevention Committee:

Hsui-Zu Ho, Ph.D.
Assistant Professor
University of California, Santa Barbara
Behavioral Genetics

T. J. Glahn, Ph.D.
Research Psychologist
University of California, Santa Barbara

Kathleen Guljé
Speech/Language
Pathologist

Appendix B

Prevention: A Challenge for the Profession

Communicative disorders constitute the nation's number one handicapped disability. It is estimated by the American Speech-Language-Hearing Association that 22 million Americans have disorders involving speech, language, or hearing. Among preschool children, speech or language disorders have the highest prevalence of any handicapping condition. Among school-age children, speech and language disorders are the second most prevalent handicapping condition. According to the 1982–1983 statistics reported by state education agencies for children receiving services under PL 94-142, 2.44% of all preschool and school-age children combined apparently exhibit speech or language disorders and 26.3% of all handicapped children exhibit such disorders. According to the same study, 71% of all preschool handicapped children are diagnosed as speech or language impaired. To illustrate the extent to which the distribution of handicapping conditions is weighted toward speech and language impairments, the second most prevalent handicap, learning disability, represents only 8.29 percent of the preschool handicapped enrollment. Hearing loss and deafness afflict about 2% of all handicapped children receiving special education services under PL 94-142 and PL 89-313, according to 1982–1983 state education agency reports.

For some populations, the prevalence of communicative disorders may be even higher. Minority and economically disadvantaged children suffer from the same types of communicative disorders as other children.

Reprinted by permission of the American Speech-Language-Hearing Association from *Asha*, 26 (1984), 35–37. Submitted by the 1983 Committee on Prevention of Speech-Language and Hearing Problems. The members of the 1983 Committee on Prevention of Speech-Language and Hearing Problems included Lorraine Cole, ex officio; Wilber Goodseal, Gail Kilburg, Kasunari Kolke, Clarence B. Sellers, Jr., Winifred Watson-Florence, and Michael Marge, Chair.

However, cross-racial and socioeconomic differences exist in epidemiology, etiology, predisposition, severity, and tolerance of communicative disorders. Because of variables associated with poverty, minority and low-income populations are often at greater risk for exposure to environmental, teratogenic, nutritional, and traumatic causes of disorders of speech, language, and hearing.

The cost to the American public for services to communicatively handicapped children is high. To illustrate, PL 94-142 accounts for less than 10% of the funding for the education of the handicapped. Appropriations for FY 1984 under PL 94-142 are $1,069,000,000. This does not include services provided under other federal health and education programs. Furthermore, it is estimated that for every dollar provided by Federal agencies for handicapped children, each state contributes $4 and local governments contribute $5. However, no dollar figure can be placed on the cost in human suffering and loss of human resources resulting from communicative disorders.

National Focus on Prevention

Prevention has been the focus of national attention since President Richard M. Nixon commissioned the President's Committee on Health Education in 1971. The committee recommended that the health problems that were influenced by behavior be identified and that "extended and intensified health education programs be developed for appropriate groups in every community to focus on health problems which apparently can be prevented, detected early or controlled through individual action."

In the decade that followed, several federal studies, public laws, and mandates were implemented. In 1974, the Bureau of Health Education was established. In 1975, the National Center for Health Education was instituted to serve as the private sector counterpart to the bureau. The Department of Health, Education and Welfare also issued its Forward Plan for Health, 1976 to 1980, that emphasized the need for and value of preventative measures in the national health strategy. In 1976, Congress backed prevention efforts by passing the Health Information and Health Promotion Act (PL 94-317). In 1977, a task force comprised of representatives from various HEW agencies was convened to review and analyze departmental activities in disease prevention and health promotion. The task force report, *Disease Prevention and Health Promotion: Federal Programs and Prospects,* certified 12 disease prevention and health promotion goals. The task force identified three prevention activities which are essential to achieve the 12 health status goals: (1) health promotion designed for population groups: (2) health protection designed for population groups: and (3) preventive health services provided to individuals. The activities can be described as follows:

1. Health promotion efforts include those that individuals and communities can undertake to promote healthy lifestyles. The areas targeted for attention that have implications for speech, language, and hearing disorders include smoking, alcohol and drug abuse, nutrition, and stress management.
2. Health protection measures include those for which control substantially is dependent upon manipulation of the environment. The areas targeted for attention that are related to communicative disorders are toxic agent control, environmental safety and health, accidental injury control, and infectious agent control.
3. Preventive health services include those usually delivered to individuals by health and allied health professionals in various clinical/educational settings. The services targeted for attention that are related to speech, language, and hearing disorders include family planning, pregnancy and infant care, immunizations, sexually transmittable disease, and high blood pressure.

A landmark document, *Healthy People: The Surgeon General's Report on Health Promotion and Disease Prevention*, released in 1979, established goals to be achieved by 1990 to reduce health problems and risks associated with problems of the principle life stages. Following an in-depth analysis of these goals, 226 national prevention objectives were developed and delineated in 1980 in *Promoting Health: Preventing Disease: Objectives for the Nation*. The objectives were placed in five categories:

1. Improved health status.
2. Reduced risk factors.
3. Increased public and professional awareness.
4. Improved services and protection.
5. Improved surveillance and evaluation.

The efforts resulting from public laws and federal initiatives and mandates are indeed commendable and undoubtedly have had a positive impact on the health of this country's children and on the reduction of the causes of some communicative disorders.

Prevention and the Profession

Paralleling government focus on prevention, there has been a limited increase in professional activity in the area of prevention of communicative disorders. Traditionally, the communicative disorders profession has emphasized secondary and tertiary prevention, with the greatest emphasis on tertiary as the major professional role of the speech-language pathologist and audiologist. Aside from screening and intervention programs, prevention activities have been practically nonexistent in the communicative disorders fields. Particularly for low-income and minority populations who are at the greatest risk for conditions that can lead to communicative disorders, increased development and implementation of primary prevention strategies are needed.

As early as 1971, ASHA established a Committee on Prevention. The Committee published a position statement entitled "Prevention of Communicative Problems in Children." The following year, ASHA conducted a project funded by the Bureau of Education for the Handicapped that focused on early childhood intervention. The purpose of this project was to disseminate information regarding language acquisition, cultural factors related to language development, language differences, and the educational implications of linguistic diversity. This information was presented to early childhood personnel during a series of conferences held within each federal region.

ASHA also published a variety of publications for parents on prevention and early identification of speech, language, and hearing disorders. *Partners in Language/Companeros en el Idioma* is an English/Spanish booklet series which provides information on speech and language development and stimulation. Two prevention brochures, "How Does Your Child Talk and Hear?" and "¿Que Tal Habla y Oye Tu Niño?" provide a checklist of age-related speech, language, and hearing behaviors.

Challenges to the Profession

Although the communicative disorders profession has developed an interest in the prevention of speech, language, and hearing disorders, it has not approached the broad range of challenges as delineated by Swift (1980).

Swift identifies seven challenges to professions interested in prevention:

1. The need to reconceptualize prevention so that it is better suited for health-related fields, such as speech-language pathology and audiology.
2. The need to separate prevention from treatment service delivery.
3. The need to decentralize prevention efforts from a central-federal government level to state levels.
4. The direction of prevention efforts to change systems which perpetuate the illness model, instead of the "wellness model."
5. The recognition of the growing constituency for prevention in the communicative disorders field.
6. The identification of new careers in prevention.

7. An emphasis on evaluation and cost-effectiveness as we proceed to implement programs of prevention in the community.

In 1981, a book entitled, Communicative Disorders, Prevention and Early Intervention, was written by Weiss and Lillywhite. Both authors are prominent researchers and scholars in the field of communicative disorders. In their introduction, they state, "There is a need for better understanding of communicative development and for a more aggressive and appropriate attempt at recognition, prevention, and early intervention in communicative disorders."

Marge (1981) describes 12 primary prevention strategies that could be applied to any disability entity, including problems leading to communicative disorders. They are immunization, prenatal care, mass public education, educational units in schools, proper health and medical care, genetic counseling, mass screening and early identification, environmental quality control, quality of life maintenance for middle-aged and elderly, family planning, governmental action and elimination of poverty.

Some of these strategies are more feasible than others for certain communicative disorders. For instance, for the primary prevention of causes of cleft lip and palate in the general population, appropriate strategies could include genetic counseling and prenatal care. For primary prevention of the causes of voice disorders in the general population, appropriate strategies could include mass public education, educational units in schools, and environmental quality control. For the primary prevention of the causes of hearing loss in the general population, appropriate strategies could include immunization, mass public education, educational units in schools, and environmental quality control.

Thus, professionals need to have a thorough understanding of (1) specific prevention strategies, (2) the strategies for a specific disorder of speech, language, or hearing and (3) their role in the application of strategies to reduce the incidence and prevalence of disorders in the population.

The application of prevention strategies must take into account the special problems of various populations. For instance, sickle cell anemia, a disorder with high prevalence in the Black population can lead to hearing loss. The most effective primary prevention strategies may be screening to determine if a couple carries sickle cell traits, genetic counseling to discuss the probability of having a child with sickle cell anemia, and, perhaps, family planning. Immunization and prenatal care, which would be effective for prevention of other causes of hearing loss, would not be the most effective strategies relative to Blacks who are at risk for having a child with sickle cell anemia. In terms of secondary prevention, a child with sickle cell anemia should have frequent hearing, speech, and language screenings, particularly following episodes of sickle cell crisis.

Likewise, for an American Indian population, which has the highest prevalence of otitis media, the most appropriate strategies for the prevention of the causes of hearing loss might be environmental quality control and proper health and medical care. Unlike the case for a Black population, genetic counseling would not be the most effective strategy for prevention of the causes of hearing impairment for American Indians.

Similarly, for the prevention of cleft lip and palate, strategies might include genetic counseling across all populations. But because the incidence of the deformity differs cross-racially, the specific counseling information should differ for each minority group. Furthermore, because genetic counseling presents certain moral considerations that may be contradictory to the cultural beliefs and values of some minority groups, professionals must be sensitive to cultural dimensions of such prevention strategies.

Effectiveness of Prevention Efforts

Prevention efforts are effective in reducing prevalence of communicative disorders and can contribute substantially to the cost containment of services to the handicapped.

Thomas Johnson of Utah State University has instituted a "Vocal Abuse Reduction Program" for the past 10 years in an effort to prevent the progress of the more common types of vocal disorders (nodules, polyps, polypoid degeneration, etc.). His program of intervention has reported 90% success in the implementation of techniques to reduce vocal abusive behaviors in children and adults.

In a recent review of early speech and language intervention programs for children with language disorders and for those who are at risk for such disorders, Leonard (1981) concluded that a number of the programs are effective, often resulting in gains that exceed the rate seen in normal development. Other studies have confirmed this finding.

In a study completed by the Bureau of Education for the Handicapped (1969), following the rubella epidemic of the early 1960's, it was estimated that if the Public Health Service had instituted a national rubella immunization program for prepubescent females in a systematic and comprehensive fashion, the strategy might have cost $10 million in 1963.

Because the strategy only was considered and not applied, a rubella epidemic left 20,000-30,000 children with serious handicapping disorders. The epidemic resulted in 5,500 becoming visually handicapped, 12,000 being hearing-impaired, 1,250 becoming deaf or blind, and 1,250 being retarded or crippled. In 1969, the average cost for special educational care for deaf-blind children was $13,500 per year, with a projected total expenditure for special educational and related services approaching $1 billion.

The Wisconsin Department of Health and Social Services developed a series of comparative cost figures for prevention, versus treatment of mental retardation, mental illness, and alcoholism. The department projected that, if the cost for maintaining one mentally retarded person for one year in a Wisconsin state facility was $24,000 and if this amount were invested in prevention programs instead, a long-range savings of over $2 million could be realized by preventing retardation in *only two cases.* According to the report, an initial investment of $5,000 to prevent mental illness through mutual support groups and school programs would result in a long-range savings of $50,000 by preventing *only one* case of mental illness.

Conclusion

The combination of (1) limited training in the area of prevention in professional education programs and (2) emphasis on secondary and tertiary prevention efforts—such as screening and early intervention—has resulted in an urgent need for a national resource development effort to prevent many of the causes of speech, language, and hearing disorders through the use of primary prevention strategies. Such an effort could result in the:

- Reduction of the incidence of communicative disorder.
- A decrease in the prevalence of communicative disorders.
- Reduction in the overall cost of services to the communicatively handicapped.
- Expansion of the role of speech-language pathologists, audiologists, and special educators in the area of health promotion or communicative "wellness."
- Reduction of the loss of human potential and human suffering that result from communicative disorders.

Goal and Objectives

While speech-language pathologists, audiologists, special educators, state education administrators, and university faculty may be aware of some factors relating to the prevention of communicative disorders, no major effort has been made to organize information about prevention and to bring this important issue to the forefront of professional awareness. Toward increased understanding and prevention of the causes of human suffering and loss of human potential the following should be considered as the primary goal and objectives of the speech-language and hearing disorders profession:

Goal: Reduce the incidence of speech, language, and hearing disorders in the general population by reducing the preventable causes of communicative disorders.

Objectives:

- To increase knowledge about the incidence and the prevalence of communicative disorders.
- To increase understanding of the characteristics and progress of diseases and disabilities that result in communicative disorders in the general population.
- To increase awareness of prevention as an important professional responsibility.
- To increase knowledge of primary prevention strategies that can reduce the preventable causes of communicative disorders.
- To develop prevention models that can be implemented at the community or state agency levels to reduce the causes of speech, language, and hearing disorders in low-income and minority populations.
- To develop an awareness of the potential for health promotion, or communicative wellness, as a service alternative.

REFERENCES

ALDERSON, MICHAEL (1977). *An Introduction to Epidemiology.* Littleton, MA: PSG Publishing Co.

ASHA COMMITTEE ON PREVENTION OF SPEECH, LANGUAGE AND HEARING PROBLEMS (1982). "Definitions of the Word 'Prevention' As It Relates to Communicative Disorders." *Asha,* 24, 425–431.

COOPER, PHILIP, KOHOE, WILLIAM, & PATRICK MURPHY (1977). *Marketing and Preventive Health Care.* Chicago: American Marketing Association.

FRIEDMAN, GARY D. (1974). *Primer of Epidemiology.* New York: McGraw-Hill.

GEISMAR, LUDWIG L. (1979). *Preventive Intervention in Social Work.* Metuchen, NJ: The Scarecrow Press, Inc.

GRAHAM, P. J. (Ed.), (1977). *Epidemiological Approaches in Child Psychiatry.* New York: Academic Press.

GRANT, MURRAY (1975). *Handbook of Community Health.* Philadelphia, PA: Lea and Febiger.

HEBER, RICK F. (1970). *Epidemiology of Mental Retardation.* Springfield, IL: Thomas.

KESSLER, IRVING & MORTON LEVIN (Ed.), (1970). *The Community as an Epidemiologic Laboratory.* Baltimore, MD: Johns Hopkins Press.

LEONARD, LAWRENCE B. (1981). "Facilitating Linguistic Skills in Children with Specific Language Impairment." *Applied Psycholinguistics,* 2, 89–118.

LILLIENFELD, ABRAHAM (1969). *Epidemiology of Mongolism.* Baltimore, MD: Johns Hopkins Press.

MARGE, MICHAEL (1981). "The Prevention of Human Disabilities: Policies and Practices for the 80's." In L. G. Perlman (Ed.), *International Aspects of Rehabilitation: Policy Guidance for the 1980s.* Alexandria, VA: National Rehabilitation Association.

MECHANIC, DAVID (1979). *Future Issues in Health Care.* New York: The Free Press.

NATIONAL INSTITUTES OF HEALTH (1976). *Health Promotion and Consumer Education.* Bethesda, MD: John E. Fogarty International Center for Advanced Study in Health Sciences.

PHILIPS, IRVING (Ed.), (1986). *Prevention and Treatment of Mental Retardation.* New York: Basic Books.

PRICE, RICHARD H., et al. (Ed.), (1980). *Prevention in Mental Health: Research, Policy and Practice.* Beverly Hills, CA: Sage Publications.

ROSEN, GEORGE (1975). *Preventive Medicine in the U.S., 1900–1975.* New York: Science History Publications.

SWIFT, CAROLYN (1980). "Primary Prevention, Policy and Practice." In Richard H. Price, et al., *Prevention in Mental Health*. Beverly Hills, CA: Sage Publications.

THE PRESIDENT'S COMMITTEE ON HEALTH EDUCATION (1973). *The Report of the President's Committee on Health Education*. Washington, DC: U.S. Department of Health, Education and Welfare.

U.S. DEPARTMENT OF HEALTH, EDUCATION AND WELFARE (1974). *Forward Plan for Health—FY 1976 to 1980*. Washington, DC: Government Printing Office.

U.S. DEPARTMENT OF HEALTH, EDUCATION AND WELFARE (1978). *Disease Prevention and Health Promotion: Federal Programs and Prospects*. Washington, DC: Government Printing Office.

U.S. DEPARTMENT OF HEALTH, EDUCATION AND WELFARE (1979). *Healthy People: The Surgeon General's Report on Health Promotion and Disease Prevention*. Washington, DC: Government Printing Office.

U.S. DEPARTMENT OF HEALTH AND HUMAN SERVICES (1980). *Promoting Health/Preventing Disease: Objectives for the Nation*. Washington, DC: Government Printing Office.

WEISS, CURTIS E. & HEROLD S. LILLYWHITE (1981). *Communicative Disorders, Prevention and Early Intervention*. St. Louis, MO: C. V. Mosby Company.

Appendix C

Materials
for the Prevention of
Speech-Language-Hearing
Problems

The Committee on Prevention of Speech, Language and Hearing Problems has selected the following materials for comment. These are but a few of the many materials for the prevention of speech, language, and hearing problems available.

The Meyer Children's Rehabilitation Institute has developed a slide-tape presentation designed to be shown to new parents who are considered to be at risk for producing a communicatively handicapped child. It emphasizes the importance of the child's early communication, what the infant is capable of accomplishing, and how the parent can best interact with the infant. This is an excellent slide-tape program that is apparently proving to be a valuable primary prevention tool.

Purchase price: $72,00
Rental price:　　$21.00
Available from:　Media Department
　　　　　　　　Meyer Children's Rehabilitation Institute
　　　　　　　　444 South 44th Street
　　　　　　　　Omaha, NE 68131
　　　　　　　　(402) 559-7467

Thomas Johnson of Utah State University has developed a Vocal Abuse Reduction Program (or VARP) which has proved to be effective in preventing further difficulties for individuals with voice disorders

Reprinted by permission of the American Speech-Language-Hearing Association from *Asha* 26 (1984), 38.

resulting from vocal abuse. VARP is a clinical management program that has undergone more than seven years of formative development. It falls under the category of secondary prevention when VARP is applied to individuals engaged in vocal abuse and who are at risk for vocal pathologies. If VARP is applied to individuals with vocal pathologies who continue to abuse their voices, it may be considered a strategy for tertiary prevention.

Available from: Department of Communicative Disorders
UMC 10, Utah State University
Logan, Utah 84322
Price per copy: $15.00
10 or more copies: $12.00

Bilsom has audiovisuals, posters, and books, all at moderate prices.
Bilsom International, Inc.
11800 Sunrise Valley Drive
Reston, VA 22091
(703) 620-3950

E.A.R. has a series of reports entitled E.A.R.LOG.
E.A.R. Corporation
7911 Zionsville Road
Indianapolis, IN 46268
(317) 293-1111

The National Technical Information Service (NTIS) has the following pamphlets for sale:
Community Noise
Effects of Noise on People
Public Health and Welfare, Criteria for Noise
Information on Levels of Environmental Noise Requisite to Protect Public Health and Welfare with an Adequate Margin for Safety

National Technical Information Service
U.S. Department of Commerce
425 13th Street, NW, Room 620
Washington, DC 20004
(202) 783-3238

The Environmental Protection Agency has a number of publications concerning noise.
Noise It Hurts
Noise: A Health Problem
Model Noise Control Ordinance
ECHO (Each Community Helps Others)

United States Environmental Protection Agency
Office of Noise Abatement and Control
Washington, D.C. 20460

The National Information Center for Quiet also has a number of pamphlets for sale:
Noise at Work
Noise Around Our Homes
Hear, here
Noise and You
Think Quietly About Noise
Noise: A Challenge to Cities
Quieting in the Homes

The National Information Center for Quiet
PO Box 571 71
Washington, DC 20037

Appendix D

The Prevention of Communication Disorders

Preventing communicative disorders should be the added new dimension to the professional responsibility of speech-language pathologists and audiologists. An overview of the field of prevention as it applies to communicative disorders is presented in this article by Michael Marge, professor in the Communicative Disorders Program in the Division of Special Education and Rehabilitation at Syracuse University, and a member of the President's National Council on the Handicapped.

It was Victor Hugo who said "Greater than the tread of mighty armies is an idea whose time has come!" The prevention of human disabilities is an idea whose time has come. For our profession, it is time to review the issue of prevention of communicative disorders and how prevention may be instituted in an organized, systematic and coordinated manner.

Prevention is not a new concept. Interest in preventive practices has long, historical roots reaching as far back as Hippocrates, the imaginative and progressive Greek physician of the fourth century B.C. Hippocrates taught that the physician should study the whole person, not just the disease, and that it is more important to prevent patients' illnesses or infirmities than to cure them. Although this concept has been in existence a long time, an organized and coordinated effort to prevent individuals in the general population from developing disabilities has not been extensively attempted by most professions in the health and health-related fields (Marge, 1981). Until recently, those engaged in psychology, social

Reprinted by permission of the American Speech-Language-Hearing Association from *Asha,* 26 (1984), 29–33, 37.

work, special education, rehabilitation counseling, nursing, and other related areas have focused primarily on the nature, diagnosis, and treatment of a disorder or disability. Currently, these professions are beginning to concentrate on their role in local and national efforts to prevent human disabilities (Price, 1980).

The profession of speech-language pathology and audiology, however, has made steady and significant contributions to the prevention of communicative disorders (Committee on Prevention, 1984). These include hearing conservation programs for preschool and school children, industrial hearing conservation programs, screening for speech-language disorders in preschool and school-aged children, screening in Project Head Start, and several national public education programs on the protection of hearing and the prevention of speech and language problems. Furthermore, through the foresight of several speech and hearing professionals, ASHA has had a Committee on Prevention since 1970. The Committee has been active in writing about prevention, sponsoring panel discussions on prevention, and reporting about professional activity in prevention at ASHA's annual conventions. In a recent survey of state associations, it was found that although our current national efforts in prevention are still quite limited in magnitude and scope, professional interest in prevention is mounting (Marge, 1983).

It was not until the development of epidemiology and preventive medicine in the 19th century that preventive practices had a decided impact on disease and disability in the United States. Since 1900, we have seen a remarkable reduction in life-threatening infectious and communicable diseases. Today, 75% of all deaths in this country are due to degenerative diseases such as heart disease, stroke, and cancer (Surgeon General's Report, 1979). The death rate has been reduced from 17 per 1,000 persons per year in 1900 to less than nine per 1,000 in 1979 (Surgeon General's Report, 1979). Therefore, we have made gains, primarily through preventive efforts.

Although we are concerned about the reduction of deaths, our primary concern in communicative disorders is the reduction of disability or what the medical field refers to as "morbidity." For example, we want to reduce smoking so as to decrease the number of deaths from cancer, emphysema, heart disease, etc. But we also are concerned about the effects of smoking on the larynx and its relationship to voice disorders. In addition, we are concerned about alcohol and drug abuse as it relates to language disorders in children born to alcoholics and drug users and to language disorders due to chronic alcoholism. Sparks (1984, p. 27) discusses the effects of Fetal Alcohol Syndrome on the neonate and the developing child. She states that FAS may account for more of the language and speech problems of children than clinicians have suspected

(Sparks, 1984). In a review of the effects of chronic undue, or low-lead absorption on the speech and language behavior of children, Mayfield (1983, p. 362) concludes that the evidence supports the presence of communicative disorders in some low-lead level children, although the severity, duration, and specific nature of the problems are not clear. The use of tobacco, drugs, and alcohol, and exposure to lead may be prevented and this should be of intensive interest to our profession because of their probable effects on the communicative behavior of individuals.

Definitions of Prevention

The ASHA Committee on Prevention of Speech, Language, and Hearing Problems published a definitional statement of prevention as it relates to communicative disorders (*Asha*, 1982). Prevention is defined, in a general sense, as the elimination of factors which interfere with the normal acquisition and development of communication skills. On the assumption that communicative problems develop in progressive stages of increasing disability, it is felt that a detailed definition of prevention should reflect this progression. Therefore, prevention is specifically defined in three phases:

1. *Primary prevention* is the elimination or inhibition of the onset and development of a communicative disorder by altering susceptibility or reducing exposure for susceptible persons. Illustrations: A patient is induced to stop smoking so as to reduce susceptibility to laryngeal and respiratory anomalies. An employee is removed from a loud, noisy work-site to prevent damage to his hearing.

2. *Secondary prevention* is the early detection and treatment of communicative disorders. Early detection may lead to the elimination of the disorder or the retardation of the disorder's progress, thereby preventing further complications. One of the major practices in secondary prevention is mass screening of persons without symptoms. Illustration: A school institutes an auditory screening program to systematically test the hearing of all children on a periodic basis and after certain illnesses, such as infectious diseases of the ear.

3. *Tertiary prevention* is the reduction of a disability by attempting to restore effective functioning. The major approach is rehabilitation of the disabled individual who has realized some residual problem as a result of the disorder. Illustration: A rehabilitation program for aphasic patients is established as soon as possible after the onset of neuropathology to prevent more serious communicative and behavioral problems (ASHA Committee on Prevention, 1982).

Causes of Disorders

Communicative disorders have been categorized generally as disorders of articulation, language, fluency, voice, and hearing. Table 1 presents lists of selected causes of communicative disorders further divided into "preventable" and "nonpreventable" causes. The lists are not exhaustive, but do include most of the better known causes. Preventable causes are those which are responsive to primary and secondary prevention measures. Nonpreventable causes are those not responsive to primary preventive measures or to early identification and screening. For example, articulation problems can be prevented in asymptomatic children who are at risk for hearing loss by educating their parents about the health of the ear, providing immediate medical intervention when necessary, and protecting the children from exposure to noise. But if a child is born with an unexpected genetic disorder which results in mental retardation and orofacial anomalies, the emerging articulation disorder probably could not have been prevented, given our current technology.

Prevention Strategies

If the major objective of a prevention program is to reduce the incidence of handicapping conditions (that is, to reduce the number of new cases which may be added to the existing handicapped population over a specified period of time), then consider the various prevention strategies which are available to meet the objective. In a review of the prevention literature, at least 13 strategies are identified. The prevention strategies represent significant activities which should be incorporated in any comprehensive community prevention effort. The speech-language pathologist and audiologist may play a direct or indirect role in the application of each strategy according to identified needs. The 13 strategies are:

1. *Immunization.* This is the most effective tool in the prevention of infectious disease. Active artificial immunization is the procedure by which we duplicate the favorable aspects of response to infection without incurring the full consequences of the specific disease (American Academy of Pediatrics, 1977). Although there are immunizing agents for 25 disorders, the American Academy of Pediatrics recommends only seven vaccines for routine use in the United States. These include vaccines for diphtheria, tetanus, pertussis, rubella, polio, common measles and mumps. Of particular interest to the profession of speech-language pathology and audiology is the protection against rubella, polio, and common measles. Rubella may damage the embryo's hearing mechanism during pregnancy; polio may affect the neuromuscular mechanism of the individual; and common measles could result in encephalitis and thereby place a child at risk for brain damage and communicative disorders.

TABLE 1 Examples of Preventable and Nonpreventable Causes of Communicative Disorders

Disorder	Preventable Causes	Nonpreventable Causes
Articulation	Hearing loss Dental abnormalities Chronic infections, esp. URI Most types of mental retardation Injuries Infectious disease (mumps, measles, encephalitis)	Developmental immaturity Neuromuscular disorders associated with unknown etiologies Some types of genetic disorders
Voice	Vocal abuse Upper respiratory infections Allergies Airborne irritants Smoking Hearing loss Trauma and injury Faulty respiration due to allergies, infections, and emphysema Drug and alcohol abuse Some genetic disorders	Constitutional factors Some cancers Viral infections Some genetic disorders
Language	Familial factors Cultural factors Most types of mental retardation Some types of hearing loss Some genetic disorders Brain damage due to prematurity, anoxia, physical trauma, Rh blood factor, infections Malnutrition Low birth weight Fetal alcohol syndrome Prenatal drugs and smoking Strokes Environmental pollutants (lead poisoning)	Some types of hearing loss Some genetic disorders Developmental immaturity Autism Progressive neurological deficits Suspected constitutional factors resulting in psychosis (schizophrenia) Some types of mental retardation
Hearing	Middle ear infections Noise Upper respiratory infections Sexually transmitted diseases Trauma Some genetic factors Prematurity at birth Rh incompatibility Ototoxic drugs Fetal alcohol syndrome Smoking Infectious diseases	Constitutional factors Some genetic factors Aging

Fluency (Stuttering)	Environmental factors:
	   General stress
	   Communicative stress
	Adverse reactions by others
	Cultural factors
		Suspected genetic factors
		Suspected neurophysiological problems

2. *Genetic Counseling.* Heredity plays an important role in a number of disabilities. It is estimated that 521 diseases result from an autosomal recessive mode of inheritance (McKusick, 1978). These include the more commonly known diseases of phenylketonuria (PKU), Tay-Sachs disease, and hypothyroidism. About 50 defined syndromes have been found to be related to hereditary hearing loss (Rand Report, 1974). To reduce the incidence of disabilities associated with genetic disorders, genetic counseling should be included in any program of prevention.

3. *Prenatal Care.* The important services needed during pregnancy include proper medical care, beginning as soon as possible; thorough assessment of any special risks because of family history or past personal medical problems; amniocentesis when needed; and medical counseling on nutrition, smoking, alcohol use, exercise, sexual activity, and family planning.

4. *Mass Screening and Early Identification.* The process of early identification and appropriate follow-up assessment and treatment is an essential preventive strategy. Since its purpose is to select individuals in the early stages of a disease or disability, this strategy is technically referred to as Secondary Prevention. Vision and hearing screening of school children is considered one of the best formal identification programs. As an example, New York State education regulations require a physical examination for all school children in kindergarten and in grades 1, 3, 7, and 10. All new students from outside New York State also are required to have the examination. The current standards and procedures, however, are decided by each school district (F. Szerba, personal communication, 1984).

5. *Early Intervention Programs.* In children who are at risk for language disorders, there is considerable evidence to support early intervention programs and environmental modification to eliminate or ameliorate disorders. In a review of the effectiveness of language intervention programs, Leonard (1981) states, "The evidence reviewed suggests that a number of training approaches are effective, often resulting in gains that exceed the rate seen in normal development." Analysis of the post-treatment usage indicated that these gains went beyond rote learning and "may even result in response classes that are different from those seen in the adult linguistic system (Leonard, 1981)."

Lazar, et al. (1977) reported on the analysis of long-term effects of 14 early intervention programs for disadvantaged children. When the children became 9 to 18 years of age, fewer were placed in special education programs and fewer were retained in grade. Implications for improved communication behavior are significant and support the importance of this strategy in any program of prevention.

6. *Family Planning.* It is reported that of the more than 4 million pregnancies a year in the United States, 1 million are terminated by legal abortion. Of the more than 3 million births each year, only one-third are planned. These statistics imply that half of all pregnancies are unplanned and many are unwanted (Surgeon General's Report, 1979). Unplanned pregnancies often lead to deleterious effects on the child, the mother, and the family. It has been observed that births which are planned are more likely to realize a higher health status and the infants become the recipients of quality parental love and support needed for healthy physical and emotional development. Speech-language pathologists are interested in this strategy because of its implications for normal speech and language acquisition.

7. *Proper Medical Care.* Whether an individual is in touch with a private physician or a health care agency, accessibility to a health care resource is essential in maintaining good health. As a prevention strategy, it is good practice to encourage each individual to maintain periodic contact with a health care provider who is aware of the patient's history and thus can keep track of pertinent developments in the health care of the individual. Again, proper medical care includes screening and early identification tests for children and adults and the role of the speech and hearing professional in screening for communicative disorders should be an important aspect of this strategy.

8. *Public Education.* This strategy refers to educating the community about prevention. The objectives are to develop a prevention-oriented person who (a) has broad knowledge of prevention strategies, (b) is strongly motivated to move from knowledge to action, in ways which lead to and will maintain good health, and (c) understand the political process and what is necessary to influence key individuals and social institutions. Information about prevention should be disseminated as widely as possible at the local, state, and national levels (Marge, 1981). Television, radio, and the press will play an important role in this if the information campaign is systematic and continuous; if the information itself is appealing and receives prime time coverage on radio and television and front page play in newspapers; and if key individuals are associated with the campaign.

9. *Children and Youth Education Programs.* This strategy refers to the introduction of information about prevention at all levels in the school system to prepare young people for a healthier life, both physically and mentally. Through instructional units, teaching aids, and observation, elementary and secondary school children should learn about health and the prevention of illness, injury, and disability. Information about hearing health, speech-language develop-

ment, and communicative disorders should be included in the school curriculum under the supervision of the school speech and hearing professional.

10. *Environmental Quality Control.* There is considerable public interest in conserving our natural and national resources and the quality of our environment. In planning for the improvement and maintenance of environmental quality, the following priorities are recognized: protection of the community water supply for consumption, recreation, and other useful purposes; control of air pollution; disposal of refuse and waste; occupational health and safety; reduction of noise; food and milk control; radiation protection; and control of toxic substances in buildings (such as lead paint, asbestos in ceilings of schools, etc.); and low cost housing (Krusé, 1976). Several of these priorities, such as noise pollution and control of toxic substances, have direct implications for the prevention of communicative disorders.

11. *Quality of Life Programs.* This strategy suggests the need for special programs for individuals at certain transitional stages in life, focusing primarily on the potential problems of adults. The purpose of the strategy is to provide assistance through education and counseling to individuals facing the prospect of stressful and disappointing experiences. Such programs could be provided by community schools, religious institutions, the courts, legislative bodies, business and industry, and other community agencies. Shadden et al. (1982) developed a program of "Pre-crisis Intervention," a management approach designed to prevent or reduce the severity of personal crises resulting from communication breakdown. It is aimed at individuals age 65 or older who are at notable risk for significant speech, language, and hearing problems. It is through such creative efforts that older Americans may realize an improved quality of life even when faced with disability.

12. *Governmental Action.* The role of local, regional, and national governments is essential in the effective implementation of a community-based prevention program. Though much can be accomplished at the community level by the concerted action of nongovernmental persons and agencies, the cooperation of government will provide a greater reservoir of resources, the establishment of regulations to protect the individual and the environment, and the legitimatization of the prevention effort.

13. *Elimination of Poverty.* There are many studies to support the observation that poverty is closely associated with poor nutrition, poor heath care, inadequate child care, and environmental factors that result in extra hazards (Hurley, 1970). To reduce these risks

governments and citizen groups should form coalitions to mount broad-based, national programs to eliminate poverty.

Models and Best Practices

The most effective prevention model is a community-based model (Marge, 1981). Using a systems approach, a plan of action is developed. Table 2 outlines the steps in the development of the community-based plan. Community is defined as a population of individuals living in a particular geographical area and having a history of social, economic, and political interests in common. The community could be a village, a neighborhood, a city or a county. Any geographical area larger than a county will defeat the purpose of the prevention effort, which should evolve and receive the support of persons at the "grass roots" (Marge, 1981).

I Prevention Program Leadership. Though one may conclude that a physician or another health provider should take the initiative to institute a community prevention program, this does not have to be the case. Any knowledgeable and determined community citizen can organize a leadership committee to plan and institute the program. The leadership committee should represent the diverse interest groups in the community. Thus, the committee should be composed of representatives from key religions, professional, educational, business, political, governmental and health provider groups.

II Development and Implementation. Once the community prevention program leadership has been identified and organized into an operating committee, a number of steps should be taken to move in a systematic and orderly fashion from intentions to implementation. These steps are as follows:

A. *Analysis of Community Prevention Needs.* First, identify the gap between current efforts in prevention and the realistic needs of the

TABLE 2 Planning and Implementing a Prevention Program

I. Identifying Prevention Program Leadership
II. Program Planning and Development
    A. Analysis of Community Needs and Resources
    B. The Development of the Long Range Plan
    C. The Need for Community Review and Approval of the Plan
    D. The Evaluation Component
III. Program Implementation
    A. Establishment of a Formal Prevention Organization
    B. The Need for Grass-Roots, Community Involvement

community. Conduct a community-wide study of the current status of prevention efforts. Second, obtain an inventory of all pertinent resources in the community. Include individuals, agencies, and groups with the potential for implementing essential prevention strategies. For example, the local society for the hearing impaired may serve in a mass screening effort for early detection of hearing loss in the population. And third, prepare a comprehensive report of the magnitude of the prevention needs in the community, projecting for at least five years ahead.

B. *The Long Range Plan.* It is at this point that the prevention program committee must decide whether to mount a comprehensive program or begin with a more modest effort, such as the selection of one area of need—the reduction in the incidence of voice disorders or the reduction in the incidence of hearing loss in the school-age population. Then, based on the analysis of needs, the planning committee should state prevention objectives in measurable terms. For example:

Objective 1. Reduce the incidence of hearing loss in the preschool and school-age population (0–17) by 40% in five years.

Strategy 1. Plan and implement a systematic television, radio, and newspaper campaign to inform the community about the prevention program and its role in implementing a successful effort (Public Education Strategy).

Strategy 2. Institute a community-wide screening program for all children 0–17 who have not been screened. The program should be systematic and on-going so that all children are periodically tested at staggered ages. All suspected of hearing impairment should be referred immediately to a center for full diagnostics and treatment (Mass Screening Strategy).

The objectives and strategies should be placed then in a timetable which tells when activities should begin and lists the milestones on the way to successful completion of objectives. Table 3 provides a Prevention Matrix for Communicative Disorders which includes information about the role of each community resource in implementing prevention strategies. Table 4 is an example of objectives and strategies in a long-range plan. According to the constraints of time, personnel, funds, and other factors, strategies are selected to be included in the plan.

C. *Community Review and Approval of Plan.* After the plan has been developed, it should be reviewed by the community. The purpose is to alert citizens to the prevention effort and their participation in the development of the plan. The community-based approach recommended here will require public participation on a periodic basis.

D. *Evaluation Component.* The plan should include a description of the procedures by which the prevention program is assessed systematically to determine progress toward the objectives. The evaluation component is essential for three reasons: (a) it allows the committee to

TABLE 3 Prevention Matrix for Communicative Disorders Prevention Strategies

Community Resources Personnel	*Immunization*	*Genetic Couns.*	*Prenatal Care*	*Mass Screening*	*Early Inter.*	*Family Planning*	*Prpr. Hlth. Care*	*Public Education*	*Educ. for Childrn.*	*Prgrms. Adults*	*Environ. Qual.*	*Govt. Action*	*Elim. Poverty*
1. Speech/Lang. Path				X	X			X	X	X	X	X	
2. Audiologists				X	X			X	X	X	X	X	
3. Physicians	X	X	X		X	X	X	X				X	
4. Nurses	X		X	X	X		X	X					
5. Public Health Prof.	X	X	X	X	X	X	X	X			X	X	X
6. Special Educators				X	X			X		X	X	X	
7. Teachers				X	X			X		X	X	X	
8. Parents	X		X	X	X	X	X	X	X	X	X	X	

Facilities and Organizations:

	Immunization	*Genetic Couns.*	*Prenatal Care*	*Mass Screening*	*Early Inter.*	*Family Planning*	*Prpr. Hlth. Care*	*Public Education*	*Educ. for Childrn.*	*Prgrms. Adults*	*Environ. Qual.*	*Govt. Action*	*Elim. Poverty*
1. Health care settings	X	X	X	X	X	X	X	X			X	X	
2. Schools	X			X	X			X		X	X	X	X
3. Unions				X			X	X			X	X	X
4. Service Clubs				X				X			X	X	X
5. Religious Org.	X	X		X	X	X		X			X	X	X
6. Public Media	X	X	X	X	X	X		X	X	X	X	X	X
7. Business/Ind.				X				X	X	X	X	X	X

determine the feasibility of the plan; (b) it allows for periodic correction of the direction of the plan if it is found that the plan is not moving successfully toward the attainment of the objectives; and (c) it develops community respect for and confidence in the plan if it is assessed systematically and the results are reported.

III Program Implementation. After the plan has been developed, reviewed, and approved by the community, it is advisable that the prevention program committee is incorporated into a committed organization (such as the Prevention Program Organization or the PPO) with a responsible and dedicated staff. The organization must collect all pertinent data during the implementation stage so that accurate reports of activities, successes, and failures are developed. Also, the evaluation of the plan must be conducted continuously and utilized to correct the plan as necessary and to inform the public about the progress of the program.

For greater detail and further information about "Planning and Implementing a Prevention Program," see "The Prevention of Human Disabilities: Recommended Policies and Practices for the 1980s" (Marge, 1981).

TABLE 4   Long Range Plan Example of Objectives and Strategies Analysis

Stated Objective: Reduce the incidence of vocal abuse in the schoolage population by 30% in five years.

Prevention Strategy: Public Education to Inform Children and Parents About Vocal Abuse Behaviors and How to Care for the Vocal Mechanism.

Coordination of Community Resources:

A. Speech-Language Pathologists:	Mount a public media campaign coordinated with other community resources; assist in the development of public announcements, pamphlets, speeches, interviews, and audiovisual materials; establish screening program in the schools for identification of children at risk.
B. Physicians:	Distribute brochures about vocal abuse to patients; assist in public media campaign.
C. Parents:	Through school communications and meetings, inform parents how to reduce vocal abuse behaviors in their children.
D. Teachers:	Through classroom instruction, teach children about vocal abuse behaviors and how to control them; focus on physical education teachers and playground activity.
E. Public Media:	Use of newspapers, television, and radio to discuss campaign and objectives and to seek public cooperation.

The Profession's Role

The time has come for the profession of speech-language pathology and audiology to take a prevention-intervention approach to communicative disorders. On the basis of what is occurring in other related professions and with our profession's history of responsiveness to citizen and community needs, one can predict that the profession will assume the new responsibility for prevention in the very near future. One can foresee the specialties of "Community Speech and Language Pathology" and "Community Audiology" emerging. In time, the titles of community speech/language pathologists and community audiologist may be used to identify those who attend to the needs of communities as they attempt to prevent the incidence and reduce the prevalence of communicative disorders in their populations.

Services, research, and training in prevention should be encouraged by ASHA and state associations. Though ASHA has had a Committee on Prevention since 1970, state associations are just beginning to focus on prevention activities. The survey of 46 state associations by Marge (1983), revealed that 20 states were engaged in one or more prevention-type activity. These include educational programming about communicative disorders, screening activities, hearing conservation programs, and legislative proposals related to prevention. These are promising signs at a time when state associations are faced with an increasing number of priorities and requests. But it is not enough to request that each state association establish its own committee on prevention. The request must be preceded by an informational program about prevention. Currently, there is a pressing need to better inform members of the profession about the area of prevention, their emerging role in conducting prevention programs and ways in which they can effectively meet their responsibilities for the reduction of the incidence and prevalence of communicative disorders.

The mark of a mature profession in health-related services is the significance of its contribution not only to the treatment but also to the prevention of specific disabilities. Let us together accept this challenge with resolve and dedication.

REFERENCES

AMERICAN ACADEMY OF PEDIATRICS (1977). *Report of the committee on infectious diseases.* Red Book, 18th Edition. Evanston, IL.

BRUST, J. C. M., SHAFER, S. Q., RICHTER, R. W., & BRUUN, B. (1976). Aphasia in acute stroke. *Stroke*, 7 (2), 167–174.

COMMITTEE ON PREVENTION OF SPEECH, LANGUAGE, AND HEARING PROBLEMS (1982). Definitions of the word "prevention" as it relates to communicative disorders. *Asha*, 24, 425–431.

COMMITTEE ON PREVENTION OF SPEECH, LANGUAGE, AND HEARING PROBLEMS (1984). Report on status of the profession in prevention. *Asha*, 26(8).

HURLEY, R. (1970). *Poverty and mental retardation: A causal relationship.* New York: Random House.

KRUSÉ, C. W. (1976). Selected environmental health problems in the United States. In W. A. Reinke and D. N. Williams (Ed.), *Health planning, qualitative aspects and quantitative techniques.* Baltimore: Waverly Press.

LAZAR, II., HUBBELL, V., MURRAY, H., ROSCHE, M., & ROYCE, J. (1977). Summary of report: The persistence of preschool effects. U.S. Department of Health, Education and Welfare. Washington, D.C.

LEONARD, L. (1981). Facilitating linguistic skills in children with specific language impairment. *Applied Psycholinguistics*, 2, 89–118.

MACMILLAN, D. L. (1977). *Mental retardation in school and society.* Boston: Little, Brown.

MARGE, M. (1981). The prevention of human disabilities: Policies and practices for the 80s. In L. G. Perlman (Ed.), *International aspects of rehabilitation: Policy guidance for the 1980s.* Alexandria, VA: National Rehabilitation Association.

MARGE, M. (1983, November). *Survey of state association activities related to prevention of communicative disorders.* Paper presented at the annual convention of the American Speech–Language–Hearing Association. Cincinnati, OH.

MAYFIELD, S. A. (1983). Language and speech behaviors in children with undue lead absorption: A review of the literature. *Journal of Speech and Hearing Research*, 26, 362–368.

MAUSNER, J. S., & BANN, A. K. (1974). *Epidemiology.* Philadelphia: Saunders.

MCKUSICK, V. A. (1978). Medelian inheritance in man: Catalogs of autosomal dominant, recessive and X-linked phenotypes. 5th Edition. Baltimore: Johns Hopkins Press.

PRICE, R. H., KETTERER, R. F., BADER, B. C., & MONAHAN, J. (Eds.), (1980). *Prevention in mental health: Research, policy and practice.* Beverly Hills, CA: Sage Publications.

RAND REPORT (1974). Improving services to handicapped children. (*DHEW* Publication No. R-1420). Santa Monica, CA: The Rand Corporation.

SANS, A. L., HARTURAU, E. C., & ARONSON, S. M. (1976). *Guidelines for stroke care.* DHEW Publication No. (HRA) 76-14017. Washington, DC.

SHADDEN, B. B., RATFORD, C. A., & SHADDEN, H. S., JR. (1982, November). *Pre-crisis intervention: Preparing older Americans to cope with communication disorders.*

Paper presented at the annual convention of the American Speech–Language–Hearing Association. Toronto, Canada.

SPARKS, S. N. (1984). Speech and language in fetal alcohol syndrome. *Asha*, 26, 27–31.

THE SURGEON GENERAL'S REPORT ON HEALTH PROMOTION AND DISEASE PREVENTION (1979). *Health People. (DHEW* (PHS) Publication No. 79-55071). Washington, DC: U.S. Government Printing Office.

Appendix E
Useful Addresses

ASHA Committee on Prevention of Speech, Language, and Hearing Problems
American Speech–Language–Hearing Association
10801 Rockville Pike
Rockville, MD 20852

Association for Retarded Citizens—United States
2501 Avenue J
Arlington, TX 76011

Association for Retarded Citizens—California
1510 J Street, Suite 180
Sacramento, CA 95814

Association for Retarded Citizens of New Mexico
8210 La Mirada NE, Suite 500
Albuquerque, NM 87109

Noble Developmental Centers
2400 North Tibbs
Indianapolis, IN 46222

March of Dimes Birth Defects Foundation
1275 Mamaroneck Avenue
White Plains, NY 10605

Office of Prevention
Department of Developmental Services
1600 9th Street
Sacramento, CA 95814

Prevention Resource Center
901 South Second
Springfield, IL 62704

President's Committee on Mental Retardation
The White House
Washington, DC 20001

Bibliography

ABEL, E. L., AND R. J. SOKOL, "Fetal Alcohol Syndrome Is Now Leading Cause of Mental Retardation," *Lancet*, 2 (1986), 1222.

ACCARDO, PASQUALE J., "Associated Deficits: The Ecology of Developmental Disabilities in Infants," *J. Dev. Beh. Peds.*, 5 (1984), 216–17.

AGRAN, PHYLLIS A., AND DEBORA E. DUNKLE, "Motor Vehicle Occupant Injuries to Children in Crash and Noncrash Events, " *Peds.*, 70 (1982), 993–96.

ALAJOUANINE, TH., AND F. LHERMITTE, "Acquired Aphasia in Children," *Brain*, 88 (1965), 653–62.

ALFORD, CHARLES A., SERGIO STAGNO, AND ROBERT F. PASS, "Natural History of Perinatal Cytomegaloviral Infection," in *Perinatal Infections*, ed. Katherine Elliot, Maeve O'Connor, and Julie Whelan, Amsterdam: Excerpta Medica, 1980.

ALLEN, DORIS A., ISABELLE RAPIN, AND MAX WIZNITZER, "Communication Disorders of Preschool Children: The Physician's Responsibility," *J. Dev. Beh. Peds.*, 9 (1988), 164–70.

AMERICAN ACADEMY OF PEDIATRICS, "Statement on Childhood Lead Poisoning," *Peds.*, 79 (1987), 457–65.

———, COMMITTEE ON GENETICS, "Prenatal Diagnosis for Pediatricians," *Peds.*, 65 (1980), 1185–86.

———, COMMITTEE ON RESEARCH, "Fetal Research," *Peds.*, 74 (1984), 440–41.

———, TASK FORCE ON PEDIATRIC AIDS, "Policy Statement: Perinatal HIV Infection (AIDS)," *AAP News*, 4(9) (1988), 6–7.

AMMANN, ARTHUR J., "Is There an Acquired Immune Deficiency Syndrome in Infants and Children?" *Peds.*, 72 (1983), 430–32.

ANDERSEN, RICHARD D., et al., *Infections in Children*. Rockville, MD: Aspen, 1986.

ANDERSSON, MEA, DAVID C. PAGE, AND ALBERT DE LA CHAPELLE, "Chromosome Y-Specific DNA Is Transferred to the Short Arm of X Chromosome in Human XX Males," *Science*, 233 (1986), 786–88.

ANDREWS, GAVIN, "The Epidemiology of Stuttering," in *Nature and Treatment of Stuttering: New Directions*, ed. Richard F. Curlee and William H. Perkins. San Diego, CA: College-Hill Press, 1984.

ANONYMOUS, "Still Some Serious Questions about Lead in Pottery," *Sunset*, July 1987, 168.

ANTHONY, B. F., AND D. M. OKADA, "The Emergence of Group B Streptococci in Infections of the Newborn Infant," *Ann. Rev. Med.*, 28 (1977), 355–69.

ARBETER, ALLAN M., et al., "Combination Measles, Mumps, Rubella and Varicella Vaccine," *Peds.*, 78, Suppl. (1986), 742–47.

ARDINGER, H. H., et al., "Further Delineation of Weaver Syndrome," *J. Peds.*, 108 (1986), 228–35.

ARONSON, ARNOLD E., *Clinical Voice Disorders*, 2nd ed. New York: Thieme, 1985.

ATKINS, JR., JOSEPH P., AND WILLIAM M. KEANE, "Embryology and Anatomy," in *Pediatric Otolaryngology*, vol. II, ed. Charles D. Bluestone and Sylvan E. Stool. Philadelphia: Saunders, 1983.

BAILEY, BYRON J., "Facial Skeletal Injuries in Children," in *Pediatric Otorhinolaryngology*, ed. Basharat Jazbi. Amsterdam: Excerpta Medica, 1979.

BALDURSSON, GYLFI, et al., "Maternal Rubella in Iceland 1963–1964," *Scand. Audiol.*, 1 (1972), 3–10.

BARGMAN, GERALD J., AND LYTT I. GARDNER, "Experimental Production of Otic Lesions with Antithyroid Drugs," in *Human Development and the Thyroid Gland: Relation to Endemic Cretinism*, ed. John B. Stanbury and Robert L. Kroc. New York: Plenum Press, 1972.

BARKER, D., et al., "Gene for Von Recklinghausen Neurofibromatosis Is in the Pericentromeric Region of Chromosome 17," *Science*, 236 (1987), 1100–102.

BARNES, DEBORAH M., "Defect in Alzheimer's Is on Chromosome 21," *Science*, 235 (1987), 846–47.

BARR, BENGT, "Teratogenic Hearing Loss," *Audiol.*, 21 (1982), 111–27.

BELL, ALEXANDER GRAHAM, *The Mechanism of Speech*, 8th ed. New York: Funk & Wagnalls, 1916.

BERGSMA, DANIEL, ed., *Birth Defects Atlas and Compendium*. Baltimore: Williams & Wilkins, 1973.

BERGSTROM, LaVONNE, et al., "Hearing Loss in Renal Disease: Clinical and Pathological Studies, *Ann. Otol., Rhinol., Laryngol.*, 82 (1973), 555–77.

———, AND PATRICIA THOMPSON, "Hearing Loss in Pediatric Renal Patients," *Intl. J. Ped. Otorhinolaryngol.*, 5 (1983), 227–34.

BERMAN, PAIGE, CLAUDE DESJARDINS, AND F. CLARKE FRASER, "The Inheritance of the Aarskog Facial-Digital-Genital Syndrome," *J. Peds.*, 86 (1975), 885–91.

BERRY, MILDRED F., AND JON EISENSON, *Speech Disorders*. New York: Appleton-Century-Crofts, 1956.

BESS, FRED H., "The Minimally Hearing-Impaired Child," *Ear and Hearing*, 6 (1984), 43–47.

———, AND ANNE MARIE THARPE, "Unilateral Hearing Impairment in Children," *Peds.*, 74 (1984), 206–16.

BILLMIRE, M. ELAINE, AND PATRICIA A. MYERS, "Serious Head Injury in Infants: Accident or Abuse?" *Peds.*, 75 (1985), 340–42.

BIRCH, HERBERT G., *Brain Damage in Children: The Biological and Social Aspects*. Baltimore: Williams & Wilkins, 1964.

BIRNHOLZ, JASON C., AND BERYL R. BENACERRAF, "The Development of Human Fetal Hearing," *Science*, 222 (1983), 516–18.

———, AND E. E. FARRELL, "Ultrasound Image of Human Development," *Amer. Scientist*, 72 (1984), 608–13.

BJERKEDAL T., et al., "Maternal Valproic Acid and Spina Bifida," *Lancet*, 2 (1982), 1096.

BLACKMAN, JAMES A., "Congenital Infections," in *Medical Aspects of Developmental Disabilities in Children Birth to Three*, ed. James A. Blackman. Rockville, MD: Aspen, 1984.

———, "Perinatal Injury," in *Medical Aspects of Developmental Disabilities in Children Birth to Three*, ed. James A. Blackman. Rockville, MD: Aspen, 1984.

BLOCH, ALAN B., et al., "Epidemiology of Measles and Its Complications, "in *Vaccinating against Brain Syndromes*, ed. Ernest M. Gruenberg, Carol Lewis, and Stephen E. Goldston. New York: Oxford University Press, 1986.

BODMER, H. C., "Delivery of Thoracopagus Twins," *J. Mich. Med. Soc.*, 152 (1953), 200.

BORDLEY, JOHN E., et al., "Observations on the Effect of Prenatal Rubella in Hearing," in *Deafness in Childhood*, ed. Freeman McConnell and Paul H. Ward. Nashville, TN: Vanderbilt University Press, 1967.

———, PATRICK E. BROOKHOUSER, AND GABRIEL FREDERICK TUCKER, JR., *Ear, Nose, and Throat Disorders in Children*. New York: Raven Press, 1986.

BRACKBILL, YVONNE, "Behavioral Teratology Comes to the Classroom," *Topics in Early Childhood Special Education*, 6 (1987), 33–48.

BRAIN, W. R., "Heredity in Simple Goiter," *Quart. J. Med.,* 20 (1927), 303.

BRASEL, JO ANNE, AND D. BARRY BOYD, "Influence of Thyroid Hormone on Fetal Brain Growth and Development," in *Perinatal Thyroid Physiology and Disease,* ed. Delbert A. Fisher and Gerard N. Burrow. New York: Raven Press, 1975.

BRICKER, DIANE, "Early Intervention: The Criteria of Success," *Allied Health and Beh. Sci.,* 1 (1978), 567–82.

BROWN, J. KEITH, "Dysarthria in Children: Neurologic Perspective," in *Speech and Language Evaluation in Neurology: Childhood Disorders,* ed. John K. Darby. Orlando, FL: Grune & Stratton, 1985.

BROWN, ROGER M., AND RACHELLE H. B. FISHMAN, "An Overview and Summary of the Behavioral and Neural Consequences of Perinatal Exposure to Psychotropic Drugs," in *Neurobehavioral Teratology,* ed. Joseph Yania. Amsterdam: Elsevier, 1984.

BROWN, W. T., et al., "Association of Fragile X Syndrome with Autism," *Lancet,* 1 (1982), 100.

——, et al., "Fragile X and Autism: A Multicenter Survey," *Amer. J. Med. Gen.,* 23 (1986), 341–52.

BUYSE, M. L., ed., *Birth Defects Encyclopedia.* New York: Alan R. Liss, 1988.

CALIFORNIA BIRTH DEFECTS MONITORING PROGRAM, CBDMP Progress Report PR2 (87). Sacramento: California Birth Defects Monitoring Program, 1987.

CANTU, E. S., AND PATRICIA A. JACOBS, "Fragile (X) Expression: Relationship to the Cell Cycle," *Human Genetics,* 67 (1984), 99–102.

CARMI, RIVKA, et al., "Fragile-X Syndrome Ascertained by the Presence of Macro-Orchidism in a 5-Month-Old Infant," *J. Peds.,* 74 (1984), 883–86.

CARREL, ROBERT E., "Epidemiology of Hearing Loss," in *Audiometry in Infancy,* ed. Sanford E. Gerber. New York: Grune & Stratton, 1977.

CASEY, ROSEMARY, STEPHEN LUDWIG, AND MARIE C. MCCORMICK, "Morbidity following Minor Head Trauma in Children," *Peds.,* 78 (1986), 497–502.

CATANZARITE, VALERIAN A., AND GARY A. AISENBERY, "Severe Malnutrition in Pregnancy: Diagnosis, Evaluation, and Management," *Perinat. / Neonat.,* 12 (1988), 11–12, 14–17.

CATLIN, FRANCIS I., "Otologic Diagnosis and Treatment of Disorders Affecting Hearing," in *Medical Audiology,* ed. Frederick N. Martin. Englewood Cliffs, NJ: Prentice Hall, 1981.

CENTERS FOR DISEASE CONTROL, *Preventing Lead Poisoning in Young Children.* Atlanta, GA: Centers for Disease Control, Center for Environmental Health, Chronic Diseases Division, 1985.

CHASNOFF, IRA J., DOUGLAS E. LEWIS, AND LIZA SQUIRES, "Cocaine Intoxication in a Breast-Fed Infant," *Peds.,* 80 (1987), 836–38.

CHECK, WILLIAM, "Nonhuman Primates Serve as Subjects in AIDS Research," *Research Resources Reporter,* 11(7) (July 1987), 13–18.

CHESS, STELLA, "Autism in Children with Congenital Rubella," *J. Autism Child. Schiz.,* 1 (1971), 33–47.

——, AND PAULINA FERNANDEZ, "Neurologic Damage and Behavior Disorder in Rubella Children," *Amer. Ann. Deaf,* 125 (1980), 998–1001.

CHRISTIAN, MILDRED S., "Statement of Problem," in *Advances in Modern Toxicology,* Vol. III: *Assessment of Reproductive and Teratogenic Hazards,* ed. Mildred S. Christian et al. Princeton, NJ: Princeton Scientific Publishers, 1983.

——, et al., eds., *Advances in Modern Toxicology,* Vol. III, *Assessment of Reproductive and Teratogenic Hazards.* Princeton, NJ: Princeton Scientific Publishers, 1983.

CHURCH, M. W., AND K. P. GERKIN, "Hearing Disorders in Children with Fetal Alcohol Syndrome: Findings from Case Reports," *Peds.,* 82 (1988), 147–54.

CLARREN, STERLING K., AND DAVID W. SMITH, "The Fetal Alcohol Syndrome," *N. Engl. J. Med.,* 298 (1978), 1063–67.

COHEN, M. MICHAEL, JR., *The Patient with Multiple Anomalies.* New York: Raven Press, 1981.

——, ROBERT J. GORLIN, AND S. LEVIN, *Syndromes of the Head and Neck,* 3rd ed. New York: Raven Press, 1988.

COHN, ARNOLD, "Etiology and Pathology of Disorders Affecting Hearing," in *Medical Audiology,* ed. Frederick N. Martin. Englewood Cliffs, NJ: Prentice Hall, 1981.

CONDON, LAWRENCE M., et al., "Cardiovocal Syndrome in Infancy," *Peds.,* 76 (1985), 22–25.

COOPER, JUDITH A., AND CHRISTY L. LUDLOW, "The Genetics of Developmental Speech and Language Disorders," in *Speech and Language Evaluation in Neurology: Childhood Disorders,* ed. John K. Darby. Orlando, FL: Grune & Stratton, 1985.

CORNBLATH, MARVIN, AND ROBERT SCHWARTZ, "Infant of the Diabetic Mother," in *Disorders of Carbohydrate Metabolism in Infancy,* Vol. III, ed. Marvin Cornblath and Robert Schwartz. Philadelphia: Saunders, 1966.

COSTELLO, JANIS M., "Treatment of the Young Chronic Stutterer: Managing Fluency," in *Nature and Treatment of Stuttering: New Directions,* ed. Richard F. Curlee and William H. Perkins. San Diego, CA: College-Hill Press, 1984.

COTTON, ROBIN T., AND JAMES S. REILLY, "Congenital Malformations of the Larynx," in *Pediatric Otolaryngology,* ed. Charles D. Bluestone and Sylvan E. Stool. Philadelphia: Saunders, 1983.

———, AND MARK A. RICHARDSON, "Congenital Laryngeal Anomalies," *Otolaryngol. Clin. N. Amer.,* 14 (1981), 203–18.

CREMERS, COR W. R. J., "Meatal Atresia and Hearing Loss. Autosomal Dominant and Autosomal Recessive Inheritance," *Intl. J. Ped. Otorhinolaryngol.,* 8 (1985), 211–13.

CROFT, C. B., et al., "The Occult Submucous Cleft Palate and the Musculus Uvulae," *Cleft Palate J.,* 15 (1978), 150–54.

CULLITON, BARBARA J., "Amniocentesis: HEW Backs Test for Prenatal Diagnosis of Disease," *Science,* 190 (1975), 537–40.

DAHLE, ARTHUR J., et al., "Subclinical Congenital Cytomegalovirus Infection and Hearing Impairment," *J. Speech Hear. Dis.,* 39 (1974), 320–29.

———, AND FAYE P. MCCOLLISTER, "Audiological Findings in Children with Neonatal Herpes," *Ear and Hearing,* 9 (1988), 256–58.

DAILY, DONNA K., "Home Oxygen Therapy for Infants with Bronchopulmonary Dysplasia," *Perinatol. /Neonatol.,* 11(3) (1987), 26, 28, 30, 32, 35–36.

DARBY, JOHN K., KENNETH K. KIDD, AND LUIGI LUCA CAVALLI-SFORZA, "Molecular Genetics in Speech and Language Disorders," in *Speech and Language Evaluation in Neurology: Childhood Disorders,* ed. John K. Darby. Orlando, FL: Grune & Stratton, 1985.

DAVENPORT, SANDRA L. H., MARGARET A. HEFNER, AND JOYCE A. MITCHELL, "The Spectrum of Clinical Features in CHARGE Syndrome," *Clin. Genetics,* 29 (1986), 298–310.

DAVIS, LARRY E., et al., "Cytomegalovirus Isolation from a Human Inner Ear," *Ann. Otol., Rhinol., Laryngol.,* 88 (1979), 424–26.

DEBRUYNE, F., M. ANDERSCHUEREN-LODEWEYCKX, AND P. BASTIJNS, "Hearing in Congenital Hypothyroidism," *Audiology,* 22 (1983), 404–9.

DEPOMPEI, ROBERTA, AND JEAN BLOSSER, "Strategies for Helping Head-Injured Children Successfully Return to School," *Lang. Speech Hear. Serv. Schools,* 18 (1987), 292–300.

DIGEORGE, ANGELO M., RICHARD W. OLSTED, AND ROBINSON D. HARLEY, "Waardenburg's Syndrome," *J. Peds.,* 57 (1960), 649–69.

DOWN, J. L. H., "Observations on an Ethnic Classification of Idiots," *London Hospital Reports,* 3 (1866), 259–62.

DREIFUSS, F. E., "The Pathology of Central Communicative Disorders in Children," in *The Nervous System.* Vol. 3, *Human Communication and Its Disorders,* ed. Eldon R. Eagles. New York: Raven Press, 1975.

DRISCOLL, SHIRLEY G., AND STELLA B. YEN, "Neonatal Pulmonary Hyaline Membrane Disease: Some Pathologic and Epidemiologic Aspects," in *Respiratory Distress Syndrome,* ed. Claude A. Villee, Dorothy B. Villee, and James Zuckerman. New York: Academic Press, 1973.

DUBLIN, WILLIAM B., *Fundamentals of Sensorineural Auditory Pathology.* Springfield, IL: Chas. C Thomas, 1976.

EDWARDS, J. H., et al., "A New Trisomic Syndrome," *Lancet,* 1 (1960), 787–90.

EHRLICH, CAROL H., et al., "Communication Skills in Five-Year-Old Children with High Risk Neonatal Histories," *J. Speech Hearing Res.,* 16 (1973), 522–29.

ELIASON, MICHELE J., "Neurofibromatosis: Implications for Learning and Behavior," *J. Dev. Beh. Peds.,* 7 (1986), 175–79.

ENGLISH, SUSAN, AND CAROL A. PRUTTING, "Teaching American Sign Language to a Normally Hearing Infant with Tracheostenosis," *Clin. Peds.,* 14 (1975), 1141, 45.

EPSTEIN, CHARLES J., AND MITCHELL S. GOLBUS, "Prenatal Diagnosis of Genetic Diseases," *Amer. Scientist,* 65 (1977), 703–11.

EPSTEIN, LEON G., et al., "Manifestations of Human Immunodeficiency Virus Infection in Children," *Peds.,* 78 (1986), 678–87.

EWING-COBBS, LINDA, et al., "Language Disorders after Pediatric Head Injury," in *Speech and Language Evaluation in Neurology: Childhood Disorders,* ed. John K. Darby. Orlando, FL: Grune & Stratton, 1985.

FARRELL, PHILIP M., "Introduction to the Preventative Approach to Perinatal Care," in *Lung Development: Biological and Clinical Perspectives,* vol. II, *Neonatal Respiratory Distress,* ed. Philip M. Farrell. New York: Academic Press, 1982.

FAZEN III, LOUIS E., FREDERICK H. LOVEJOY, JR., AND ROBERT K. CRONE, "Acute Poisoning in a Children's Hospital: A 2-Year Experience," *Peds.,* 77 (1986), 144–51.

FERGUSON, CHARLES F., "Congenital Malformations," in *Pediatric Otolaryngology.* Vol. II, *Disorders of the Respiratory Tract in Children,* eds. Charles F. Ferguson and Edwin L. Kendig, Jr. Philadelphia: Saunders, 1972.

FIELD, TIFFANY, JEAN DEMPSEY, AND H. H. SHUMAN, "Five-Year Follow-Up of Preterm Respiratory Distress Syndrome and Post-Term Postmaturity Syndrome Infants," in *Infants Born at Risk,* eds. Tiffany Field and Anita Sostek. New York: Grune & Stratton, 1983.

FISCH, ROBERT O., "Long-Term Consequences of Survivors of Respiratory Distress Syndrome," in *Pulmonary Development: Transition from Intrauterine to Extrauterine Life,* ed. George H. Nelson. New York: Marcel Dekker, 1985.

FISCHLER, RONALD S., "The Pediatrician's Role in Early Identification," in *Hearing-Impaired Children and Youth with Developmental Disabilities,* ed. Evelyn Cherow. Washington, DC: Gallaudet College Press, 1985.

FISHER, DELBERT A., AND GERARD N. BURROW, eds., *Perinatal Thyroid Physiology and Disease.* New York: Raven Press, 1975.

FLEISCHER, M., et al., "Environmental Impact of Cadmium: A Review by the Panel on Hazardous Trace Substances," *Env. Health Perspectives,* 29 (1974), 253–323.

FLETCHER, JACK M., et al., "Cognitive and Psychosocial Sequelae of Head Injury in Children: Implications for Assessment and Management," in *The Injured Child,* ed. Benjy Frances Brooks. Austin: University of Texas Press, 1985.

FLINT, EWEN F., "Severe Childhood Deafness in Glasgow, 1965–1979," *J. Laryngol. Otol.,* 97 (1983), 421–25.

FLOWER, WILDA M., AND C. DANIEL SOOY, "AIDS: An Introduction for Speech-Language Pathologists and Audiologists," *Asha,* 29(11) (1987), 25–30.

FORD, C. E., et al., "A Sex-Chromosome Anomaly in a Case of Gonadal Dysgenesis (Turner's Syndrome)," *Lancet,* 1 (1959), 711–13.

FOUSHEE, D., Personal communication, 1987.

FRASER, GEORGE R., *The Causes of Profound Deafness in Childhood.* Baltimore: Johns Hopkins University Press, 1976.

FRIED, PETER A., et al., "Neonatal Neurological Status in a Low-Risk Population after Prenatal Exposure to Cigarettes, Marijuana, and Alcohol," *J. Dev. Beh. Peds.,* 8 (1987), 318–26.

FREIDMAN, ELLEN M., et al., "Sickle Cell Anemia and Hearing," *Ann. Otol.,* 89 (1980), 342–47.

GABEL, STEWART, AND MARILYN T. ERICKSON, *Child Development and Developmental Disabilities.* Boston: Little, Brown, 1980.

GALABURDA, ALBERT M., "Definition of the Anatomical Phenotype," in *Genetic Aspects of Speech and Language Disorders,* ed. Christy L. Ludlow and Judith A. Cooper. New York: Academic Press, 1983.

GARVEY, MAUREEN, AND DAVID E. MUTTON, "Sex Chromosome Aberrations and Speech Development," *Arch. Dis. Childhood,* 48 (1973), 937–41.

GATOT, ALBERT, FERIT TOVI, AND ABRAHAM MOSHIASHVILI, "Periorbital Cellulitis: Presenting Feature of Undiagnosed Old Maxillary Fracture," *Intl. J. Ped. Otorhinolaryngol.,* 11 (1986), 129–34.

GEISMAR, L. L., *Preventive Intervention in Social Work.* Metuchen, NJ: Scarecrow Press, 1969.

GERBER, SANFORD E., "Cerebral Palsy and Hearing Loss," *Cerebral Palsy J.,* 6 (1966), 6–7.

———, "The Deaf Dalmatian," *The Voice,* 17 (1968), 12–14.

———, "Asphyxia Neonatorum and Subsequent Communicative Disorders," paper presented at the XVth International Congress of Audiology, Krakow, Poland, 1980.

———, ed., *Audiometry in Infancy.* New York: Grune & Stratton, 1977.

———, "Acoustical Analyses of Neonates' Vocalizations," *Intl. J. Ped. Otorhinolaryngol.,* 10 (1985), 1–8.

———, "Congenital Conductive Hearing Impairment in Noonan Syndrome," *Human Comm. Canada,* 10 (1986), 21–3.

———, "The State of the Art in Pediatric Audiology," in *International Perspectives on Communication Disorders,* eds. Sanford E. Gerber and George T. Mencher. Washington, D.C.: Gallaudet University Press, 1988.

———, CONSTANCE J. LYNCH, AND WILLIAM S. GIBSON, JR., "The Acoustic Characteristics of the Cry of an Infant with Unilateral Vocal Fold Paralysis," *Intl. J. Ped. Otorhinolaryngol.,* 13 (1987), 1–9.

———, AND GEORGE T. MENCHER, *Auditory Dysfunction.* Houston: College-Hill Press, 1980.

———, "Is There an Increased Incidence of Congenital Deafness?" Unpublished mini-seminar presented to the annual convention of the American Speech–Language–Hearing Association, 1983.

———, eds., *Early Diagnosis of Hearing Loss.* New York: Grune & Stratton, 1978.

———, MAURICE I. MENDEL, AND MONICA GOLLER, "Progressive Hearing Loss Subsequent to Congenital Cytomegalovirus Infection," *Human Comm. Canada,* 4 (1979), 231—34.

———, ELIZABETH WILE, AND NANCY T. HAMAI, "Central Auditory Dysfunction in Deaf Children," *Human Communication Canada,* 9 (1985), 39–44.

GITLIN, JONATHAN D., et al., "Randomized Controlled Trial of Exogenous Surfactant for the Treatment of Hyaline Membrane Disease," *Peds.,* 79 (1987), 31–37.

GODAI, U., R. TATARELLI, AND G. BONNANI, "Stuttering and Tics in Twins," *Acta Geneticae Medicae et Gomellologiae,* 25 (1976), 369–75.

GOIN, DONALD W., "Otospongiosis," in *Otolaryngology: A Textbook,* ed. Gerald M. English. New York: Harper & Row, 1976.

GOLDING-KUSHNER, K., G. WELLER, AND ROBERT J. SHPRINTZEN, "Velo-Cardio-Facial Syndrome: Language and Psychological Profiles," *J. Craniofacial Genet. Devel. Biol.,* 5 (1985), 259–66.

GOLDSON, EDWARD, "Bronchopulmonary Dysplasia: Its Relation to Two-Year Developmental Functioning in the Very Low Birth Weight Infants," in *Infants Born at Risk,* ed. Tiffany Field and Anita Sostek. New York: Grune & Stratton, 1983.

———, "Severe Bronchopulmonary Dysplasia in the Very Low Birth Weight Infant: Its Relationship to Developmental Outcome," *J. Dev. Beh. Peds.,* 5 (1984), 165–68.

GOLDSTEIN, ARTHUR I., et al., "Perinatal Outcome in the Diabetic Pregnancy," *J. Reproductive Med.,* 20 (1978), 61–66.

GOLDSTEIN, S., et al., "Correction of Deficient Sleep Entrained Growth Hormone Release and Obstructive Sleep Apnea by Tracheostomy in Achondroplasia," *Birth Defects Original Article Series,* 21(2) (1985), 85–92.

GORLIN, ROBERT, JENS J. PINDBORG, AND M. MICHAEL COHEN, JR., *Syndromes of the Head and Neck.* New York: McGraw-Hill, 1976.

GRAHAM, JOHN M., JR., et al., "Oral and Written Language Abilities of XXY Boys: Implications for Anticipatory Guidance," *Peds.,* 81 (1988), 795–806.

GRANT, MURRAY, *Handbook of Community Health,* 3rd ed. Philadelphia: Lea and Febiger, 1981.

GRASS, F., et al., "Reproduction in XYY Males: Two New Cases and Implications for Genetic Counseling," *Amer. J. Med. Genetics,* 19 (1984), 553–60.

GRAY, LINCOLN, et al., "Fourier Analysis of Infantile Stridor," *Intl. J. Ped. Otorhinolaryngol.,* 10 (1985), 191–99.

GREENOUGH, WILLIAM T., "Experiential Modification of the Developing Brain," *Amer. Scientist,* 63 (1975), 37–46.

GREGG, N. M., "Congenital Cataract following German Measles in the Mother," *Trans. Ophth. Soc. (Austral.),* 3 (1941), 35–46.

GREGORY, HUGO H., "Prevention of Stuttering: Management of Early Stages," in *Nature and Treatment of Stuttering: New Directions*, ed. Richard F. Curlee and William H. Perkins. San Diego, CA: College-Hill Press, 1984.

GRIFFITH, F., "The Significance of Pneumococcal Types," *J. Hygiene*, 27 (1928), 113–59.

GRUNDFAST, KENNETH M., "The Role of the Audiologist and Otologist in the Identification of the Dysmorphic Child," *Ear and Hearing*, 4 (1983), 24–30.

GUTTMACHER, A. F., AND B. L. NICHOLS, "Teratology of Conjoined Twins," *Birth Defects Original Article Series*, 3 (1967), 3–9.

HAGBERG, BENGT, "Rett Syndrome: Swedish Approach to Analysis of Prevalence and Cause," *Brain and Development*, 7 (1985), 277–80.

———, et al., "A Progresive Syndrome of Autism, Dementia, Ataxia, and Loss of Purposeful Hand Use in Girls: Rett's Syndrome. Report of 35 Cases," *Ann. Neurol.*, 14 (1983), 471–79.

HANSHAW, JAMES B., "Perinatal Infections: Prevention of Long–Term Sequelae," in *Perinatal Infections*, ed. Katherine Elliot, Maeve O'Connor, and Julie Whelan. Amsterdam: Excerpta Medica, 1980.

HANSON, JAMES W., KENNETH L. JONES, AND DAVID W. SMITH, "Fetal Alcohol Syndrome: Experience with 41 Patients," *J. Amer. Med. Assn.*, 235 (1976), 1458–60.

HARRIS, STEN, et al., "Congenital Cytomegalovirus Infections and Sensorineural Hearing Loss," *Ear and Hearing*, 5 (1984), 352–55.

HARRISON, MICHAEL R., MITCHELL S. GOLBUS, AND ROY A. FILLY, *The Unborn Patient*. Orlando, FL: Grune & Stratton, 1984.

HAVRANKOVA, JANA, M. BROWNSTEIN, AND J. ROTH, "Insulin and Insulin Receptors in Rodent Brain," *Diabetologia*, 29 (1981), 268–73.

HAYES, E., R. BABIN, AND C. PLATZ, "The Otologic Manifestations of Mucopolysaccharidoses," *Amer. J. Otology*, 2, 65–69.

HECHT, FREDERICK, AND BARBARA KAISER HECHT, "Autosomal Fragile Sites Not a Current Indication for Prenatal Diagnosis," *Human Genetics*, 67 (1984), 352–53.

HEINONEN, OLLI P., "Risk Factors for Congenital Heart Disease," in *Birth Defects: Risks and Consequences*, ed. Sally Kelly et al. New York: Academic Press, 1976.

HEMENWAY, W. GARTH, ISAMU SANDO, AND D. MCCHESNEY, "Temporal Bone Pathology following Maternal Rubella," *Arch. Klin. Exp. Ohren-, Nasen-, Kehlk. Heilk.*, 193 (1969), 287–300.

HERRMANN, J., AND J. M. OPITZ, "The Stickler Syndrome (Hereditary Arthro-Ophthalmopathy)," *Birth Defects Original Article Series*, 11(2) (1975), 76–103.

HETZEL, BASIL S., "Similarities and Differences between Sporadic and Endemic Cretinism," in *Human Development and the Thyroid Gland (Relation to Endemic Cretinism)*, ed. John Stanbury and Robert L. Kroc. New York: Plenum Press, 1972.

HICKMAN, MARY LU, et al., *Prevention 1990: California's Future*. Sacramento: California Department of Developmental Services, 1985.

HICKS, SAMUEL P., AND CONSTANCE J. D'AMATO, "Effects of Ionizing Radiation on Developing Brain and Behavior," in *Studies on the Development of Behavior and the Nervous System*, Vol. 4, *Early Influences*, ed. Gilbert Gottlieb. New York: Academic Press, 1978.

HILL, R. M., et al., "Infants Exposed *in Utero* to Antiepileptic Drugs. A Prospective Study," *Am. J. Dis. Child.*, 127 (1974), 645–53.

HIRSCHBERG, J., AND T. SZENDE, *Pathological Cry, Stridor, and Cough in Infants*, trans. L. Elias. Budapest: Adademiai Klado, 1982.

HIRSCHOWITZ, BASIL I., A. GROLL, AND RICHARD CEBALLOS, "Hereditary Nerve Deafness in Three Sisters with Absent Gastric Motility, Small Bowel Diverticulitis and Ulceration, and Progressive Sensory Neuropathy," *Birth Defects*, 8 (1972), 27–41.

HO, HSIU-ZU, T. J. GLAHN, AND JU-CHANG HO, "The Fragile-X Syndrome," *Dev. Med. Child Neurol.*, 30 (1988), 252–65.

HOAR, RICHARD M., "Pharmaceuticals, Drugs and Birth Defects," in *Advances in Modern Environmental Toxicology*, Vol. III, *Assessment of Reproductive and Teratogenic Hazards*, ed. Mildred S. Christian et al. Princeton, NJ: Princeton Scientific Publishers, 1985.

HOCKEY, A., AND J. CROWHURST, "Early Manifestations of the Martin-Bell Syndrome Based on a Series of Both Sexes from Infancy," *Amer. J. Med. Gen.*, 30 (1988), 61–71.

HOGNESTAD, S., "Hereditary Nerve Deafness Associated with Diabetes," *Acta Oto-Laryngol.*, 64 (1967), 219–25.

HOLINGER, LAUREN D., "Etiology of Stridor in the Neonate, Infant and Child," *Ann. Otol., Rhinol., Laryngol.*, 89 (1980), 397–400.

HOLINGER, PAUL H., AND W. T. BROWN, "Congenital Webs, Cysts, Laryngoceles and Other Anomalies of the Larynx," *Ann. Otol., Rhinol., Laryngol.*, 76 (1967), 744.

HOPKINS-ACOS, PATRICIA, AND KAREN BUNKER, "A Child with Noonan Syndrome," *J. Speech Hear. Dis.*, 44 (1979), 495–503.

HOSKING, D. J., "Autonomic Neuropathy," in *The Diabetes Annual/3*, ed. K. G. M. M. Alberti and L. P. Krall. Amsterdam: Elsevier, 1987.

HOWARD-PEEBLES, PATRICIA N., GAYLE R. STODDARD, AND MILDRED G. MIMS, "Familial X-Linked Mental Retardation, Verbal Disability, and Marker X Chromosomes," *Amer. J. Human Genetics*, 31 (1979), 214–22.

HUNTER, C., "A Rare Disease in Two Brothers," *Proc. R. Soc. Med.*, 10 (1917), 104.

HURLEY, LUCILLE S., "Nutritional Deficiencies and Excesses," in *Handbook of Teratology*, vol. 1, *General Principles and Etiology*, ed. James G. Wilson and F. Clarke Fraser. New York: Plenum Press, 1977.

HUTCHINGS, DONALD E., "Behavioral Teratology: Embryopathic and Behavioral Effects of Drugs during Pregnancy," in *Studies on the Development of Behavior and the Nervous System*, vol. 4, *Early Influences*, ed. Gilbert Gottlieb. New York: Plenum Press, 1978.

INFURNA, ROBERT, AND BERNARD WEISS, "Neonatal Behavioral Toxicity in Rats following Prenatal Exposure to Methanol," *Teratol.*, 33 (1986), 259–65.

INGHAM, ROGER J., "Stuttering: Recent Trends in Research and Therapy," in *Human Communication and Its Disorders*, ed. Harris Winitz. Norwood, NJ: Ablex, 1987.

IOSUB, SILVIA, et al., "More on Human Immunodeficiency Virus Embryopathy," *Peds.*, 80 (1987), 512-16.

JACOBS, PATRICIA A., et al., "Aggressive Behaviour, Mental Subnormality and the XYY Male," *Nature*, 208 (1965), 1351–52.

JAFFE, BURTON F., "Topographical Signs Associated with Congenital Hearing Loss," in *Early Diagnosis of Hearing Loss*, ed. Sanford E. Gerber and George T. Mencher. New York: Grune & Stratton, 1978.

——, "Deformities of the External Ear Associated with Middle Ear, Inner Ear, or Distant Malformations," *Clin. Plastic Surg.*, 5 (1978), 413–18.

——, ed., *Hearing Loss in Children*. Baltimore: University Park Press, 1977.

JANOWSKY, JERI S., AND RUTH NASS, "Early Language Development in Infants with Cortical and Subcortical Perinatal Brain Injury," *J. Dev. Beh. Peds.*, 8 (1987), 3–7.

JILEK, L., E. TRAVNICKOVA, AND S. TROJAN, "Characteristic Metabolic and Functional Responses to Oxygen Deficiency in the Central Nervous System," in *Physiology of the Perinatal Period*, vol. 2, ed. Uwe Stave. New York: Appleton-Century-Crofts, 1970.

JOHNSON, RICHARD T., AND DIANE E. GRIFFIN, "The Neuropsychiatric Sequelae of Measles," in *Vaccinating against Brain Syndromes*, eds. Ernest M. Gruenberg, Carol Lewis, and Stephen E. Goldston. New York: Oxford University Press, 1986.

JOHNSON, SALLY J., et al., "Prevalence of Sensorineural Hearing Loss in Premature and Sick Term Infants with Perinatally Acquired Cytomegalovirus Infection," *Ear and Hearing*, 7 (1986), 325–27.

JOHNSON, WENDELL, "The Indians Have No Word for It," *Quart. J. Speech*, 30 (1944), 330–37.

——, "Speech Disorders and Remedial Speech Services," in *Speech Handicapped School Children*, 3rd ed., eds. Wendell Johnson and Dorothy Moeller. New York: Harper & Row, 1967.

JOINT COMMITTEE ON INFANT HEARING, "Position Statement, 1982," *Peds.*, 70 (1982), 496–97.

JONATHA, W., "Amniocentesis in Early Pregnancy under Ultrasonic Visual Control," *Electromedica*, 42 (1974), 94–6.

JONES, KENNETH L., AND DAVID W. SMITH, "Recognition of the Fetal Alcohol Syndrome in Early Infancy," *Lancet*, 2 (1973), 999–1001.

——, et al., "Pattern of Malformation in Offspring of Chronic Alcoholic Mothers," *Lancet*, 1 (1973), 1267–71.

————, et al., "Outcome in Offspring of Chronic Alcoholic Women," *Lancet*, 1 (1974), 1076–78.
KAMINSKI, M., C. RUMEAU, AND D. SCHWARTZ, "Alcohol Consumption in Pregnant Women and the Outcome of Pregnancy," *Alcoholism: Clin. Exp. Res.*, 2 (1978), 155–63.
KANE, DOROTHY NOYES, *Environmental Hazards to Young Children*. Phoenix, AZ: Oryx Press, 1985.
KARAGAN, N. J., AND HANS U. ZELLWEGER, "Early Verbal Disability in Children with Duchenne Muscular Dystrophy," *Dev. Med. Child Neurol.*, 20 (1978), 435–41.
KARCHMER, M. A., M. N. MILONE, AND S. WOLK, "Educational Significance of Hearing Loss at Three Levels of Severity," *Amer. Ann. Deaf*, 124 (1979), 97–109.
KARMODY, COLLIN S., "Developmental Anomalies of the Neck," in *Pediatric Otolaryngology*, ed. Charles D. Bluestone and Sylvan E. Stool. Philadelphia: Saunders, 1983.
KASTNER, TED, AND DEBORAH FREIDMAN, "Pediatric Acquired Immune Deficiency Syndrome and the Prevention of Mental Retardation," *J. Dev. Beh. Peds.*, 9 (1988), 47–48.
KELEMEN, GEORGE, "Hurler's Syndrome and the Hearing Organ," *J. Laryngol. Otol.*, 80 (1966), 791–803.
————, "Morquio's Disease and the Hearing Organ," *ORL*, 39 (1977), 233–40.
KELLY, THADDEUS E., *Clinical Genetics and Genetic Counseling*. Chicago: Year Book Medical Publishers, 1980.
————, *Clinical Genetics and Genetic Counseling*, 2nd ed. Chicago: Year Book Medical Publishers, 1986.
KHOURY, MUIN J., et al., "Congenital Malformations and Intrauterine Growth Retardation: A Population Study," *Peds.*, 82 (1988), 83–89.
KIDD, KENNETH K., "Recent Progress on the Genetics of Stuttering," in *Genetic Aspects of Speech and Language Disorders*, ed. Christy L. Ludlow and Judith A. Cooper. New York: Academic Press, 1983.
————, "Stuttering as a Genetic Disorder," in *Nature and Treatment of Stuttering: New Directions*, ed. Richard F. Curlee and William H. Perkins. San Diego, CA: College-Hill Press, 1984.
KILENY, P., C. CONNELLY, AND C. ROBERTSON, "Auditory Brainstem Responses in Perinatal Asphyxia," *Intl. J. Ped. Otorhinolaryngol.*, 2 (1980), 147–59.
KINSBOURNE, MARCEL, AND PAULA J. CAPLAN, *Children's Learning and Attention Problems*. Boston: Little, Brown, 1979.
KLEIN, RONALD, et al., "The Wisconsin Epidemiological Study of Diabetic Retinopathy. II. Prevalence and Risk of Diabetic Retinopathy When Age at Diagnosis Is Less Than 30 Years," *Arch. Ophthalmol.*, 102 (1984), 520–526.
————, et al., "An Epidemiologic Study of Diabetic Retinopathy in Younger Insulin-Taking Patients," in *Childhood and Juvenile Diabetes Mellitus*, ed. Goro Mimura. Amsterdam: Excerpta Medica, 1985.
KLINEFELTER, H. F., E. C. REIFENSTEIN, AND F. ALBRIGHT, "Gynecomastia, Aspermatogenesis without Aleydigism and Increased Excretion of Follicle-Stimulating Hormone," *J. Clin. Endocrinol.*, 2 (1942), 615–27.
KLINGBERG, MARCUS A., et al., "The Etiology of Central Nervous System Defects," in *Neurobehavioral Teratology*, ed. Joseph Yanai. Amsterdam: Elsevier, 1984.
KOENIG, M. P., AND M. NEIGER, "The Pathology of the Ear in Endemic Cretinism," in *Human Development and the Thyroid Gland (Relation to Endemic Cretinism)*, eds. John B. Stanbury and Robert L. Kroc. New York: Plenum Press, 1972.
KONIGSMARK, BRUCE W., "Hereditary Congenital Severe Deafness Syndromes," in *The Clinical Delineation of Birth Defects: Part IX, Ear*, ed. D. Bergsma. Baltimore: Williams & Wilkins, 1971.
————, "Hereditary Congenital Severe Deafness Syndromes," *Ann. Otol., Rhinol., Laryngol.*, 80 (1971), 269–88.
————, AND ROBERT J. GORLIN, *Genetic and Metabolic Deafness*. Philadelphia: Saunders, 1976.
KORNER, ANNELIESE F., "Preventive Intervention with High-Risk Newborns: Theoretical, Conceptual, and Methodological Perspectives," in *Handbook of Infant Development*, 2nd ed., ed. Joy Doniger Osofsky. New York: Wiley, 1987.
KRYNSKI, S., et al., "Perinatal Anoxia and Mental Retardation," *Acta Paedopsychiatrica*, 39 (1973), 347–55.

KUHL, CLAUS, AND LARS MOLSTED-PEDERSEN, "Pregnancy and Diabetes: Gestational Diabetes," in *The Diabetes Annual/3*, eds. K. G. M. M. Alberti and L. P. Krall. Amsterdam: Elsevier, 1987.

KWONG, MELINDA, AND EDMUND A. EGAN, "Reduced Incidence of Hyaline Membrane Disease in Extremely Premature Infants Following Delay of Delivery in Mother with Preterm Labor: Use of Ritodrine and Betamethasone," *Peds.*, 78 (1986), 767–74.

LAMPERT, R. P., "Dominant Inheritance of Femoral Hypoplasia—Unusual Facies Syndrome," *Clin. Genet.*, 17 (1980), 255–58.

LANDRIGAN, PHILIP J., AND JOHN W. GRAEF, "Pediatric Lead Poisoning in 1987: The Silent Epidemic Continues," *Peds.*, 79 (1987), 582–83.

LAURENCE, K. MICHAEL, "Prenatal Diagnosis of Anencephaly and Spina Bifida," in *Birth Defects: Risks and Consequences*, ed. Sally Kelly et al. New York: Academic Press, 1976.

LEATHWOOD, PETER, "Influence of Early Undernutrition on Behavioral Development and Learning in Rodents," in *Studies on the Development of Behavior and the Nervous System*, vol. 4, *Early Influences*, ed. Gilbert Gottlieb. New York: Academic Press, 1978.

LECLERC, JACQUES E., AND BLAIR FEARON, "Choanal Atresia and Associated Anomalies," *Intl. J. Ped. Otorhinolaryngol.*, 13 (1987), 265–72.

LEDERER, FRANCIS L., "Granulomas and Other Specific Diseases of the Ear and Temporal Bone," in *Otolaryngology*, vol. 2, *Ear*, ed. Michael M. Paparella and Donald A. Shumrick. Philadelphia: Saunders, 1973.

LEGRAND, JACQUES, "Effects of Thyroid Hormones on Central Nervous System Development," in *Neurobehavioral Teratology*, ed. Joseph Yanai. Amsterdam: Elsevier, 1984.

LEIBERMAN, ALBERTO, ARNON COHEN, AND ASHER TAL, "Digital Signal Processing of Stridor and Snoring in Children," *Intl. J. Ped. Otorhinolaryngol.*, 12 (1986), 173–85.

LEJEUNE, JEROME, MARTHE GAUTIER, AND RAYMOND TURPIN, "Etude des Chromosomes Somatiques de Neuf Enfants Mongoliens," *C. R. Acad. Sci.*, 248 (1959), 1721–22.

LEROY, J. G., AND A. C. CROCKER, "Clinical Definition of the Hunter-Hurler Phenotype, A Review of 50 Patients," *Am. J. Dis. Child.*, 112, 518–530.

LESTER, BARRY M., "A Biosocial Model of Infant Crying," in *Advances in Infancy Research*, ed. L. Lipsett. Norwood, NJ: Ablex, 1984.

———, "Developmental Outcome Prediction from Acoustic Cry Analysis in Term and Preterm Infants," *Peds.*, 80 (1987), 529–34.

LEVITAS, ANDREW, et al., "Autism and the Fragile X Syndrome," *J. Dev. Beh. Peds.*, 4 (1983), 151–58.

LEVY, S., et al., "Communication and Neuropsychologic Dysfunction in Children with Neurofibromatosis," unpublished paper given at the Second Annual Williamsburg meeting of the Society for Developmental Pediatrics, 1986.

LEWIN, M. L., C. B. CROFT, AND ROBERT J. SHPRINTZEN, "Velopharyngeal Insufficiency Due to Hypoplasia of the Musculus Uvulae and Occult Submucous Cleft Palate," *Plast. Reconstr. Surg.*, 65 (1980), 585–91.

LILEY, A. W., "Liquour Amnii Analysis in the Management of the Pregnancy Complicated by Rhesus Sensitization," *Amer. J. Obs. Gyn.*, 82 (1961), 1359–70.

LINDSAY, JOHN R., "Profound Childhood Deafness: Inner Ear Pathology," *Ann. Otol., Rhinol., Laryngol.*, 82 (1973), suppl. 5.

LITCH, SUZANNE, "Prevention Curriculum in the Public Schools," paper presented at the Conference on Tomorrow's Child, Irvine, CA, 1984.

LLOYD, DAVID J., AND THOMAS M. S. REID, "Group B Streptococcal Infection in the Newborn. Criteria for Early Detection and Treatment," *Acta Ped. Scand.*, 65 (1976), 585–91.

LONGO, L. D., AND G. G. POWER, "Fetal Physiology: A Primer for the 70s," *Doctor*, 3 (1975), 10–14.

LOWE, C. R., "Congenital Malformations among Infants Born to Epileptic Women," *Lancet*, 1 (1973), 9–10.

LUDLOW, CHRISTY L., AND JUDITH A. COOPER, "Genetic Aspects of Speech and Language Disorders: Current Status and Future Directions," in *Genetic Aspects of Speech and Language Disorders*, eds. Christy L. Ludlow and Judith A. Cooper. New York: Academic Press, 1983.

LUGO, JAMES O., AND GERALD L. HERSHEY, *Human Development,* 2nd ed. New York: Macmillan, 1979.

MACKENZIE-STEPNER, L., et al., "Abnormal Carotid Arteries in the Velocardiofacial Syndrome: A Report of Three Cases," *Plast. Reconstr. Surg.,* 80 (1987), 347–51.

MADDEN, JOHN D., TERRENCE F. PAYNE, AND SUE MILLER, "Maternal Cocaine Abuse and Effect on the Newborn," *Peds.,* 77 (1986), 209–11.

MAGENIS, R. E., et al., "Parental Origin of the Extra Chromosome in Down's Syndrome," *Human Genetics,* 37 (1977), 7–16.

MAISEL, ROBERT H., AND ROBERT H. MATHOG, "Injuries of the Mouth, Pharynx, and Esophagus," in *Pediatric Otolaryngology,* eds. Charles D. Bluestone and Sylvan E. Stool. Philadelphia: Saunders, 1983.

MAJEWSKI, F., AND T. GOECKE, "Alcohol Embryopathy," in *Fetal Alcohol Syndrome,* vol. II: *Human Studies,* ed. E. L. Abel. Cleveland: CRC Press, 1982.

MALLING, H. V., AND J. S. WASSOM, "Action of Mutagenic Agents," in *Handbook of Teratology,* vol. 1: *General Principles and Etiology,* eds. James G. Wilson and F. Clarke Fraser. New York: Plenum Press, 1977.

MCCABE, BRIAN F., "The Etiology of Deafness," *Volta Review,* 65 (1963), 471–77.

MCGAHAN, JOHN P., AND ALAN R. OSBORN, "Sonographic Evaluation of the Large-for-Dates Pregnancy," *Perinatol./Neonatol.,* 9(4) (1985), 45–52.

MCKUSICK, VICTOR A., *Mendelian Inheritance in Man,* 5th ed. Baltimore: Johns Hopkins University Press, 1983.

———, *Mendelian Inheritance in Man,* 6th ed. Baltimore: Johns Hopkins University Press, 1986.

MCLOUGHLIN, E., et al., "Project Burn Prevention: Outcome and Implications," *Amer. J. Pub. Health,* 72 (1982), 241–47.

MALVERN, JOHN, "Perinatal Infections: The Obstetrician's Viewpoint," in *Perinatal Infections,* ed. Katherine Elliot, Maeve O'Connor, and Julie Whelan. Amsterdam: Excerpta Medica, 1980.

MAN, EVELYN B., "Maternal Hypothyroxinemia: Development of 4- and 7-Year-Old Offspring," in *Perinatal Thyroid Physiology and Disease,* ed. Delbert A. Fisher and Gerard N. Burrow. New York: Raven Press, 1975.

MARGE, MICHAEL M., "The Prevention of Communication Disorders," *Asha,* 26 (1984), 29–33.

MARLOWE, FRANK I., "Injuries of the Nose, Facial Bones, and Paranasal Sinuses," in *Pediatric Otolaryngology,* ed. Charles D. Bluestone and Sylvan E. Stool. Philadelphia: Saunders, 1983.

MARX, JEAN L., "Cytomegalovirus: A Major Cause of Birth Defects," *Science,* 190 (1975), 1184–86.

MATHOG, ROBERT H., "Otologic Manifestations of Retrocochlear Disease," in *Otolaryngology,* vol. 2, *Ear,* ed. Michael M. Paparella and Donald A. Shumrick. Philadelphia: Saunders, 1973.

MAUSNER, JUDITH S., AND ANITA K. BAHN, *Epidemiology: An Introductory Text.* Philadelphia: Saunders, 1974.

MEDEARIS, JR., D. N., "Observations concerning Human Cytomegalovirus Infection and Disease," *Bull. Johns Hopkins Hosp.,* 114 (1964), 181–211.

MELNICK, MICHAEL, DAVID BIXLER, AND EDWARD D. SHIELDS, eds., *Progress in Clinical and Biological Research,* vol. 46, *Etiology of Cleft Lip and Cleft Palate.* New York: Alan R. Liss, 1980.

MENCHER, GEORGE T., GYLFI BALDURSSON, AND LENORE S. MENCHER, "Prologue: The Way We Were," in *Early Management of Hearing Loss,* ed. George T. Mencher and Sanford E. Gerber. New York: Grune & Stratton, 1981.

MENDELSON, TERRIE, AND ALAN SALAMY, "Maturational Effects on the Middle Components of the Averaged Electroencephalic Response," *J. Speech Hear. Res.,* 24 (1981), 140–44.

MENTIS, MICHELLE, "The Study of Aphasia and Closed Head Injury from a Philosophy of Science Perspective," unpublished monograph, University of California Santa Barbara, 1987.

———, AND CAROL A. PRUTTING, "Cohesion in the Discourse of Normal and Head-Injured Adults," *J. Speech Hear. Res.,* 30 (1987), 88–98.

MILISEN, ROBERT, "The Incidence of Speech Disorders," in *Handbook of Speech Pathology,* ed. Lee E. Travis. New York: Appleton-Century-Crofts, Inc., 1957.

MIMURA, GORO, "The Present Status of Immunogenetic Research in Japan," in *Childhood and Juvenile Diabetes Mellitus,* ed. Goro Mimura. Amsterdam: Excerpta Medica, 1985.

MINKOFF, HOWARD, et al., "Pregnancies Resulting in Infants with Acquired Immunodeficiency Syndrome or AIDS-Related Complex," *Obst. Gynecol.,* 69 (1987), 285–87.

———, et al., "Pregnancies Resulting in Infants with Acquired Immunodeficiency Syndrome or AIDS-Related Complex: Follow-up of Mothers, Children, and Subsequently Born Siblings," *Obst. Gynecol.,* 69 (1987), 288–91.

MOESCHLER, JOHN B., et al., "Rett Syndrome: Natural History and Management," *Peds.,* 82 (1988), 1–10.

MOON, MARY ANN, "Research Highlights," *Research Resources Reporter,* 11 (1987), 10–12.

MOSES, KENNETH, AND M. V. VAN HECKE-WULATIN, "The Socio-Emotional Impact of Infant Deafness: A Counselling Model," in *Early Management of Hearing Loss,* ed. George T. Mencher and Sanford E. Gerber. New York: Grune & Stratton, 1981.

MOTULSKY, ARNO G., "Pharmacogenetics, Enzyme Polymorphisms, and Teratogenesis," in *Methods for Detection of Environmental Agents that Produce Congenital Defects,* ed. Thomas H. Shepard, James R. Miller, and Maurice Marois. Amsterdam: North-Holland Publishing, 1975.

MYERS, EUGENE N., AND SYLVAN E. STOOL, "Cytomegalic Inclusion Disease of the Inner Ear," *Laryngoscope,* 78 (1968), 1904–14.

———, AND PETER J. KOBLENZER, "Congenital Deafness, Spiny Hyperkeratosis, and Universal Alopecia," *Arch. Otolaryngol.,* 93 (1971), 68–74.

MYKLEBUST, HELMER R., *Auditory Disorders in Children.* New York: Grune & Stratton, 1954.

MYRIANTHOPOLOUS, NTINOS C., "The Human Population Data: Critique II," in *Progress in Clinical and Biological Research,* vol. 46, *Etiology of Cleft Lip and Cleft Palate,* ed. Michael Melnick, David Bixler, and Edward D. Shields. New York: Alan R. Liss, 1980.

NAEYE, RICHARD L., "Epidemiology of Hyaline Membrane Disease. Selective Aspects," in *Respiratory Distress Syndrome,* ed. Claude A. Villee, Dorothy B. Villee, and James Zuckerman. New York: Academic Press, 1973.

NANCE, WALTER E., AND ANNE SWEENEY, "Genetic Factors in Deafness of Early Life," *Otolaryngol. Clin. N. Amer.,* 8 (1975), 19–48.

NATIONAL INSTITUTE OF CHILD HEALTH AND HUMAN DEVELOPMENT, *Antenatal Diagnosis,* NIH Publ. No. 79–1973. Bethesda, MD: National Institutes of Health, 1979.

NEEDLEMAN, HERBERT L., "Environmental Pollutants," in *Childhood Learning Disabilities and Prenatal Risk,* ed. Catherine Caldwell Brown. Skillman, NJ: Johnson & Johnson Baby Products, 1983.

NELSON, SEVERINA E., "The Role of Heredity in Stuttering," *J. Peds.,* 14 (1939), 642–54.

———, NAOMI HUNTER, and MARJORIE WALTER, "Stuttering in Twin Types," *J. Speech Dis.,* 10 (1945), 335–43.

NEMAN, RONALD, *Prevention: If Not You, Who? If Not Now, When?* Arlington, TX: Association for Retarded Citizens, 1984.

NETLEY, C., "Sex Chromosome Abnormalities and the Development of Verbal and Nonverbal Abilities," in *Genetic Aspects of Speech and Language Disorders,* ed. Christy L. Ludlow and Judith A. Cooper. New York: Academic Press, 1983.

NIELSEN, KAREN BRONDUM, "Diagnosis of the Fragile X Syndrome (Martin-Bell Syndrome). Clinical Findings in 27 Males with the Fragile Site at Xq28," *J. Ment. Defic. Res.,* 27 (1983), 211–26.

NOONAN, JACQUELINE A., AND DOROTHY A. EHMKE, "Associated Noncardiac Malformations in Children with Congenital Heart Disease," *J. Peds.,* 63 (1963), 468–70.

NORA, JAMES J., et al., "The Ullrich Noonan Syndrome (Turner Phenotype)," *Amer. J. Dis. Child.,* 127 (1974), 48–55.

NORTHERN, JERRY L., AND MARION P. DOWNS, *Hearing in Children,* 4th ed. Baltimore: Williams & Wilkins, 1984.

NUSSBAUM, ELIEZER, AND J. CARLOS MAGGI, "Pentobarbital Therapy Does Not Improve Neurologic Outcome in Nearly Drowned, Flaccid-Comatose Children," *Peds.,* 8 (1988), 630–34.

NYHAN, WILLIAM L., AND NADIA O. SAKATI, *Genetic and Malformation Syndromes in Clinical Medicine.* Chicago: Year Book Medical Publishers, 1976.

OGATA, EDWARD S., "Diabetes-Related Problems of the Newborn," *Perinatol./Neonatol.,* 8 (1984), 48–53.

O'LOUGHLIN, E. V., AND D. LILLYSTONE, "Ear Anomalies, Deafness and Facial Nerve Palsy in Infants of Diabetic Mothers," *Austral. Ped. J.,* 19 (1983), 109–11.

OMENN, GILBERT S., "Prenatal Diagnosis of Genetic Disorders," *Science,* 200 (1978), 952–58.

OPITZ, JOHN M., "Genetic Malformation Syndromes Associated with Mental Retardation," in *Congenital Mental Retardation,* ed. William M. McIsaac, James Claghorn, and Gordon Farrell. Austin: University of Texas Press, 1969.

ORENSTEIN, WALTER A., et al., "Epidemiology of Rubella and Its Complications," in *Vaccinating Against Brain Syndromes,* ed. Ernest M. Gruenberg, Carol Lewis, and Stephen E. Goldston. New York: Oxford University Press, 1986.

ORNITZ, EDWARD M., DONALD GUTHRIES, AND ARTHUR J. FARLEY, "The Early Development of Autistic Children," *J. Autism Child Schiz.,* 7 (1977), 207–29.

PADMANABHAN, R., "Abnormalities of the Ear Associated with Exencephaly in Mouse Fetuses Induced by Maternal Exposure to Cadmium," *Teratol.,* 35 (1987), 9–18.

PAINE, RICHMOND S., "Phenylketonuria," *Clin. Proc.,* 20 (1964), 143–52.

PAINTER, MICHAEL J., "Neurologic Disorders of the Mouth, Pharynx, and Esophagus," in *Pediatric Otolaryngology,* ed. Charles D. Bluestone and Sylvan E. Stool. Philadelphia: Saunders, 1983.

PAPARELLA, MICHAEL M., "Surgery of the Middle Ear, Eustachian Tube and Mastoid," in *Otolaryngology,* vol. 2, *Ear,* ed. Michael M. Paparella and Donald A. Shumrick. Philadelphia: Saunders, 1973.

———, AND MARY JANE CAPPS, "Sensorineural Deafness in Children—Genetic," in *Otolaryngology,* vol. 2, *Ear,* ed. Michael M. Paparella and Donald A. Shumrick. Philadelphia: Saunders, 1973.

PAPIERNIK, E., et al., "Prevention of Preterm Births: A Perinatal Study in Haguenik, France," *Peds.,* 76 (1985), 154–58.

PAPPAS, DENNIS G., "A Study of the High-Risk Registry for Sensorineural Hearing Impairment," *Otol.—Head and Neck Surg.,* 91 (1983), 41–44.

———, *Diagnosis and Treatment of Hearing Impairment in Children.* San Diego, CA: College-Hill Press, 1985.

———, AND MARY SCHAIBLY, "A Two-Year Diagnostic Report of Bilateral Sensorineural Hearing Loss in Infants and Children," *Amer. J. Otol.,* 5 (1984), 339–43.

PARISIER, SIMON C., "Injuries of the Ear and Temporal Bone," in *Pediatric Otolaryngology,* eds. Charles D. Bluestone and Sylvan E. Stool. Philadelphia: Saunders, 1983.

PATAU, K., et al., "Multiple Congenital Anomaly Caused by an Extra Autosome," *Lancet,* 1 (1960), 790–93.

PECK, JAMES E., "Hearing Loss in Hunter Syndrome—MPS II." Paper given at the meeting of the American Auditory Society, 1982.

PENDRED, VAUGHAN, "Deaf-Mutism and Goitre," *Lancet,* 2 (1896), 532.

PERSAUD, T. V. N., "Brief History of Teratology," in *Basic Concepts in Teratology,* eds. T. V. N. Persaud, A. E. Chudley, and R. G. Skalko. New York: Alan R. Liss, 1985.

———, "Classification and Epidemiology of Developmental Defects," in *Basic Concepts in Teratology,* ed. T. V. N. Persaud, A. E. Chudley, and R. G. Skalko. New York: Alan R. Liss, 1985.

———, "Causes of Developmental Defects," in *Basic Concepts in Teratology,* ed. T. V. N. Persaud, A. E. Chudley, and R. G. Skalko. New York: Alan R. Liss, 1985.

PLUMRIDGE, DIANE, AND JUDITH HYLTON, *Smooth Sailing into the Next Generation.* Clackamas County, OR: Association for Retarded Citizens, 1987.

PROUJAN, BARBARA J., "AIDS in Children," *Research Resources Reporter,* 12 (1988), 1–5.

REAL, RANDY, MICHELLE THOMAS, AND JOHN M. GERWIN, "Sudden Hearing Loss and Acquired Immunodeficiency Syndrome," *Otol.—Head and Neck Surg.,* 97 (1987), 409–12.

RECORDS, MARY ANN, KENNETH K. KIDD, AND JUDITH R. KIDD, "The Family Clustering of Stuttering," paper presented at the Annual Meeting of the American Speech and Hearing Association, 1977.

REGEHR, SONYA M., "The Genetic Aspects of Developmental Dyslexia," *Can. J. Beh. Sci.,* 19 (1987), 240–53.

———, AND BONNIE J. KAPLAN, "Reading Disability with Motor Problems May Be an Inherited Subtype," *Peds.,* 82 (1988), 204–10.

REID, THOMAS M. S., AND DAVID J. LLOYD, "Neonatal Group B Streptococcal Infection," in *Perinatal Infections,* ed. Katherine Elliot, Maeve O'Connor, and Julie Whelan. Amsterdam: Excerpta Medica, 1980.

REINWEIN, D., "Treatment of Diminished Thyroid Hormone Formation," in *Diminished Thyroid Formation: Possible Causes and Clinical Aspects,* ed. D. Reinwein and E. Klein. Stuttgart: Schattauer Verlag, 1982.

RESNICK, MICHAEL B., SUSAN ARMSTRONG, AND RANDY L. CARTER, "Developmental Intervention Program for High-Risk Premature Infants: Effects on Development and Parent-Infant Interactions," *J. Dev. Beh. Peds.,* 9 (1988), 73–78.

REYNOLDS, DAVID W, et al., "Inapparent Congenital Cytomegalovirus Infection with Elevated Cord IgM Levels," *New Engl. J. Med.,* 290 (1974), 291–96.

RHINE, SAMUEL A., "The Most Important Nine Months," *The Science Teacher,* October 1983, 46–51.

RICCARDI, V. M., AND J. E. EICHNER, *Neurofibromatosis: Phenotype, Natural History, and Pathogenesis.* Baltimore: Johns Hopkins University Press, 1986.

RIDING, KEITH H., AND CHARLES D. BLUESTONE, "Burns and Acquired Strictures of the Esophagus," in *Pediatric Otolaryngology,* ed. Charles D. Bluestone and Sylvan E. Stool. Philadelphia: Saunders, 1983.

RIEDNER, ERWIN D., AND STEFAN LEVIN, "Hearing Patterns in Morquio's Syndrome (Mucopolysaccharidosis IV)," *Arch. Otolaryngol.,* 103 (1977), 518–20.

RIVARA, FREDERICK P., AND MELVIN BARBER, "Demographic Analysis of Childhood Pedestrian Injuries," *Peds.,* 76 (1985), 375–81.

ROBERT, K. E., AND P. GULBRAND, "Maternal Valproic Acid and Congenital Neural Tube Defects," *Lancet,* 2 (1982), 937.

ROBERTSON, CHARLENE, "Pediatric Assessment of the Infant at Risk for Deafness," in *Early Diagnosis of Hearing Loss,* ed. Sanford E. Gerber and George T. Mencher. New York: Grune & Stratton, 1978.

———, AND LILLIAN WHYTE, "Prospective Identification of Infants with Hearing Loss and Multiple Handicaps: The Role of the Neonatal Follow-Up Clinic," in *The Multiply Handicapped Hearing Impaired Child,* ed. George T. Mencher and Sanford E. Gerber. New York: Grune & Stratton, 1983.

ROGERS, BLAIR O., "Some Congenital and Acquired Deformities Causing Facial Disfigurement," in *Facial Disfigurement,* ed. Blair O. Rogers. Washington, DC: U.S. Department of Health, Education, and Welfare, 1963.

ROSA, FRANZ W., ANN L. WILK, AND FRANCES O. KELSEY, "Teratogen Update: Vitamin A Congeners," *Teratol.,* 33 (1986), 355–64.

ROSEN, ZVI, AND ELI DAVIS, "Microangiopathy in Diabetics with Hearing Disorders," *EENT Monthly,* 50 (1971), 31, 33–35.

ROSENBLOOM, ARLAN L., "Diabetes in Children," in *The Diabetes Annual /3,* ed. K. G. M. M. Albertia and L. P. Krall. Amsterdam: Excerpta Medica, 1987.

ROSETTI, LOUIS M., *High-Risk Infants: Identification, Assessment, and Intervention.* Boston: Little, Brown, 1986.

ROSMAN, N. PAUL, "The Neuropathology of Congenital Hypothyroidism," in *Human Development and the Thyroid Gland: Relation to Endemic Cretinism,* eds. John B. Stanbury and Robert L. Kroc. New York: Plenum Press, 1972.

ROSS, MARK, AND THOMAS G. GIOLAS, *Auditory Management of Hearing-Impaired Children.* Baltimore: University Park Press, 1978.

ROSS, S. M., et al., "The Genesis of Amniotic Fluid Infections," in *Perinatal Infections,* eds. Katherine Elliot, Maeve O'Connor, and Julie Whelan. Amsterdam: Excerpta Medica, 1980.

ROVET, JOANNE F., ROBERT M. EHRLICH, AND DONNA-LEE SORBARA, "Outcome in Neonatally Identified Thyroid Hormone Deficient Children: Persistent Deficits and Associated Risk Factors." Paper presented at the Fifth Annual Meeting of the Society for Behavioral Pediatrics, Anaheim, CA, 1987.

———, "Intellectual Outcome in Children with Fetal Hypothyroidism," *J. Peds.,* 110 (1987), 700–704

RUBEN, ROBERT J., AND THOMAS R. VAN DE WATER, "Recent Advances in the Developmental Biology of the Inner Ear," in *The Development of Auditory Behavior,* ed. Sanford E. Gerber and George T. Mencher. New York: Grune & Stratton, 1983.

RUSH, DAVID, "Cigarette Smoking During Pregnancy: The Relationship with Depressed Weight Gain and Birthweight," in *Birth Defects: Risks and Consequences,* ed. Sally Kelly, et al. New York: Academic Press, 1976.

RUTTER, MICHAEL, "Continuities and Discontinuities from Infancy," in *Handbook of Infant Development*, 2nd ed., ed. Joy Doniger Osofsky. New York: John Wiley, 1987.

——, OLIVER CHADWICK, AND DAVID SHAFFER, "Head Injury," in *Developmental Neuropsychiatry*, ed. Michael Rutter. New York: Guildford Press, 1983.

SADEWITZ, VICKI L., AND ROBERT J. SHPRINTZEN, *Pierre Robin: A New Look at an Old Disorder*, video production, March of Dimes, 1986.

——, *Syndrome Identification and Communication Impairment*, video production, March of Dimes, 1987.

SAHU, S., "Birthweight, Gestational Age, and Neonatal Risks," *Perinatol./Neonatol.*, 8(1) (1984), 28–30, 32–33, 36.

SANDO, ISAMU, et al., "Temporal Bone Histopathological Findings in Trisomy 13 Syndrome," *Ann. Otol., Rhinol., Laryngol.*, 84, suppl. 21 (1975), 1–20.

——, SUSUMO SUEHIRO, AND RAYMOND P. WOOD, II, "Congenital Anomalies of the External and Middle Ear," in *Pediatric Otolaryngology*, ed. Charles D. Bluestone and Sylvan E. Stool. Philadelphia: Saunders, 1983.

SATZ, PAUL, AND CAROL BULLARD-BATES, "Acquired Aphasia in Children," in *Acquired Aphasia*, ed. Martha Taylor Sarno. New York: Academic Press, 1981.

SCHARDEIN, JAMES L., *Drugs as Teratogens*. Cleveland, OH: CRC Press, 1976.

SCHOR, DAVID P., "Teratogens," in *Medical Aspects of Developmental Disabilities in Children Birth to Three*, ed. James A. Blackman. Rockville, MD: Aspen, 1984

SCHREINER, C. A., "Petroleum and Petroleum Products: A Brief Review of Studies to Evaluate Reproductive Effects," in *Advances in Modern Experimental Toxicology*, vol. III, *Assessment of Reproductive and Teratogenic Hazards*, ed. Mildred S. Christian et al. Princeton, NJ: Princeton Scientific Publishers, 1983.

SCHULTZ, FREDERICK R., "Phenylketonuria and Other Metabolic Diseases," in *Medical Aspects of Developmental Disabilities in Children Birth to Three*, ed. James A. Blackman. Rockville, MD: Aspen, 1984.

——, "Respiratory Distress Syndrome," in *Medical Aspects of Developmental Disabilities in Children Birth to Three*, ed. James A. Blackman. Rockville, MD: Aspen, 1984.

SEESSEL, THOMAS V., ed., *National School Health Services Program*. Princeton, NJ: Robert Wood Johnson Foundation, 1985.

SEID, ALLAN B., AND ROBIN COTTON, "Tumors of the Larynx, Trachea, and Bronchi," in *Pediatric Otolaryngology*, ed. Charles D. Bluestone and Sylvan E. Stool. Philadelphia: Saunders, 1983.

SEIZINGER, BERND R., et al., "Common Pathogenetic Mechanism for Three Tumor Types in Bilateral Acoustic Neurofibromatosis," *Science*, 236 (1987), 317–19.

SEPE, STEPHEN J., et al., "Genetic Services in the United States 1979–80," *J. Amer. Med. Assn.*, 248 (1982), 1733–35.

SEVER, JOHN L., "Maternal Infections," in *Childhood Learning Disabilities and Prenatal Risk*, ed. Catherine Caldwell Brown. Skillman, NJ: Johnson & Johnson Baby Products Co., 1983.

——, et al., "Toxoplasmosis: Maternal and Pediatric Findings in 23,000 Pregnancies," *Peds.*, 82 (1988), 181–192.

SHAPIRO, SAM, et al., "Changes in Infant Morbidity Associated with Decreases in Neonatal Mortality," *Peds.*, 72 (1983), 408–14.

SHEA, ROBERT D., et al., *Childhood Hearing Impairment*. Ottawa: Health Services Directorate, Health Services and Promotion Branch, Health and Welfare Canada, 1984.

SHEFTEL, DAVID N., ROBERT H. PERELMAN, AND PHILIP M. FARRELL, "Long-Term Consequences of Hyaline Membrane Disease," in *Lung Development: Biological and Clinical Perspectives*, vol. II, *Neonatal Respiratory Distress*, ed. Philip M. Farrell, New York: Academic Press, 1982.

SHER, AARON E., ROBERT J. SHPRINTZEN, AND M. J. THORPY, "Endoscopic Observations of Obstructive Sleep Apnea in Children with Anomalous Upper Airways: Predictive and Therapeutic Value," *Intl. J. Ped. Otorhinolaryngol.*, 11 (1986), 135–46.

SHIH, LUCY, BARBARA CONE-WESSON, AND BRUCE REDDIX, "Effects of Maternal Cocaine Abuse on the Neonatal Auditory System," *Intl. J. Ped. Otorhinolaryngol.*, 15 (1988), 245–51.

SHPRINTZEN, ROBERT J., "Palatal and Pharyngeal Anomalies in Craniofacial Syndromes," *Birth Defects Original Article Series*, 18(1) (1982), 53–78.

——, "Reply from Dr. Shprintzen," *Amer. J. Med. Genet.*, 28 (1987), 753–55.

————, "Pierre Robin, Micrognathia, and Airway Obstruction: The Dependency of Treatment on Accurate Diagnosis," *Intl. Anesthes. Clin.*, 26 (1988), 84–91.

————, and R. B. Goldberg, "Male-to-Male Transmission of the Velo-Cardio-Facial Syndrome: A Case Report and Review of 60 Cases," *J. Craniofacial Genet. Devel. Biol.*, 5 (1985), 175–80.

————, "Velo-Cardio-Facial Syndrome," in *Birth Defects Encyclopedia*, ed. M. L. Buyse. New York: Alan R. Liss, 1988.

———— et al., "A New Syndrome Involving Cleft Palate, Cardiac Anomalies, Typical Facies, and Learning Disabilities: Velo-Cardio-Facial Syndrome," *Cleft Palate J.*,15 (1978), 56–62.

———— et al., "Pharyngeal Hypoplasia in the Treacher Collins Syndrome," *Arch. Otolaryngol.*, 105 (1979), 127–31.

———— et al.,"The Velo-Cardio-Facial Syndrome: A Clinical and Genetic Analysis," *Peds.*, 67 (1981), 167–72.

SIEGEL-SADEWITZ, VICKI AND ROBERT J. SHPRINTZEN, "The Relationship of Communication Disorders to Syndrome Identification," *J. Speech Hear. Dis.*, 47 (1982), 338–54.

SILVERMAN, FREDERIC N., "Child Abuse: The Conflict of Underdetection and Overreporting," *Peds.*, 80 (1987), 440–43.

SINEX, F. MAROT, AND CARL R. MERRILL, eds., *Alzheimer's Disease, Down's Syndrome, and Aging*. New York: The New York Academy of Sciences, 1982.

SMEETS, D. F. C. M., J. M. J. C. SCHERES, AND T. W. J. HUSTINX, "The Fragile Site on Chromosome 3," *Human Genetics*, 67 (1984), 351.

SMITH, ALEXANDER BROWNLIE, "Unilateral Hereditary Deafness," *Lancet*, 2 (1939), 1172–73.

SMITH, DAVID W., *Recognizable Patterns of Human Malformation: Genetic, Embryologic, and Clinical Aspects*, 2nd ed. Philadelphia: Saunders, 1976.

————, *Recognizable Patterns of Human Deformation*. Philadelphia: Saunders, 1981.

————, *Recognizable Patterns of Human Malformation*, 2nd ed. Philadelphia: W.B. Saunders Co., 1976.

————, *Recognizable Patterns of Human Malformation*, 3rd ed. Philadelphia: Saunders, 1982.

SMITH, S. E., et al., "A Genetic Analysis of Specific Reading Disability," in *Genetic Aspects of Speech and Language Disorders*, eds. Christy L. Ludlow and Judith A. Cooper. New York: Academic Press, 1983.

SOLER, N. G., C. H. WALSH, AND J. M. MALINS, "Congenital Malformations in Infants of Diabetic Mothers," *Q. J. Med.*, 45 (1976), 303–13.

SOLOMONS, N. B. AND C. A. J. PRESCOTT, "Laryngomalacia: A Review and theSurgical Management for Severe Cases,"*Intl. J. Ped. Otorhinolaryngol.*, 13 (1987), 31–9.

SOUTHALL, D. P., "Role of Apnea in the Sudden Infant Death Syndrome," *Peds.*, 80 (1988), 73–84.

SPARKS, SHIRLEY N., *Birth Defects and Speech-Language Disorders*. San Diego, CA: College–Hill Press, 1984.

STANBURY, JOHN B., "The Pathogenesis of Endemic Retardation Associated with Endemic Goiter," in *Diminished Thyroid Hormone Formation: Possible Causes and Clinical Aspects*, eds. D. Reinwein and E. Klein. Stuttgart: Schattauer Verlag, 1982.

STARLE, LINDA, ed., *Screening and Counseling for Genetic Conditions*. Washington, DC: President's Commission for the Study of Ethical Problems in Medicine and Biomedical and Behavioral Research, 1983.

STEELE, MARK W. AND W. ROY BREG, JR., "Chromosome Analysis of Human Amniotic Fluid Cells," *Lancet*, 1 (1966), 383.

STEIN, ZENA AND MERVYN SUSSER, "Maternal Starvation and Birth Defects," in *Birth Defects: Risks and Consequences*, eds. Sally Kelly et al. New York: Academic Press, 1976.

STEIS, RONALD AND SAMUEL BRODER, "AIDS: A General Overview," in *AIDS: Etiology, Diagnosis, Treatment, and Prevention*, ed. Vincent T. DeVita, Jr., Samuel Hellman, and Steven A. Rosenberg. Philadelphia: Lippincott, 1985.

STICKLER, GUNNAR B. et al., "Hereditary Progressive Arthro-Ophthalmopathy," *Mayo Clin. Proc.*, 40 (1965), 433–35.

STOOL, SYLVAN E. AND ROBERT HOULIHAN, "Otolaryngologic Management of Craniofacial Anomalies," *Otolaryngol. Clin. N. Amer.*, 10 (1977), 41–4.

STUBBS, E. G., "Autistic Symptom in a Child with Congenital Cytomegalovirus Infection," *J. Autism Child. Schiz.*, 8 (1978), 37–43.

SUMMITT, ROBERT L., "Familial Goldenhaar Syndrome," *Birth Defects Original Article Series,* 5 (1969), 106–109.

SWANN, C., "Congenital Malformations in Infants following Maternal Rubella during Pregnancy: Review of Investigations Carried Out in South Australia," *Trans. Ophthal. Soc. (Austral.),* 4 (1944), 132–41.

SWISHER, LINDA, "Language Disorders in Children," in *Speech and Language Evaluation in Neurology: Childhood Disorders,* ed. John K. Darby. Orlando, FL: Grune & Stratton, 1985.

TATTERSALL, ROBERT AND IAN PEACOCK, "Assessment of Diabetic Control," in *The Diabetes Annual/3,* ed. K. G. M. M. Alberti and L. P. Krall. Amsterdam: Elsevier, 1987.

TAUSSIG, H. B., "A Study of the German Outbreak of Phocomelia. The Thalidomide Syndrome," *J. Am. Med. Assn.,* 180 (1962),1106–14.

THEISSING, G. AND G. KITTEL, "Die Bedeutung der Toxoplasmose in der Atiologie der Connatalen und Fruh Erworbenen Horstorungen," *Arch. Ohren-, Nasen-, Kehlk. Heilk.,* 180, (1962), 219.

THOMPSON, JAMES S., AND MARGARET W. THOMPSON, *Genetics in Medicine,* 3rd ed. Philadelphia: Saunders. 1980.

THOMPSON, MARGARET W., *Genetics in Medicine,* 4th ed. Philadelphia: Saunders. 1986.

THOMPSON, R.W., J. E. PETERS, AND S. D. SMITH, "Intellectual, Behavioral, and Linguistic Characteristics of Three Children with 18p- Syndrome," *J. Dev. Beh. Peds.,* 7 (1986), 1–7.

THOMSEN, J., P. BECH, AND W. SZPIRT, "Otologic Symptoms in Chronic Renal Failure," *Arch. Oto-Rhino-Laryngol.,* 214 (1976), 71–79.

TODRES, I. DAVID, "Respiratory Disorders of the Newborn," in *Pediatric Otolaryngology,* ed. Charles D. Bluestone and Sylvan E. Stool. Philadelphia: Saunders, 1983.

TOWBIN, ABRAHAM, "The Depressed Newborn: Pathogenesis and Neurologic Sequels," *Perinatol./Neonatol.,* 11(3)(1987), 16–18.

TRON, V. A., V. J. BALDWIN, AND G. E. PIRIE, "Hot Tub Drownings," *Peds.,* 75 (1985), 789–90.

TUNCBILEK, E., C. YALCIN, AND M. ATASU, "Aglossia-Adactylia Syndrome (Special Emphasis on the Inheritance Pattern)," *Clin. Genet.,* 11 (1977), 421–32.

TURNER, HENRY H., "A Syndrome of Infantilism, Congenital Webbed Neck, and Cubitus Valgus," *Endocrinol.,* 23 (1938), 566–74.

UNITED STATES DEPARTMENT OF EDUCATION, *Annual Report on Public Law 94–142.* Washington, DC: Department of Education, 1984.

UNITED STATES NATIONAL INSTITUTE OF CHILD HEALTH AND HUMAN DEVELOPMENT, *Antenatal Diagnosis: Report of a Consensus Development Conference.* Bethesda, MD: National Institutes of Health, 1979.

USHER, C. H., "On the Inheritance of Retinitis Pigmentosa, with Notes of Cases," *Royal London Ophthal.Hosp.Report,* 9 (1914), 130–236.

VAN DER HOEVE, J., "Abnorme Lange der Tranenrohrchen mit Ankeloblepharon," *Klin. Mbl. Augenheilk.,* 56 (1916), 232.

VAN DONGEN, H. R., AND M. C. B. LOONEN, "Factors Related to Prognosis of Acquired Aphasia in Children," *Cortex,* 13 (1977), 131–36.

VAN HATTUM, ROLLAND J., "Research Priorities in Speech," *Ann. Otol., Rhinol., Laryngol.,* 89 (1980), Suppl. 74, 161–64.

VAN RIPER, CHARLES, *Speech Correction.* Englewood Cliffs, NJ: Prentice Hall, 1939.

————, *Speech Correction,* 4th ed. Englewood Cliffs, NJ: Prentice Hall, 1963.

VARLEY, CHRISTOPHER K., VANJA A. HOLM, AND MUAZZEZ O. EREN, "Cognitive and Psychiatric Variability in Three Brothers with Fragile X Syndrome," *J. Dev. Beh. Peds.,* 6 (1985), 87–90.

VARTIAINEN, EERO, SEPPO KARJALAINEN, AND JUHANI KARJI, "Vestibular Disorders following Head Injury in Children," *Intl. J. Ped. Otorhinolaryngol.,* 9 (1985), 135–41.

VENKATESAM, M., "Preventive Health: Positive Aspects," in *Marketing in Preventative Health Care: Interdisciplinary and Interorganizational Perspectives,* ed. P. D. Copper, W. J. Kehoe, and P. E. Murphy. Chicago: American Marketing Association, 1978.

VERNON, MCCAY, "Usher's Syndrome: Problems and Some Solutions," *Hearing and Speech Action,* 44 (1976), 6–13.

VINING, EILEEN P. G. et al., "Psychologic and Behavioral Effects of Antiepileptic Drugs in Children: A Double-Blind Comparison between Phenobarbitol and Valproic Acid," *Peds.,* 80 (1987), 165–74.

VORHEES, CHARLES V., AND ELIZABETH MOLLNOW, "Behavioral Teratogenesis: Long-Term Influences on Behavior from Early Exposure to Environmental Agents," in *Handbook of Infant Development*, 2nd ed. ed. Joy Doniger Osofsky. New York: John Wiley, 1987.

WAARDENBURG, P. J., *Des Menschliche Auge und Seine Erbanlagen*. The Hague: Nijoff, 1932.

———, "Dystopia Punctorum Lacrimalium, Blepharophimosis, en Partiele Irisatrophia bij een Doofstomme," *Ned. Tijdschr. Geneeskd.*, 92 (1948), 3463–66.

———, "A New Syndrome Combining Developmental Anomalies of the Eyelids, Eyebrows and Nose Root with Pigmentary Defects of the Iris and Head Hair and with Congenital Deafness," *Amer. J. Human Genetics*, 3 (1951), 195–253.

WAGENAAR, ALEXANDER C., AND DANIEL W. WEBSTER, "Preventing Injuries to Children Through Compulsory Automobile Safety Seat Use," *Peds.*, 78 (1986), 662–72.

WEBSTER, DOUGLAS B., AND MOLLY WEBSTER, "Effects of Neonatal Conductive Hearing Loss on Brain Stem Auditory Nuclei," *Ann. Otol., Rhinol., Laryngol.*, 88 (1979), 684–88.

WEGMAN, MYRON E., "Annual Summary of Vital Statistics—1987," *Peds.*, 82 (1988), 817–27.

WELLER, T. H., AND F. A. NEVA, "Propagation in Tissue Culture of Cytopathic Agents from Patients with Rubella-Like Illness," *Proc. Soc. Exp. Biol. Med.*, 111 (1962), 215–25.

WENTHOLD, ROBERT J., "Neurochemistry of the Auditory System," *Ann. Otol., Rhinol., Laryngol.*, 89 (1980), Suppl. 74, 121–31.

WEST, ROBERT, "An Agnostic's Speculations about Stuttering," in *Stuttering: A Symposium*, ed. Jon Eisenson. New York: Harper & Row, 1958.

———, MERLE ANSBERRY, AND ANNA CARR, *The Rehabilitation of Speech*, 3rd ed. New York: Harper & Row, 1957.

WETHERBY, AMY MILLER, "Speech and Language Disorders in Children—An Overview," in *Speech and Language Evaluation in Neurology: Childhood Disorders*, ed. John K. Darby. Orlando, FL: Grune & Stratton, 1985.

WEVER, ERNEST G., AND MERLE LAWRENCE, *Physiological Acoustics*. Princeton, NJ: Princeton University Press, 1954.

WHITE HOUSE CONFERENCE ON CHILD HEALTH AND PROTECTION, *Special Education, Report of the Committee on Special Classes*. New York: Appleton-Century-Crofts, 1931.

WILLIAMS, MICHAEL A., 1987. "Head and Neck Findings in Pediatric Acquired Immune Deficiency Syndrome," *Laryngoscope*, 97, 713–716.

WILSON, JAMES G., "Teratologic Causation in Man and Its Evaluation in Non-Human Primates," in *Birth Defects*, ed. A. G. Motulsky and W. Lenz. Amsterdam: Excerpta Medica, 1974.

———, "Environmental Chemicals," in *Handbook of Teratology*, vol. 1, *General Principles and Etiology*, ed. James G. Wilson and R. Clarke Fraser. New York: Plenum Press, 1977.

———, "Embryotoxicity of Drugs in Man," in *Handbook of Teratology*, vol. 1, *General Principles and Etiology*, ed. James G. Wilson and R. Clarke Fraser. New York: Plenum Press, 1977.

WILSON, JOHN, "Prevention of Deafness in Developing Countries," paper presented at the 17th International Congress of Audiology, Santa Barbara, 1984.

WILSON, MARGO, AND ALICE DYSON, "Noonan Syndrome: Speech and Language Characteristics," *J. Comm. Dis.*, 15 (1982), 347–52.

WILSON, RICHARD, AND E. A. C. CROUCH, "Risk Assessment and Comparisons: An Introduction," *Science*, 236 (1987), 267–70.

WITT-ENGERSTROM, INGEGERD, AND CHRISTOPHER GILLBERG, "Rett Syndrome in Sweden," *J. Autism Dev. Dis.*, 17 (1987), 149–50.

WIZNITER, MAX, ISABELLE RAPIN, AND THOMAS R. VAN DE WATER, "Neurologic Findings in Children with Ear Malformations," *Intl. J. Ped. Otorhinolaryngol.*, 13 (1987), 41–55.

WOLF-SCHEIN, ENID G., et al., "Speech-Language and the Fragile X Syndrome: Initial Findings," *Asha*, 29 (1987), 35–8.

WOLFSON, ROBERT J., ALI M. AGHAMOHAMADI, AND STEVEN E. BERMAN, "Disorders of Hearing," in *Child Development and Developmental Disabilities*, ed. Stewart Gabel and Marilyn T. Erickson. Boston: Little, Brown, 1980.

WOOD, ROBERT E., "Physiology of the Larynx, Airways, and Lungs," in *Pediatric Otolaryngology*, ed. Charles D. Bluestone and Sylvan E. Stool. Philadelphia: Saunders, 1983.

WOODS, BRYAN T., AND SUSAN CAREY, "Language Deficits after Apparent Clinical Recovery from Childhood Aphasia," *Ann. Neurol.*, 6 (1979), 405–409.

WOOLF, ALAN, et al., "Prevention of Childhood Poisoning: Efficacy of an Educational Program Carried Out in an Emergency Clinic," *Peds.*, 80 (1987), 359–63.

WRIGHT, MARY INGLE, *The Pathology of Deafness.* Manchester, England: Manchester University Press, 1971.

YARINGTON, JR., C. THOMAS, "Maxillofacial Trauma in Children," *Otolaryngol. Clin. N. Amer.*, 10 (1977), 25–32.

YOGMAN, M. W., et al., "Behavior of Newborns of Diabetic Mothers," *Infant Beh. Dev.*, 5 (1982), 331–40.

YOUNG, PATRICK, *Drugs and Pregnancy.* New York: Chelsea House, 1987.

ZADIG, JEAN M. AND ALLEN C. CROCKER, "A Center for Study of the Young Child with Developmental Delay," in *Exceptional Infant,* vol. 3: *Assessment and Intervention,* ed. Bernard Z. Friedlander, Graham M. Sterritt, and Girvin E. Kirk. New York: Brunner/Mazel, 1975.

ZAMENHOF, S. AND E. VAN MARTHENS, "Nutritional Influences on Prenatal Brain Development," in *Studies on the Development of Behavior and the Nervous System,* vol. 4, *Early Influences,* ed. Gilbert Gottlieb. New York: Academic Press, 1978.

ZOLLER, MICHAEL, et al., "Detection of Syphilitic Hearing Loss," *Arch. Otolaryngol.,* 104 (1978), 63–65.

ZWIREN, GERALD T., H. GIBBS ANDREWS, AND THOMAS RODERICK HESTER, JR., "Progress in Treating Lye Burn Injuries of the Esophagus in Children," in *The Injured Child,* ed. Benjy Frances Brooks. Austin: University of Texas Press, 1985.

Name Index

Subject Index

АА8-1817